PEPFAR IMPLEMENTATION

PROGRESS AND PROMISE

Committee for the Evaluation of the President's Emergency Plan for AIDS Relief (PEPFAR) Implementation

Board on Global Health
Board on Children, Youth, and Families

Jaime Sepúlveda, Charles Carpenter, James Curran, William Holzemer, Helen Smits, Kimberly Scott, and Michele Orza, *Editors*

INSTITUTE OF MEDICINE
OF THE NATIONAL ACADEMIES

THE NATIONAL ACADEMIES PRESS
Washington, D.C.
www.nap.edu

THE NATIONAL ACADEMIES PRESS 500 Fifth Street, N.W. Washington, DC 20001

NOTICE: The project that is the subject of this report was approved by the Governing Board of the National Research Council, whose members are drawn from the councils of the National Academy of Sciences, the National Academy of Engineering, and the Institute of Medicine. The members of the committee responsible for the report were chosen for their special competences and with regard for appropriate balance.

This project was supported by Contract No.SAQMPD05D1147 between the National Academy of Sciences and the U.S. Department of State. Any opinions, findings, conclusions, or recommendations expressed in this publication are those of the author(s) and do not necessarily reflect the view of the agency that provided support for this project.

Library of Congress Cataloging-in-Publication Data

Institute of Medicine (U.S.). Committee for the Evaluation of the President's Emergency Plan for AIDS Relief (PEPFAR) Implementation.

PEPFAR implementation : progress and promise / Committee for the Evaluation of the President's Emergency Plan for AIDS Relief (PEPFAR) Implementation, Board on Global Health, Board on Children, Youth, and Families ; Jaime Sepúlveda ... [et al.] editors.

p. ; cm.

Includes bibliographical references.

ISBN-13: 978-0-309-10982-6 (hardback : alk. paper)

ISBN-10: 0-309-10982-5 (hardback : alk. paper) 1. AIDS (Disease)—Prevention—Government policy—United States. 2. HIV infections—Prevention—Government policy—United States. 3. AIDS (Disease)—Prevention—International cooperation.

[DNLM: 1. Government Programs—organization & administration—United States. 2. HIV Infections—prevention & control—United States. 3. Disease Outbreaks—prevention & control—United States. 4. Emergencies—United States. 5. International Cooperation—United States. 6. World Health—United States. WC 503.6 I585p 2007] I. Sepúlveda Amor, Jaime. II. Title.

RA643.83.I57 2007

362.196′9792—dc22

2007023493

Additional copies of this report are available from the National Academies Press, 500 Fifth Street, N.W., Lockbox 285, Washington, DC 20055; (800) 624-6242 or (202) 334-3313 (in the Washington metropolitan area); Internet, http://www.nap.edu.

For more information about the Institute of Medicine, visit the IOM home page at: www.iom.edu.

Printed in the United States of America.

The serpent has been a symbol of long life, healing, and knowledge among almost all cultures and religions since the beginning of recorded history. The serpent adopted as a logotype by the Institute of Medicine is a relief carving from ancient Greece, now held by the Staatliche Museen in Berlin.

COVER: The flags of the 15 PEPFAR focus countries are overlaying the global symbol of the red ribbon for HIV/AIDS awareness arranged in alphabetical order by country.

Suggested citation: IOM (Institute of Medicine). 2007. *PEPFAR Implementation: Progress and Promise.* Washington, DC: The National Academies Press.

"Knowing is not enough; we must apply.
Willing is not enough; we must do."
—Goethe

INSTITUTE OF MEDICINE
OF THE NATIONAL ACADEMIES

Advising the Nation. Improving Health.

THE NATIONAL ACADEMIES

Advisers to the Nation on Science, Engineering, and Medicine

The **National Academy of Sciences** is a private, nonprofit, self-perpetuating society of distinguished scholars engaged in scientific and engineering research, dedicated to the furtherance of science and technology and to their use for the general welfare. Upon the authority of the charter granted to it by the Congress in 1863, the Academy has a mandate that requires it to advise the federal government on scientific and technical matters. Dr. Ralph J. Cicerone is president of the National Academy of Sciences.

The **National Academy of Engineering** was established in 1964, under the charter of the National Academy of Sciences, as a parallel organization of outstanding engineers. It is autonomous in its administration and in the selection of its members, sharing with the National Academy of Sciences the responsibility for advising the federal government. The National Academy of Engineering also sponsors engineering programs aimed at meeting national needs, encourages education and research, and recognizes the superior achievements of engineers. Dr. Charles M. Vest is president of the National Academy of Engineering.

The **Institute of Medicine** was established in 1970 by the National Academy of Sciences to secure the services of eminent members of appropriate professions in the examination of policy matters pertaining to the health of the public. The Institute acts under the responsibility given to the National Academy of Sciences by its congressional charter to be an adviser to the federal government and, upon its own initiative, to identify issues of medical care, research, and education. Dr. Harvey V. Fineberg is president of the Institute of Medicine.

The **National Research Council** was organized by the National Academy of Sciences in 1916 to associate the broad community of science and technology with the Academy's purposes of furthering knowledge and advising the federal government. Functioning in accordance with general policies determined by the Academy, the Council has become the principal operating agency of both the National Academy of Sciences and the National Academy of Engineering in providing services to the government, the public, and the scientific and engineering communities. The Council is administered jointly by both Academies and the Institute of Medicine. Dr. Ralph J. Cicerone and Dr. Charles M. Vest are chair and vice chair, respectively, of the National Research Council.

www.national-academies.org

COMMITTEE FOR THE EVALUATION OF PEPFAR IMPLEMENTATION

Jaime Sepúlveda (*Chair*), 2007 University of California, San Francisco Presidential Chair and Visiting Professor
Helen Smits (*Vice Chair*), Former Faculty of Medicine, Eduardo Mondlane University, Mozambique
Charles Carpenter (*Treatment Subcommittee Chair*), Professor of Medicine, Director of the Brown University AIDS Center, Brown University, Providence, Rhode Island
James Curran (*Prevention Subcommittee Chair*), Dean, Professor of Epidemiology, Rollins School of Public Health, Emory University, Atlanta, Georgia
William L. Holzemer (*Care Subcommittee Chair*), Professor of Nursing and Associate Dean, International Programs, School of Nursing, University of California, San Francisco
Stefano M. Bertozzi, Director of Health Economics, National Institutes of Health, Mexico
Geoff Garnett, Professor of Microparasite Epidemiology, Faculty of Medicine, Imperial College, London, United Kingdom
Ruth Macklin, Head, Division of Bioethics, Department of Epidemiology and Population Health, Albert Einstein College of Medicine, New York
Affette McCaw-Binns, Professor, Reproductive Health Epidemiology, Section of Community Health, University of the West Indies, Jamaica
A. David Paltiel, Professor, Yale School of Medicine, Yale School of Management, New Haven, Connecticut
Priscilla Reddy, Director, Health Promotion Research and Development Unit, Medical Research Council of South Africa
David Ross, Director, Public Health Informatics Institute, Decatur, Georgia
Heather Weiss, Director, Harvard Family Research Project, Harvard University, Boston, Massachusetts

Subcommittee Members, Liaisons, and Study Consultants

Maureen Black, John A. Scholl Professor of Pediatrics, University of Maryland School of Medicine, Baltimore
Hoosen Coovadia, Victor Daitz Professor of HIV/AIDS Research, Centre for HIV/AIDS Networking, Doris Duke Medical Research Institute, University of Kwazulu/Natal, Durban, South Africa
Henry Fomundam, Regional Director, Howard University/PACE Centre, Washington DC/South Africa
Paul Gertler, Professor of Economics, Haas School of Business, Professor of Health Services Finance, School of Public Health, University of California, Berkley

Carl A. Latkin, Professor, Department of Health, Behavior, and Society, Johns Hopkins University Bloomberg School of Public Health, Baltimore, Maryland

James Ntozi, Professor, Department of Population Studies, Makerere University, Uganda

James Sherry, Professor of Global Health, School of Public Health and Health Services, The George Washington University, Washington, D.C.

Olaitan Soyannwo, Professor of Anesthesia and Consultant Anesthetist, College of Medicine, University of Ibadan and University College Hospital, Ibadan, Nigeria

Burton Wilcke, Jr., Chair and Associate Professor, Department of Medical Laboratory and Radiation Sciences, University of Vermont, Burlington

Michael Merson (*Board on Global Health Liaison*), Founding Director, Global Health Institute, Duke University, North Carolina

Elena O. Nightingale (*Board on Children, Youth, and Families Liaison*), Scholar-in-Residence, Institute of Medicine, The National Academies, Washington, D.C.

Julia Coffman (*Consultant*), Independent Evaluation Consultant, Alexandria, Virginia

Thomas Denny (*Consultant*), Research Associate Professor, Chief Operating Officer, Duke Human Vaccine Institute and Center for HIV/AIDS Vaccine Immunology, Duke University Medical Center, Durham, North Carolina

Florencia Zulberti (*Consultant*), Assistant Director for Global Health, National Institutes of Health, Mexico

Study Staff

Patrick Kelley, Board Director, Global Health

Rosemary Chalk, Board Director, Children, Youth and Families

Michele Orza, Study Director

Kimberly Scott, Senior Program Officer

Lucía Fort, Program Officer (through November 2006)

J. Alice Nixon, Program Officer (through November 2006)

Angela Mensah, Senior Program Assistant

Kimberly Weingarten, Senior Program Assistant (through September 2006)

Sheyi Lawoyin, Senior Program Assistant (May 2006 through July 2006)

Jessica Manning, Mirzayan Science and Technology Policy Fellow (May 2006 through August 2006)

Keren Ladin, Mirzayan Science and Technology Policy Fellow (June 2006 through August 2006)

Reviewers

This report has been reviewed in draft form by individuals chosen for their diverse perspectives and technical expertise, in accordance with procedures approved by the National Research Council's (NRC) Report Review Committee. The purpose of this independent review is to provide candid and critical comments that will assist the institution in making its published report as sound as possible and to ensure that the report meets institutional standards for objectivity, evidence, and responsiveness to the study charge. The review comments and draft manuscript remain confidential to protect the integrity of the deliberative process. We wish to thank the following individuals for their review of this report:

Roberto Arduino, Division of Infectious Diseases, The University of Texas Health Science Center at Houston

Solomon R. Benatar, Department of Medicine, University of Cape Town, South Africa

Alan Berkman, Mailman School of Public Health, Columbia University, New York

Jo Ivey Boufford, Robert F. Wagner Graduate School of Public Service, New York University

Fred Carden, International Development Research Centre, Ottawa, Canada

Ambassador Johnnie Carson, National Intelligence Council of the Office of the National Director of Intelligence, Washington, District of Columbia

Thomas J. Coates, David Geffen School of Medicine, University of California, Los Angeles

Susan A. Cohen, Guttmacher Institute, Washington, District of Columbia
Carlos del Rio, Emory AIDS International Training and Research, Rollins School of Public Health of Emory University and Grady Memorial Hospital, Atlanta, Georgia
Christopher J. Elias, PATH, Seattle, Washington
Helene Gayle, CARE, Atlanta, Georgia
Geeta Rao Gupta, International Center for Research on Women, Washington, District of Columbia
Grace John-Stewart, Department of Medicine, International AIDS Research and Training Program, University of Washington, Seattle, Washington
James W. Kazura, Center for Global Health and Diseases, Case Western Reserve University, Cleveland, Ohio
Mary Anne Koda-Kimble, School of Pharmacy, University of California, San Francisco
Adel A. F. Mahmoud, Merck Vaccines, Merck & Co., Inc., Whitehouse Station, New Jersey
Anne Mills, London School of Hygiene & Tropical Medicine, London
Roeland Monasch, United Nations Children's Fund, Harare, Zimbabwe
J. Stephen Morrison, HIV/AIDS Task Force, Center for Strategic & International Studies, Washington, District of Columbia
Anne Peterson, World Vision International, Washington, District of Columbia
Robert Redfield, Institute of Human Virology/Microbiology and Immunology, University of Maryland School of Medicine, Baltimore, Maryland
Catherine M. Wilfert, Duke University Medical Center, Duke University, Chapel Hill, North Carolina; The Elizabeth Glaser Pediatric AIDS Foundation

Although the reviewers listed above have provided many constructive comments and suggestions, they were not asked to endorse the conclusions or recommendations nor did they see the final draft of the report before its release. The review of this report was overseen by **Bernard Guyer,** Bloomberg School of Public Health, Johns Hopkins University, Baltimore, Maryland, and **Charles E. Phelps,** University of Rochester, New York. Appointed by the National Research Council and Institute of Medicine, they were responsible for making certain that an independent examination of this report was carried out in accordance with institutional procedures and that all review comments were carefully considered. Responsibility for the final content of this report rests entirely with the authoring committee and the institution.

Preface

Only a quarter of a century after first reported, HIV/AIDS has become one of the largest global health scourges of all times. This preventable viral disease caused the death of almost 3 million people last year alone, while over 4 million others became infected. The majority of this disease burden occurs in the developing world, with sub-Saharan Africa carrying the largest burden. As a result, life expectancy in that region has decreased, causing enormous human suffering and long-lasting demographic, social, and economic consequences.

The very rapid scientific discoveries on the etiology and modes of transmission, and later the development of effective treatment against HIV/AIDS are a tribute to human ingenuity. Our collective social response, however, has taken longer to get organized. Although still far from adequate, the global response to the epidemic is finally growing and progress is evident on a number of fronts. Hope has been restored based on a broad awakening of international commitment and strong evidence that the technical challenges can be met on a large scale.

A major factor in the increasing global response is "The President's Emergency Plan for AIDS Relief," or PEPFAR. This plan derives from novel legislation, passed by the U.S. Congress in 2003, which also mandated an evaluation of progress on this initiative. It has been the challenge and privilege of our Institute of Medicine to be charged with the conduct of this independent evaluation.

The Emergency Plan set ambitious goals. It seeks to support the prevention of 7 million HIV infections, the treatment of 2 million people with

AIDS, and the care of 10 million orphans and others affected by this epidemic. PEPFAR has focused on 15 countries, which collectively represent around 50 percent of the HIV infections worldwide (12 countries of Africa plus Vietnam, Haiti, and Guyana). Our IOM committee has found its work to evaluate such a multidimensional plan to be a unique challenge. Not only are the programs focused on different activities of prevention, treatment, and care, but within the 15 countries they are also conducted by a variety of public- and private-sector organizations, with various degrees of expertise. Some programs were started shortly after the first funds started to flow in 2004 and others more recently. Few, if any, of the programs observed could be described as mature. Yet, the Committee found evidence to guide future planning and policy. The bulk of this report communicates that evidence and presents the Committee's conclusions and recommendations.

It is in our human nature to better respond to emergencies than to sustain efforts over time. HIV/AIDS, however, is a chronic infection that requires life-long treatment. The continuity of the support is a medical and moral imperative, and therefore PEPFAR will need to make the transition from an emergency plan to a sustained effort that invests in building the capacity within countries to eventually take full responsibility for responding to their epidemics. Constant learning should be at the center of such a transition considering the need to economically and effectively replicate these programs in so many places. The energy, empathy, perseverance, and technical competence of those implementing PEPFAR will be needed for many years into the future.

The number of newly infected people with HIV vastly outpaces the capacity to treat patients with AIDS. Treatment of patients is not only a humanitarian imperative; it is also an indivisible component of prevention. But let us make no mistakes here: the only way to eventually control this pandemic is by preventing new cases. The epidemiologic facts are clear. The past occurrence of still largely invisible HIV infections will generate a deluge of new AIDS cases needing treatment over the next decade. Even more sobering is the fact that the rate of new HIV infections continues to grow. Proud as we should be of PEPFAR's success in providing medication to many of those already ill, it needs to urgently put the accent on preventive measures of proven efficacy on a much larger scale.

Nothing is as persuasive as success. A proof of concept is required to make a case; to the usual skeptics, PEPFAR has successfully demonstrated that programs of quality can be implemented, even in resource-thin settings. The many heroic professionals working in suboptimal conditions in the field have proven that large-scale HIV/AIDS prevention services, care, and treatment are feasible. However, many more like them will need to be trained and supported if quality care is to be continued, as it needs to be, over the decades to come.

Indeed, one area of special concern for sustainability of efforts in affected countries is the local health workforce. Human resource capacity is projected to be a critical rate-limiting factor for all future HIV prevention and treatment initiatives. These capacities take time to build. Health infrastructures are being impaired as worker death and worker morbidity from AIDS, migration to more favorable and high-paying work environments (i.e., the brain drain), and retirements deplete the already thin workforce. The epidemic also has many negative collateral impacts on other health initiatives—such as maternal and reproductive health, vaccination, or malaria—as human, laboratory, and financial resources become overwhelmed by HIV/AIDS-specific needs and resources are diverted to AIDS from other health programs. Building human capacity will need to be an even more essential element of future global AIDS initiatives.

"Learning by doing" is a necessary corollary to this unprecedented scale-up of a complex global public health initiative. The Office of the Global AIDS Coordinator has increasingly been making investments into monitoring, evaluation, and various forms of operational research to this end. The IOM committee would like to see its work as part of this evaluative continuum and encourages transparency and wide dissemination of the findings from the ongoing program evaluations of the U.S. Global AIDS Initiative. Creative and accountable action needs to continue unabated, and quality must always be at the forefront. The citizens of the United States expect this, those in need deserve it, and our call to be humanitarians demands no less. The United States has taken a critical leadership role in responding to the HIV/AIDS pandemic but since it can not provide all the necessary resources, the lessons learned from PEPFAR will be critical leverage to motivate other donor nations to follow its lead with deeper investments.

The IOM evaluation of the implementation of PEPFAR reflects many months of work not only by 22 uncompensated committee and subcommittee members, but also dozens of consultants, staff members, editors, board liaisons, and reviewers. The committee members enjoyed and were honored by the professionalism of hundreds of individuals who gave candid testimony about how PEPFAR is working in the field and at the management level in Washington, DC. While opinions varied about specific scientific and management approaches and priorities, it became clear that PEPFAR represents a notable achievement not only in its conceptualization but also in its implementation.

Global security is profoundly influenced by our increasing health interdependence. No one is safe from the international transfer of risks, and no one should be left out of the international transfer of opportunities, in the form of knowledge, resources and technology. The PEPFAR initiative should be seen not only as an important investment in the lives of many individuals and their families, but also as an investment in global security.

This is a good example of the kind of health diplomacy needed on a global scale.

PEPFAR is a vertical program. Much debate has existed in the past around the relative merits of vertical versus horizontal approaches to health care. To me, this is a false dilemma and an unnecessary dichotomy, for we should aim to have the best of both. A diagonal approach is one in which explicit intervention priorities—such as HIV/AIDS—is used to drive the desired improvements into the health system. AIDS is certainly not the only health problem in sub-Saharan Africa, nor can we tackle all problems at once. PEPFAR is laying the grounds for a unique opportunity—by contributing to the necessary capacity building—to incrementally incorporate other selected health priorities in the different countries' agendas.

While the Committee approached its task to conduct the evaluation in a dispassionate manner, it feels passionate about the problem and the potential solutions. It could not be otherwise; after all, the progress of PEPFAR is measured in real people—men, women, and children supported with vital HIV/AIDS services; health care workers trained to provide HIV/AIDS care; people enabled to change themselves, their communities, and their nations to better respond to the epidemic. Though the programs evaluated are still young, it was clear that millions of people are being served and life-saving medical care is being delivered on a large scale in some of the world's most challenging settings. As a Foreign Associate member of the Institute of Medicine who had the distinct privilege of leading this evaluation, I strongly believe that the American people, acting through PEPFAR, are to be complimented for supporting this remarkable humanitarian undertaking.

I would like to express my deep appreciation to the Institute of Medicine's authorities for the trust deposited in us, and to the heroic staff for all their hard work; and my perennial gratitude to all our Committee members, from whom I learned so much. The Committee hopes that the recommendations presented herein will be a constructive contribution to the current and future U.S. Global AIDS Initiatives.

Jaime Sepúlveda, M.D., Dr.Sc.
Chair

Acknowledgments

The Committee is deeply appreciative of the valuable contributions to this project of many knowledgeable and experienced people. Appendix A lists the many people and organizations who generously assisted the Committee with its study.

The Committee would like to thank the Office of the U.S. Global AIDS Coordinator—in particular Ambassador Mark Dybul, Dr. Kathy Marconi, and Dr. Nadine Rogers for their assistance throughout the project.

The Committee expresses its admiration for and gratitude to its dedicated, hard-working staff, ably led by Dr. Michele Orza—particulary Kimberly Scott and Angela Mensah who saw this book through to completion. Thanks also to the many IOM staff not listed in the following pages including Bronwyn Schrecker, Janice Mehler, Lara Andersen, Allison Brantley, Elizabeth Sharp, Bethany Hardy, and Tyjen Tsai. Special thanks to Hellen Gelband for assistance in drafting background chapters of the report and to Rona Briere and Alisa Decatur for editorial assistance.

Contents

Tables, Figures, and Boxes

TABLES

FIGURES

BOXES

Abstract

The Institute of Medicine (IOM) undertook this short-term evaluation of the implementation of the President's Emergency Plan for AIDS Relief (PEPFAR) to inform Congress about the program's progress 3 years after its authorizing legislation was passed. The IOM committee found that PEPFAR has supported the expansion of HIV/AIDS prevention, treatment, and care services in the focus countries. For continued progress toward its 5-year targets and longer-term goals, PEPFAR should transition from a focus on emergency relief to an emphasis on the long-term strategic planning and capacity building necessary for sustainability. The committee identifies a number of opportunities for improvement that would support this transition, including

- Greater emphasis on prevention of HIV infection generally, and better linkage between the program planning process and improved data on prevalence and populations at risk in particular.
- Increased attention to the factors that heighten the vulnerability of women and girls to HIV infection and its consequences, such as their legal, economic, educational, and social status.
- Continued commitment to and additional emphasis on harmonization—a concept based on the importance of each country's leadership of its response to its epidemic. All three aspects of harmonization—alignment between donor and country plans, coordination with national AIDS coordinating agencies, and support for national monitoring and evaluation frameworks—need strengthening. Of particular importance is to transition

from the current requirement to use medications approved by the U.S. Food and Drug Administration to support for World Health Organization prequalification as the accepted global standard for assuring the quality of generic medications.

- Enhanced ability to tailor interventions to the nature of the epidemic in each country and the countries' national plans through removal of the limitations imposed by congressional budget allocations for particular activities. Alternative mechanisms that allow for spending to be directly linked with the efforts necessary to achieve performance targets would improve the necessary accountability for results.
- Expansion and better integration of services to meet the needs of all people living with HIV/AIDS, and to both improve prevention, treatment, and care interventions and capitalize on the synergy among them.
- Strengthened and expanded country capacity to provide services—particularly the necessary human resources—through implementation of HIV/AIDS programs in a manner that strengthens systems overall.
- Enhanced knowledge about what works against the pandemic, to be gained by increasing the emphasis on learning from experience with the program and on conducting operations research and program evaluations.

The Committee concludes that PEPFAR has made a promising start, but the need for U.S. leadership in the effort to control the HIV/AIDS pandemic continues.

Summary

INTRODUCTION

On May 27, 2003, the U.S. Congress passed the United States Leadership against HIV/AIDS, Tuberculosis, and Malaria Act of 2003 (the Leadership Act) and launched the U.S. Global AIDS Initiative. Among other things, this broad legislation required the President to establish a comprehensive, integrated 5-year strategy to combat global HIV/AIDS. The initiative is commonly known by the title of this strategy: "The President's Emergency Plan for AIDS Relief," or PEPFAR. The legislation also required the President to establish the position of U.S. Global AIDS Coordinator (the Coordinator) within the U.S. Department of State, with primary responsibility for oversight and coordination of all U.S. international activities to combat the HIV/AIDS pandemic.

As mandated by the Leadership Act, the U.S. Institute of Medicine (IOM) undertook a short-term evaluation of the implementation of PEPFAR to inform Congress about the initiative's progress 3 years after passage of the legislation. The IOM Committee for the Evaluation of PEPFAR Implementation (the Committee) began its work on this short-term evaluation in February 2005. Although the Leadership Act was passed in May 2003, Congress first appropriated funds for the program in January 2004, and the majority of the first year's funding was not obligated until September 2004. Thus at the close of the Committee's short-term evaluation, PEPFAR had been supporting the implementation of programs in the focus countries for less than 2 years.

The U.S. Global AIDS Initiative is working in more than 120 countries around the world, but concentrates resources in 15 focus countries so as to have an impact on their epidemics at the national level.[1] The scope of this evaluation is limited to the implementation of PEPFAR in the focus countries and does not include the U.S. contribution to the Global Fund to Fight AIDS, Tuberculosis and Malaria, which is also overseen by the Coordinator. Although direct evaluation of the Leadership Act was beyond its scope, the Committee examined and reached conclusions about factors that appeared to be having a pronounced effect on the implementation of PEPFAR, some of which have their roots in the legislation.

PEPFAR's 5-year performance targets for the focus countries are to support the prevention of 7 million HIV infections; treatment for 2 million people with HIV/AIDS with antiretroviral therapy (ART); and care for 10 million people infected with and affected by HIV/AIDS, including orphans and other vulnerable children (United States Leadership against HIV/AIDS, Tuberculosis, and Malaria Act of 2003, P.L. 108-25, 108th Cong., 1st Sess.; OGAC, 2004). The Committee intended its evaluation to be appropriate for a program early in its implementation, and to provide insight into whether PEPFAR is making reasonable progress toward meeting these targets and positioning the U.S. Global AIDS Initiative to achieve the ultimate goal of the Leadership Act—sustainable gains against the HIV/AIDS pandemic.

At the core of the complex structure and approach of PEPFAR—which involves numerous U.S. government agencies and is centrally coordinated by the Office of the U.S. Global AIDS Coordinator (OGAC), but implemented by the U.S. teams in the focus countries (Country Teams)—is the U.S. commitment to the principles of harmonization (The Rome Declaration, 2003; UN, 2003; Tobias, 2003a, 2004; UNAIDS, 2004a; OGAC, 2005a; The Paris Declaration, 2005). The central tenet of harmonization is that sustainable gains against the HIV/AIDS pandemic will require that each country own and lead its response to its epidemic. The role of donors is to support and participate in the three country-determined elements critical for an effective response—one national AIDS plan, one national AIDS coordinating mechanism, and one national AIDS monitoring and evaluation framework (UNAIDS, 2004a). Therefore, the Committee evaluated the implementation of PEPFAR primarily through the lens of harmoniza-

[1]The 15 focus countries are the Republic of Botswana, the Republic of Côte d'Ivoire, the Federal Democratic Republic of Ethiopia, the Cooperative Republic of Guyana, the Republic of Haiti, the Republic of Kenya, the Republic of Mozambique, the Republic of Namibia, the Federal Republic of Nigeria, the Republic of Rwanda, the Republic of South Africa, the United Republic of Tanzania, the Republic of Uganda, the Socialist Republic of Vietnam, and the Republic of Zambia. With the exception of Vietnam, these countries are named in the Leadership Act.

tion and sought to determine how effectively the program is meeting its commitment to support the focus countries' responses to their HIV/AIDS epidemics (IOM, 2005b).

THE PROGRESS OF PEPFAR

PEPFAR Has Supported the Expansion of HIV/AIDS Services in the Focus Countries

In the 15 focus countries, the U.S. Global AIDS Initiative has, as intended, supported HIV/AIDS activities and programs on a national scale, and OGAC reports substantial early progress toward its targets. In roughly 2 years, OGAC reports that PEPFAR has supported ART for more than 800,000 adults and children; HIV testing and counseling for nearly 19 million people; services to prevent mother-to-child transmission of HIV to women during more than 6 million pregnancies, including preventive antiretroviral medications (ARVs) for more than half a million women found to be HIV-positive (estimated by OGAC to have resulted in the prevention of HIV infection in more than 100,000 infants); public education campaigns, school curricula, and other types of information and education community outreach that are estimated to have reached more than 140 million adults and children; care and support services for approximately 4.5 million adults, orphans, and other vulnerable children; training in HIV/AIDS care and support services for well over a million people, including physicians, nurses, clinical officers, pharmacists, laboratory workers, epidemiologists, community workers, teachers, midwives, birth attendants, and traditional healers; and expansion and strengthening of clinical laboratories, supply chain management systems, blood supply systems, safe medical practices, and monitoring and evaluation systems (OGAC, 2005b, 2006a,b, 2007). Although data are not yet available with which to determine the quality or impact of these services, the Committee believes this substantial expansion of services represents inroads into the HIV/AIDS epidemics in the focus countries. Thus the primary early accomplishment of the U.S. Global AIDS Initiative has been to demonstrate that HIV/AIDS services, particularly treatment, can be rapidly scaled up in resource-constrained and otherwise severely challenged environments such as those existing in the focus countries—something many had doubted could be done (UNAIDS, 2001; WHO, 2003a,b; IOM, 2005a).

Transition from Emergency to Sustainability Is Essential to Achieve the Goals of the Leadership Act

Hallmarks of PEPFAR have been its continued sense of urgency and the rapidity with which it has supported the implementation of programs and delivery of services—not only ART, but across the spectrum of HIV/AIDS care and support (Nieburg et al., 2004). Although its emergency response has allowed PEPFAR to support rapid expansion of services in the focus countries, it has not necessarily facilitated coordination with global partners, harmonization with the strategies and plans of partner countries, services that are comprehensive and integrated at the community level, sustainable programs, or adequate monitoring and evaluation. Yet the Coordinator has described "building capacity for sustainable, effective, and widespread HIV/AIDS responses" as one of the cornerstones of the PEPFAR strategy (OGAC, 2004). According to the Leadership Act, as well as PEPFAR documents and official statements, the program has from the beginning been aimed at strengthening and expanding the capacity of the focus countries to develop HIV/AIDS programs and provide services (Tobias, 2003b; OGAC, 2004). PEPFAR has provided funding and technical assistance to help focus country governments develop national plans and monitoring and evaluation systems; improve existing and build new facilities; develop curricula for and train health workers; strengthen and expand laboratory, blood supply, and medical waste management systems; improve and expand supply chains; and strengthen existing and foster new community-based organizations.

> ***The continuing challenge for the U.S. Global AIDS Initiative is to simultaneously maintain the urgency and intensity that have allowed it to support a substantial expansion of HIV/AIDS services in a relatively short time while also placing greater emphasis on long-term strategic planning and increasing the attention and resources directed to capacity building for sustainability.*** **The U.S. Global AIDS Coordinator should continue to focus on planning for the next decade of the U.S. Global AIDS Initiative, taking full advantage of the knowledge gained from the early years of PEPFAR about the focus countries' epidemics and how best to address them. The next strategy should squarely address the needs and challenges involved in supporting sustainable country HIV/AIDS programs, thereby transitioning from a focus on emergency relief.** (8.1)[2]

The Committee's recommendations for improvement are premised on the assumption that Congress will reauthorize the U.S. Global AIDS Initiative and directed toward helping PEPFAR continue the transition from

---

[2]The first digit of each recommendation number refers to the chapter in which the recommendation is discussed in full.

emergency response to sustainability, and thus to make further progress toward both its 5-year performance targets and the ultimate goal of the Leadership Act. None of the issues raised by the Committee or its recommendations for enabling PEPFAR to progress more effectively should be construed as a lack of support for the U.S. Global AIDS Initiative or its authorizing legislation.

THE PROMISE OF PEPFAR

Successful Prevention Is Key for Sustainability

If countries do not succeed in stemming the tide of new infections, the need for treatment will continue to increase and outpace their ability to develop the capacity to meet it (Mathers and Loncar, 2006). PEPFAR is currently supporting a wide range of programs directed at preventing the spread of HIV. Partly in response to legislative mandates, however, it has supported some preventive interventions that are not firmly evidence-based, addressed sources of HIV transmission in disproportion to their expected contribution to the ultimate goal of preventing new infections, and not fully capitalized on opportunities to integrate prevention activities optimally with each other and into treatment and care programs. To help countries sustain and expand their gains against their HIV/AIDS epidemics, the U.S. Global AIDS Initiative will need to emphasize effective, evidence-based prevention with the same urgency and intensity it has focused on treatment. Moreover, the initiative cannot afford to conceptualize prevention narrowly or as distinct from treatment and care, and needs to support countries in seizing the abundant opportunities for prevention throughout people's lives and regardless of their HIV status; across the full spectrum of health and social services; and in all settings, from the street to the school to the home to the clinic (Salomon et al., 2005; UNAIDS, 2005c).

The U.S. Global AIDS Initiative should enhance and intensify HIV prevention through a planning process that links timely national information on the epidemic to the selection of the most appropriate intervention packages and to the optimal targeting of interventions to populations in whom infections are most likely to occur. The U.S. Global AIDS Coordinator should enhance current data on HIV prevalence by supporting quality behavioral surveys to identify patterns of risk. The Coordinator should support country plans to identify where infections are to be averted to achieve prevention targets and should track progress toward achieving prevention goals by measuring risk behaviors, the prevalence and incidence of other sexually transmitted infections, and ultimately the prevalence and incidence of HIV. (4.1)

Increasing Focus on the Status of Women and Girls Is Critical for Sustainability

The Leadership Act calls for a focus on women and girls, articulates the need to address their particular vulnerability if the fight against the HIV/AIDS pandemic is to succeed, and requires that the PEPFAR strategy address their unique needs. The strategy is largely responsive to this mandate, and PEPFAR is currently supporting numerous programs and services directed at reducing the risks faced by women and girls. These efforts are focused in five areas: increasing gender equity, addressing male norms, reducing violence and sexual coercion, increasing income generation for both women and girls, and ensuring legal protection and property rights (OGAC, 2005b, 2006b). However, no information is available with which to determine either the individual or collective impact of these activities on the status of and risks to women and girls. To the extent possible with data collection systems that do not always identify the sex of the person receiving services, PEPFAR has been able to demonstrate that women and girls are receiving PEPFAR-supported prevention, treatment, and care services in seemingly appropriate proportions to men and boys.

> ***Most of the factors that contribute to the increased vulnerability of women and girls to HIV/AIDS cannot be readily addressed in the short term. The Leadership Act appropriately views these factors as priorities on the agenda for the fight against HIV/AIDS. In the transition from emergency response to sustainability, these factors will require increased emphasis and support, and the U.S. Global AIDS Initiative will need to keep gender issues at the core of its efforts.*** **The U.S. Global AIDS Initiative should continue to increase its focus on the factors that put women at greater risk of HIV/AIDS and to support improvements in the legal, economic, educational, and social status of women and girls.** (8.2)

Improved Harmonization and Coordination Are Needed to Strengthen the Foundation for Sustainability

Countries' ownership and leadership of their responses to their HIV/AIDS epidemics are recognized as essential for success and sustainability (The Rome Declaration, 2003; Tobias, 2003b; UN, 2003; The Paris Declaration, 2005). Because no single approach can work in the context of harmonization, the PEPFAR Country Teams need maximum flexibility to work closely with and within the framework and priorities of the partner countries. The PEPFAR Country Teams have been largely successful in aligning their plans with the partner countries' national HIV/AIDS strategies, coordinating with national AIDS coordinating agencies, and supporting national monitoring and evaluation frameworks (OGAC, 2005c, 2006g). However, particularly as the partner countries improve their national programs and become more directive with donors, there is room for the U.S. Global AIDS Initiative to improve on all three aspects of harmonization, and greater flexibility would facilitate this improvement.

Closer coordination and cooperation with other international donors at both the global and country levels is also necessary for harmonization to succeed in empowering countries. As the number of donors and the amount of available resources increase, so, too, will the need for coordination. As highlighted by the Leadership Act, a key feature of U.S. leadership is commitment to coordination at all levels. At the global level, it is essential for the United States to continue to work closely with other multilateral and bilateral donors to ensure that the comparative strengths of each are maximized and have a positive, synergistic impact on countries, rather than a duplicative, inefficient, and disempowering one (OECD, 2003; UNAIDS, 2005a; GIST, 2006).

> **To support country leadership, the U.S. Global AIDS Coordinator should seek to identify and remove barriers to coordination with partner governments and other donors, with a particular focus on promoting transparency and participation throughout the annual planning process.** (3.1)

During the Committee's visits to the focus countries, the most frequently cited example of an impediment to coordination and harmonization was PEPFAR's requirement for U.S. Food and Drug Administration (FDA) approval of ARVs. A previous IOM Committee strongly endorsed "a rigorous, standardized international mechanism to support national quality assurance programs for antiretroviral drugs" (IOM, 2005a, p. 8). The international mechanism on which most other donors and the majority of the PEPFAR focus countries rely is the World Health Organization (WHO) Prequalification of Medications Project (WHO, 2006b). When PEPFAR was initiated, however, the Coordinator determined that FDA approval would be the standard for ensuring the quality of PEPFAR-provided ARVs (OGAC, 2004). This standard posed a major challenge to implementation because most of the focus countries had selected generic versions of ARVs for their formularies, and no generic ARVs had FDA approval (GAO, 2005). Subsequently, the Coordinator has fostered and supported an expedited FDA review process for generic ARVs, and since December 2004, more than 30 generic versions of the first-line ARVs have been FDA-approved for purchase by PEPFAR (DHHS, 2004; FDA, 2006; OGAC, 2006c). However, many of these medications, including some of the fixed-dose combination ARVs that are most desirable in the focus countries, were approved only within the past year (FDA, 2006). According to OGAC, only 10 percent of total PEPFAR-supported ARV purchases were for FDA-approved generics in fiscal year 2005, increasing to 27 percent in 2006 (OGAC, 2006c, 2007). In addition, because some focus countries rely on WHO prequalification, they require it in addition to FDA approval. Thus, PEPFAR's strategy for ensuring the quality of the ARVs it provides has impeded harmonization and the rapid availability of PEPFAR-supported first-line ARVs.

To support countries' ownership of their responses to their HIV/AIDS epidemics, the U.S. Global AIDS Initiative should maintain its commitment to harmonization and participate fully in the development of harmonized procedures. To this end, the U.S. Global AIDS Coordinator should work to support World Health Organization (WHO) prequalification as the accepted global standard for assuring the quality of generic medications. Specifically, the Coordinator should provide an analysis of WHO prequalification that determines whether it can adequately assure the quality of generic antiretroviral medications for purchase under PEPFAR. If the analysis shows that WHO prequalification needs strengthening to provide a sufficient guarantee of quality for PEPFAR, the U.S. Global AIDS Initiative should work with other donors to support strengthening of the process, and work to transition from U.S. Food and Drug Administration approval to WHO prequalification as rapidly as feasible. (5.2)

Budget Allocations Reduce Flexibility and Impede Harmonization and Program Implementation

One of the strengths of the U.S. Global AIDS Initiative is its orientation toward and accountability for specified results. The Coordinator's annual reports to Congress have shown progress toward the defined, measurable performance targets set forth in the legislation and the PEPFAR strategy (OGAC, 2005b, 2006b). Appropriately for a program this early in implementation, most of the results reported at this stage are for targets that can be measured in the short term, and thus they reveal more about the program's implementation than its impact.

However, one set of the Leadership Act's short-term targets—its budget allocations—has adversely affected implementation of the U.S. Global AIDS Initiative. In mandating the strategy that was eventually to become known as PEPFAR, Congress wisely required that the "strategy shall maintain sufficient flexibility and remain responsive to the ever-changing nature of the HIV/AIDS pandemic." However, Congress also required that the program adhere to a fairly large set of specific budget allocations.[3] At the

[3]The budget allocations include 55 percent for "therapeutic medical care of individuals infected with HIV, of which such amount at least 75 percent should be expended for the purchase and distribution of antiretroviral pharmaceuticals and at least 25 percent should be expended for related care"; 20 percent for "HIV/AIDS prevention, of which such amount at

time the Leadership Act was passed, little information existed with which to determine precisely how resources should be allocated to achieve the performance targets across the focus countries; thus the budget allocations could not be evidence-based. Furthermore, Congress established these allocations so that they become more, not less, restrictive over time as the pandemic evolves and the program gains experience and knowledge.[4] Contrary to basic principles of good management and accountability, the budget allocations have made spending money in a particular way an end in itself rather than a means to an end—in this instance, the vitally important end of saving lives today and in the future.

In the Committee's judgment, the Coordinator and the Country Teams have made reasonable attempts to both respect the congressional budget allocations and implement within these constraints an effective program that can achieve its ambitious targets. However, their task is to implement a comprehensive, integrated, evidence-based program to address the HIV/AIDS epidemics in 15 unique, resource-constrained countries within the framework of harmonization. Particularly because Congress demonstrated no relationship between the budget allocations and the performance targets—prevention of 7 million infections, provision of ART to 2 million people, and provision of care for 10 million people—the budget allocations have further complicated this already daunting task and thus have been counterproductive. It is readily apparent that PEPFAR's approach to and mechanisms for planning, implementing, and measuring the initiative are to a large extent structured to be able to adhere to and report on the budget allocations. PEPFAR staff, both in headquarters and on the Country Teams, have explained to the Committee and others their frustration with these allocations and have illustrated how they thwart rational and strategic planning to meet the performance targets (GAO, 2006). Thus the manner in which Congress has required resources to be allocated, rather than what is necessary to have an impact, is having an unwarranted influence on PEPFAR. The U.S. Global AIDS Initiative needs maximum flexibility and agility not only to adapt to a changing pandemic and be harmonized with the efforts of 15 different focus countries, but also to be able to incorporate what is learned through program implementation about how to have the greatest impact. Resource allocation that is the consequence of rather than

least 33 percent should be expended for abstinence-until-marriage programs"; 15 percent for "palliative care of individuals with HIV/AIDS"; and 10 percent for "assistance for orphans and vulnerable children affected by HIV/AIDS, of which such amount at least 50 percent shall be provided through non-profit, nongovernmental organizations, including faith-based organizations, that implement programs on the community level."

[4]Many of the budget allocations became mandatory beginning with fiscal year 2006.

the precursor for adaptive, evidence-based programming, would better enable the initiative to have an optimal impact.

> ***Although they may have been helpful initially in ensuring a balance of attention to activities within the four categories of prevention, treatment, care, and orphans and vulnerable children, the Committee concludes that rigid congressional budget allocations among categories, and even more so within categories, have also limited PEPFAR's ability to tailor its activities in each country to the local epidemic and to coordinate with the level of activities in the countries' national plans.*** **Congress should remove the budget allocations and replace them with more appropriate mechanisms that ensure accountability for results from Country Teams to the U.S. Global AIDS Coordinator and to Congress. These mechanisms should also ensure that spending is directly linked to and commensurate with necessary efforts to achieve both country and overall performance targets for prevention, treatment, care, and orphans and vulnerable children.** (3.3)

Expansion, Improvement, and Better Integration of Services Are Needed for Sustainability

If the U.S. Global AIDS Initiative is to succeed, it is essential that PEPFAR support programs and services that are evidence-based; strategically planned using the best data available; and implemented equitably, efficiently, and effectively (UNAIDS, 1998, 2004b). Although PEPFAR does not necessarily categorize activities in accordance with global norms, it is supporting all of the major components of a comprehensive HIV/AIDS program recommended by global consensus (UNAIDS, 2001, 2005b; WHO, 2004). The Committee observed much promise in the programs PEPFAR supports, as well as room for improvement and a need for expansion. Of particular importance is for PEPFAR to support programs in a manner that fosters integration both within and among the program categories of prevention, treatment, care, and orphans and vulnerable children—or, more appropriately, regardless of categorization. Neither the congressional budget allocations discussed above nor the budgeting, planning, and reporting mechanisms the Coordinator established to ensure that PEPFAR complies with these allocations facilitate integration. Optimal integration is critical to achieve not only the success of individual interventions and services, but also to realize the additional benefits that derive from the synergy among them (Salomon et al., 2005). The Committee's recommendation for improving PEPFAR's approach to prevention was discussed earlier; recommendations for improving its approach to treatment, care, and services for orphans and vulnerable children, as well as to ensuring equity, are presented below.

Treatment

The U.S. Global AIDS Coordinator should ensure that adequate medications are available to place 2 million people on sustained antiretroviral therapy to achieve PEPFAR's stated 5-year treatment target. To achieve this target, the Coordinator should also ensure that adequate linkages are established among prevention, treatment, and care programs and rapidly expand the availability of antiretroviral therapy to both children and adults. (5.1)

Care

The U.S. Global AIDS Coordinator should continue to promote and support a community-based, family-centered model of care in order to enhance and coordinate supportive care services for people living with HIV/AIDS, with special emphasis on orphans, vulnerable children, and people requiring end-of-life care. This model should include integration as appropriate with prevention and treatment programs and linkages with other public-sector and nongovernmental organization services within and outside of the health sector, such as primary health care, nutrition support, education, social work, and the work of agencies facilitating income generation. (6.1)

Orphans and Other Vulnerable Children

***The needs of orphans and other children made vulnerable by AIDS cover a wide spectrum that cuts across all of PEPFAR's categories of prevention, treatment, and care and extends well beyond the health sector. It is essential for an HIV/AIDS response to address these needs adequately—not only to support these children in living healthy and productive lives, but also to protect them from becoming the next wave of the pandemic.* The U.S. Global AIDS Initiative should continue to support countries in the development of national plans that address the needs of orphans and other children made vulnerable by AIDS, as well as to support the priorities delineated in these plans. To ensure adequate focus on and accountability for addressing the needs of orphans and other vulnerable children, the U.S. Global AIDS Coordinator should work with Congress to set a distinct and meaningful performance target for this population. This target should be developed in a manner that both builds on the improvements PEPFAR has made in its indicator for children served and enhances its ability to support comprehensive and integrated HIV/AIDS programming. (7.1)**

Equity

The commitment of the U.S. Global AIDS Initiative to work toward reducing stigma and discrimination against people living with HIV/AIDS requires that marginalized and difficult-to-reach groups receive prevention, treatment, and care services. These groups include sex workers, prisoners, those who use injection drugs, and men who have sex with men—groups that not only are characterized by their high-risk behavior, but also tend to be stigmatized and subject to discrimination. **The U.S. Global AIDS Coordinator should document how these groups are included in the program planning, implementation, and evaluation of PEPFAR activities.** (3.2)

Expanded Capacity Is Necessary to Meet Current and Future Needs

Severe human resource shortages are a continuing challenge to PEPFAR implementation (OGAC, 2005b, 2006b; WHO, 2006c). Plans for ART scale-up that have been developed by some partner countries and are now being formulated in others include specific efforts to increase the health care workforce, with an emphasis on increasing the numbers of nurses, clinical officers, and pharmacists, among others. Training periods for these vital personnel are typically 2 to 3 years. Expansion of class sizes and repetition of existing programs are, in some partner countries, easily identified and cost-effective means for workforce expansion. In other countries, the lack of clinical faculty mirrors the lack of overall personnel, and increases in the numbers of teachers are badly needed (UNAIDS, 2006).

PEPFAR's initial emergency approach to meeting personnel needs has been to focus on HIV-specific training of existing clinicians and other health care workers (OGAC, 2006d). Support for expansion of the professional clinical workforce has been limited, even when such expansion is an explicit part of the country's HIV/AIDS plan, and the effort is endorsed and supported by other donors (OGAC, 2005c, 2006g). During its visits to the focus countries, the Committee saw many programs of all varieties—particularly ART programs—that were overflowing their capacity, had long waiting lists, and had insufficient numbers of staff who were highly stressed. PEPFAR Country Teams often expressed concern that they were not allowed to fund activities unless those activities were specifically part of the HIV/AIDS effort and so could not support, for example, the training of new clinical officers, who in some countries are the mainstay of the treatment effort.

PEPFAR reports that its response to the shortage of health workers to date has been to provide support, within national plans and priorities and the principles of harmonization, for policy reform to promote task shifting from physicians and nurses to community health workers; for the development of information systems; for human resource assessments; for training for health workers, including community health workers; for retention strategies; and for twinning partnerships (OGAC, 2006d). One mainstay of this approach—task shifting—is not possible in countries with few health personnel because the nurses and clinical officers to whom tasks could be shifted are not available. A refocus on new personnel, with use of twinning to expand the numbers of faculty available, is needed to enable task shifting.

If focus countries' plans for expanding their health workforce are not supported, PEPFAR may also exacerbate national shortages by shifting a disproportionate share of the workforce to efforts against HIV/AIDS, with the result that other health priorities would be neglected. To ameliorate this potential negative consequence of PEPFAR's disease-specific focus, Country Teams need to work closely with governments and other donors to determine a reasonable proportion of PEPFAR funding to be allocated to the education of new health professionals. Also, to ensure that PEPFAR itself is not drawing workers out of the public system through disproportionate incentives and salaries, it is important that the Coordinator continue to study the impact of the program's hiring practices and compensation policies and act quickly and decisively to address any problems identified. Finally, evaluation of PEPFAR's impact needs to include indicators for areas of the public health system likely to be sensitive to the loss of personnel, such as maternal and child health and immunization programs.

To meet existing targets for prevention, treatment, and care, the U.S. Global AIDS Initiative should increase the support available to expand workforce capacity in heavily affected countries. These efforts should include education of new health care workers in addition to AIDS-related training for existing health care workers. Such support should be planned in conjunction with other donors to ensure that comparative advantages are maximized and be provided in the context of national human resource strategies that include relevant stakeholders, such as the ministries of health, labor, and education; other ministries; employers; regulatory bodies; professional associations; training institutions; and consumers. (8.3)

Knowledge About What Works Against the HIV/AIDS Pandemic Is Essential for Sustainability

Because of its magnitude and reach, the U.S. Global HIV/AIDS Initiative represents a golden opportunity to learn about what works best in addressing the pandemic, and such learning is in turn essential to the program's success. The Leadership Act emphasizes the importance of both basic and applied research, and requires that research be an integral part of the initiative. In addition, because of the many gaps in the knowledge base for addressing HIV/AIDS, the initiative has an obligation to "learn by doing" (IOM, 2005a). In doing so, the initiative can help the global community learn not only about what approaches are cost-effective for preventing infection and caring for people affected by HIV/AIDS and its consequences, but also about how to scale up effective programs, how to implement programs in a manner that builds capacity and strengthens health systems overall, how best to manage such global initiatives, and how to work most effectively within the framework of harmonization to empower countries to own and lead their responses to their HIV/AIDS epidemics.

Functioning as a Learning Organization

Beginning with its strategy, PEPFAR has been committed to learning, and the program has displayed many of the characteristics of a successful learning organization. The PEPFAR strategy envisioned OGAC as a "small organization focused on leadership, coordination, learning, and oversight" that would "strive to remain flexible and innovative in its approaches" (OGAC, 2004, p. 67). The Committee has seen many examples of OGAC's success in realizing this vision and encourages OGAC to continue in this vein. However, OGAC currently does not formally evaluate or provide information about its performance on critical aspects of program management—such as coordination—and would benefit from doing so.

Research

The PEPFAR strategy also commits to building the evidence base on what works against HIV/AIDS and fostering innovation (OGAC, 2004), and the initiative is indeed helping to expand knowledge about the implemention of HIV/AIDS programs and services in resource-constrained countries. The U.S. Global AIDS Initiative supports the full spectrum of global AIDS research, from basic to operations research, through several entities in addition to OGAC, including the National Institutes of Health, the Centers for Disease Control and Prevention, and the U.S. Agency for International Development. OGAC directly funds targeted evaluations to support the programs and policies of the initiative and is currently providing about $22 million for these evaluations, primarily in the focus countries. The evaluations cover a wide range of topics related to prevention, treatment, and care (OGAC, 2006e,f). However, many Country Teams and implementing partners believe that using PEPFAR funds for research of any kind is prohibited and thus have not rountinely incorporated operations research into their programs. Yet there are still more questions than answers about how best to respond to the HIV/AIDS epidemics in these countries, and the Committee highlights some of these in the ensuing chapters.

The U.S. Global AIDS Initiative should increase its contribution to the global evidence base for HIV/AIDS interventions by better capitalizing on the opportunity PEPFAR represents to learn about and share what works. The U.S. Global AIDS Coordinator should further emphasize the importance of and provide additional support for operations research and program evaluation in particular—not as the primary aim but as an integral component of programs. All programs should include robust monitoring and evaluation that factors into decisions about whether and in what manner the programs are to continue. The initiative should maintain its appropriate openness to new and innovative approaches and programs, but unproven programs in particular should be required to have an evaluation component to determine their effectiveness. (8.4)

Key to understanding what works against the HIV/AIDS pandemic will be to learn whether PEPFAR has succeeded—that is, to understand its long-term impact. To measure what really matters—reductions in disability, disease, and death from HIV/AIDS; increases in the capacity of partner countries to sustain and expand HIV/AIDS programs without setbacks in other aspects of their public health systems; and improvements in the lives of the people living in these countries—the United States and other donors will be heavily dependent on the capabilities of the partner countries. To understand whether countries are achieving these ultimate goals and what contributions the U.S. Global AIDS Initiative is making to their achievement, the initiative will need to study national trends, such as rates of new HIV and other infections; rates of survival from HIV/AIDS and other diseases; child survival, development, and well-being; and the general health status of the population and key subpopulations. Particularly within the agreed framework of harmonization, the data and analyses necessary to study these trends will have to come primarily from the partner countries themselves (UNAIDS, 2004a). Thus it is essential that the United States, in conjunction with other donors, continue to place priority on helping to strengthen the monitoring and evaluation systems of the partner countries.

The Need for U.S. Leadership Against the HIV/AIDS Pandemic Continues

The Committee found that the U.S. Global AIDS Initiative has made a strong start, is progressing toward its 5-year targets, and is increasingly well positioned to support countries in controlling their epidemics. At the same time, however, PEPFAR has not yet reached the half-way mark for any of its targets, each focus country still faces an enormous challenge in controlling its epidemic, and the HIV/AIDS pandemic continues to grow. The Joint United Nations Programme on HIV/AIDS has estimated that more than 4 million people worldwide became newly infected with HIV in 2006, and, unless prevention efforts are highly successful, millions more will become infected every year (UNAIDS, 2006). Of the nearly 7 million people in low- and middle-income countries now estimated to need ART or to face an early death, fewer than one-quarter are receiving the therapy (WHO, 2006a), and millions more of those already infected with HIV will eventually need it. Fewer than 1 in 10 pregnant women infected with HIV in low- and middle-income countries are benefiting from ARVs to prevent transmission to their babies, and at most 12 percent of the children born to these women who require ART are receiving it (WHO, 2006a). With ART and appropriate care, AIDS is a chronic disease—it can be managed but not cured—and people receiving ART will need to be on it for the rest of their lives. Only a fraction of the legions of devastated families and orphaned children are currently receiving the support services they need, and the number of children orphaned by AIDS globally is projected to exceed 20 million by 2010 (UNICEF, 2006).

The Committee believes that continued commitment by the United States, along with all other donors, to supporting the fight against the HIV/AIDS pandemic will be required until countries have developed sustainable programs, and that continued U.S. leadership is necessary to prevent complacency and battle fatigue and to bring the virus under control.

REFERENCES

DHHS (Department of Health and Human Services). 2004. *HHS proposes rapid process for review of fixed dose combination and co-packaged products.* http://www.hhs.gov/news/press/2004pres/20040516.html (accessed September 6, 2006).

FDA (Food and Drug Administration). 2006. *President's Emergency Plan for AIDS Relief approved and tentatively approved antiretrovirals in association with the President's emergency plan.* http://www.fda.gov/oia/pepfar.htm (accessed January 11, 2007).

GAO (Government Accountability Office). 2005. *Global HIV/AIDS epidemic: Selection of antiretroviral medications provided under U.S. emergency plan is limited* (GAO-05-133). Washington, DC: GAO.

GAO. 2006. *Global health: Spending requirement presents challenges for allocating prevention funding under the President's Emergency Plan for AIDS Relief* (GAO-06-395). Washington, DC: GAO.

GIST (Global Implementation Support Team). 2006. *Fact sheet: The Global Implementation Support Team: Coordinating UN action and provision of technical support for accelerating HIV/AIDS responses in countries.* http://data.unaids.org/pub/BrochurePamphlet/2006/2006_gist_en.pdf (accessed January 12, 2007).

IOM (Institute of Medicine). 2005a. *Scaling up treatment for the global AIDS pandemic: Challenges and opportunities.* Washington, DC: The National Academies Press.

IOM. 2005b. *Plan for a short-term evaluation of PEPFAR implementation.* Washington, DC: The National Academies Press.

Mathers, C., and D. Loncar. 2006. Projections of global mortality and burden of disease from 2002 to 2030. *PLoS Medicine* 3(11):e442.

Nieburg, P., J. Kates, and J. S. Morrison. 2004. *Enhancing the rapid response capacity of the U.S. global AIDS coordinator: Lessons from other U.S. emergency responses. A report of the CSIS HIV/AIDS Task Force in collaboration with the Kaiser Family Foundation.* Washington, DC: Center for Strategic and International Studies.

OECD (Organisation for Economic Co-operation and Development). 2003. *Harmonising donor practices for effective aid delivery good practice papers: A DAC reference document.* Paris, France: OECD.

OGAC (Office of the Global AIDS Coordinator). 2004. *The President's Emergency Plan for AIDS Relief: U.S. five-year global HIV/AIDS strategy.* Washington, DC: OGAC.

OGAC. 2005a. *The President's Emergency Plan for AIDS Relief: Defining U.S. support for national strategies* (PowerPoint Presentation, July 2005). Washington, DC: OGAC.

OGAC. 2005b. *PEPFAR first annual report to Congress.* Washington, DC: OGAC.

OGAC. 2005c. *FY2005 Country Operational Plans.* Washington, DC: OGAC.

OGAC. 2006a. *PEPFAR semi-annual report, FY2006.* Washington, DC: OGAC.

OGAC. 2006b. *PEPFAR second annual report to Congress.* Washington, DC: OGAC.

OGAC. 2006c. *Bringing hope: Supplying antiretroviral drugs for HIV/AIDS treatment: The President's Emergency Plan for AIDS Relief report on antiretroviral drugs for HIV/AIDS treatment.* Washington, DC: OGAC.

OGAC. 2006d. *PEPFAR report on work force capacity and HIV/AIDS.* Washington, DC: OGAC.

OGAC. 2006e. *PEPFAR: Technical considerations for the FY2007 Country Operational Plans.* Washington, DC: OGAC.

OGAC. 2006f. *PEPFAR FY2007 COP resource guide.* Washington, DC: OGAC.

OGAC. 2006g. *FY2006 Country Operational Plans.* Washington, DC: OGAC.

OGAC. 2007. *PEPFAR third annual report to Congress.* Washington, DC: OGAC.

Salomon, J., D. Hogan, J. Stover, K. Stanecki, N. Walker, P. D. Ghys, and B. Schwartlander. 2005. Integrating HIV prevention and treatment: From slogans to impact. *PLoS Medicine* 2(1):e16.

The Paris Declaration on aid effectiveness: Ownership, harmonization, alignment, results and mutual accountability. 2005. High level forum on harmonization, February 28–March 2, 2005, Paris, France. http://www.aidharmonization.org (accessed November 10, 2006).

The Rome Declaration on Harmonization. 2003. High level forum on harmonization, February 24–25, 2003, Rome, Italy. http://www.aidharmonization.org (accessed November 10, 2006).

Tobias, R. 2003a. *Remarks at InterAction annual CEO retreat at the Washington Terrace Hotel, Washington, DC.* http://www.pepfar.gov (accessed December 9, 2003).

Tobias, R. 2003b. *Remarks at Woodrow Wilson Center of the U.S. Global AIDS Coordinator at the Ronald Reagan Building, Washington, DC.* http://www.pepfar.gov (accessed December 11, 2003).

Tobias, R. 2004. *Remarks on the five-year strategy for the President's Emergency Plan for AIDS Relief, Washington, DC.* http://www.pepfar.gov (accessed February 23, 2004).

UN (United Nations). 2003. *Monterrey Consensus of the International Conference on Financing for Development: The final text of agreements and commitments adopted at the International Conference on Financing for Development, Monterrey, Mexico, 18–22 March 2002.* Geneva, Switzerland: UN.

UNAIDS (Joint United Nations Programme on HIV/AIDS). 1998. *UNAIDS best practice collection: Guide to the strategic planning process for a national response to HIV/AIDS, modules 1–4.* Geneva, Switzerland: UNAIDS.

UNAIDS. 2001. *The global strategy framework on HIV/AIDS.* Geneva, Switzerland: UNAIDS.

UNAIDS. 2004a. *"Three ones" key principles.* Conference paper 1, Washington consultation of April 4, 2004. Geneva, Switzerland: UNAIDS. http://www.unaids.org/NetTools/Misc/DocInfo.aspx?LANG=en&href=http://gva-doc-owl/WEBcontent/Documents/pub/UNA-docs/Three-Ones_KeyPrinciples_en.pdf (accessed September 20, 2006).

UNAIDS. 2004b. *Clearing the common ground for the "three ones": A report of a consulation process.* Conference paper 2. Geneva, Switzerland: UNAIDS.

UNAIDS. 2005a. *Global task team on improving AIDS coordination among multilateral institutions and international donors.* Geneva, Switzerland: UNAIDS.

UNAIDS. 2005b. *Resource needs for an expanded response to AIDS in low- and middle-income countries.* Geneva, Switzerland: UNAIDS.

UNAIDS. 2005c. *Policy position paper: Intensifying HIV prevention.* Geneva, Switzerland: UNAIDS.

UNAIDS. 2006. *2006 report on the global AIDS epidemic.* Geneva, Switzerland: UNAIDS.

UNICEF (United Nations Children's Fund). 2006. *Africa's orphaned and vulnerable generations: Children affected by AIDS.* New York: UNICEF.

WHO (World Health Organization). 2003a. *A public health approach for scaling up antiretroviral (ARV) treatment.* http://www.who.int/hiv/toolkit/arv/en/index.jsp (accessed September 7, 2006).

WHO. 2003b. *Treating 3 million by 2005, making it happen: The WHO strategy.* http://www.who.int/hiv/toolkit/arv/en/index.jsp (accessed September 7, 2006).

WHO. 2004. *Guide to monitoring and evaluating HIV/AIDS care and support.* Geneva, Switzerland: WHO.

WHO. 2006a. *Fact sheet: Progress in scaling up access to HIV treatment in low- and middle-income countries.* Geneva, Switzerland: WHO.

WHO. 2006b. *Prequalification project: Ensuring the quality, safety and efficacy of HIV/AIDS medicines and diagnostics.* http://mednet3.who.int/prequal/ (accessed September 1, 2006).

WHO. 2006c. *Working together for health: The world health report 2006.* Geneva, Switzerland: WHO.

Part I

The U.S. Global AIDS Initiative

1

Introduction

HIV/AIDS has evolved into one of the world's greatest public health crises. More than 39 million people are estimated to be living with HIV/AIDS worldwide, over 60 percent of them in sub-Saharan Africa (UNAIDS, 2006). HIV prevalence among adults aged 15–49 now exceeds 15 percent in many countries and has approached nearly 25 percent in Botswana, Lesotho, Swaziland, and Zimbabwe. In 2006 alone, more than 4 million people are estimated to have become infected with HIV, including nearly 2 million women and over half a million children under the age of 14. The Joint United Nations Programme on HIV/AIDS (UNAIDS) has estimated that nearly 3 million people died of AIDS worldwide in 2006, and that AIDS has reversed the gains in life expectancy that had been achieved by Africa over the past 50 years (UNAIDS, 2004a, 2006).

By 2006, an estimated 12 million children had been orphaned in sub-Saharan Africa as a result of HIV/AIDS (UNICEF, 2006). The status of girls and women makes them especially vulnerable to HIV, and they now account for nearly half of people living with HIV worldwide and 59 percent of those in sub-Saharan Africa (UNAIDS, 2006). In addition, HIV/AIDS has severely strained national economies and contributed to political instability in many of the countries experiencing an epidemic (UN, 2003b; CSIS, 2005; Rice, 2006). Chapter 2 provides more background about the HIV/AIDS pandemic.

BACKGROUND

The U.S. Leadership Against HIV/AIDS, Tuberculosis, and Malaria Act

Global funding in response to HIV/AIDS has increased dramatically since 2001 (Kates and Lief, 2006; UNAIDS, 2006). On May 27, 2003, the U.S. Congress passed the United States Leadership against HIV/AIDS, Tuberculosis, and Malaria Act of 2003 (the Leadership Act)[1] and launched the U.S. Global AIDS Initiative. The provisions of the legislation that pertain most directly to the initiative (1) required the President to establish a comprehensive, integrated 5-year strategy to combat global HIV/AIDS, including specific objectives, strategies, and approaches related to prevention, treatment, and care; (2) assigned priorities for relevant executive branch agencies; (3) required improved coordination among such agencies; and (4) projected general levels of resources needed to achieve the stated goals. The legislation emphasized the establishment of programs focused on national HIV/AIDS strategies of recipient countries, the needs of women and children, strengthening of countries' health care infrastructure and workforce, and effective monitoring and evaluation to assess programmatic success. The legislation also required the President to establish within the U.S. Department of State the position of Global AIDS Coordinator (the Coordinator), who would have primary responsibility for oversight and coordination of all U.S. international activities to combat the HIV/AIDS pandemic. On October 6, 2003, Randall Tobias was sworn in as the first Coordinator, with the rank of ambassador. On February 23, 2004, Ambassador Tobias presented the required presidential strategy, the U.S. 5-year Global HIV/AIDS Strategy, to Congress.

The President's Emergency Plan for AIDS Relief (PEPFAR)

The U.S. Global AIDS Initiative is commonly known by the title given to the U.S. 5-year Global HIV/AIDS Strategy: "The President's Emergency Plan for AIDS Relief," or PEPFAR. To measure the progress of the initiative, the PEPFAR strategy establishes three overarching goals (OGAC, 2004):

- To encourage bold leadership at every level to fight HIV/AIDS.
- To apply best practices within bilateral HIV/AIDS prevention, treatment, and care programs, in concert with the objectives and policies of host governments' national HIV/AIDS strategies.

---

[1]United States Leadership against HIV/AIDS, Tuberculosis, and Malaria Act of 2003, P.L. 108-25, 108th Cong., 1st Sess. (2003).

- To encourage partners, including multilateral organizations and other host governments, to coordinate at all levels to strengthen response efforts, to embrace best practices, to adhere to principles of sound management, and to harmonize monitoring and evaluation efforts to ensure the most effective and efficient use of resources.

The PEPFAR strategy also sets forth guiding principles for achieving the initiative's mission and goals, including responding with urgency to the crisis; seeking new approaches; coordinating U.S. government oversight and direction of PEPFAR activities; drawing on the scientific evidence base in developing interventions; establishing and ensuring accountability for measurable goals; harmonizing program development and implementation with the host countries; integrating prevention, treatment, and care programs; building national capacity; encouraging national leadership; and coordinating with other partners (OGAC, 2004).

The U.S. Global AIDS Initiative, while encompassing activities in more than 120 countries, is focused on the development of comprehensive and integrated prevention, treatment, and care programs in 15 countries selected largely because they are heavily affected by HIV/AIDS (OGAC, 2004). Of the $15 billion authorized under the Leadership Act, $10 billion is to be allocated to efforts in these 15 countries over a 5-year period (OGAC, 2004). The remainder of the funding goes predominantly to the Global Fund to Fight AIDS, Tuberculosis and Malaria (Global Fund); international HIV/AIDS research at the National Institutes of Health; and HIV/AIDS activities in other, nonfocus countries. The 15 PEPFAR focus countries, 14 of which were named in the Leadership Act, are the Republic of Botswana (Botswana), the Republic of Côte d'Ivoire (Côte d'Ivoire), the Federal Democratic Republic of Ethiopia (Ethiopia), the Cooperative Republic of Guyana (Guyana), the Republic of Haiti (Haiti), the Republic of Kenya (Kenya), the Republic of Mozambique (Mozambique), the Republic of Namibia (Namibia), the Federal Republic of Nigeria (Nigeria), the Republic of Rwanda (Rwanda), the Republic of South Africa (South Africa), the United Republic of Tanzania (Tanzania), the Republic of Uganda (Uganda), the Socialist Republic of Vietnam (Vietnam), and the Republic of Zambia (Zambia). PEPFAR has established specific targets for its prevention, treatment, and care programs in these countries to support prevention of 7 million new HIV infections; treatment of 2 million HIV-infected people with antiretroviral therapy (ART); and care of 10 million people living with and affected by HIV/AIDS, including orphans and other children made vulnerable by HIV/AIDS.[2] Chapter 2 provides more background information about the Leadership Act, the PEPFAR strategy, PEPFAR funding, and the focus countries.

STUDY GOALS AND APPROACH

Study Mandate and Scope

The Leadership Act mandates that the Institute of Medicine (IOM) evaluate PEPFAR and directs the President to consider the IOM's findings. Specifically, Section 101(c)(1) of the Leadership Act states:

> Not later than 3 years after the date of the enactment of this Act, the Institute of Medicine shall publish findings comparing the success rates of the various programs and methods used under the [PEPFAR] strategy.
>
> In prioritizing the distribution of resources under the [PEPFAR] strategy, the President shall consider the findings published by the Institute of Medicine under this subsection.

This mandate is somewhat ambiguous as to whether the IOM should conduct macro-level comparisons (considering the relative success of PEPFAR and other approaches to aid, such as the Global Fund, for example) or micro-level comparisons (looking, for instance, at the comparative success of different PEPFAR-supported ART or prevention programs). Consultations between the IOM and cognizant congressional staff and State Department officials who were involved in structuring the original mandate and study contract indicated that the true "success" of PEPFAR needed to be judged in terms of real impact—both on the lives of people and on the nature of the epidemics in the affected countries. Recognizing that an in-depth assessment of the impact of PEPFAR would not be feasible within the time frame and resources allocated for the IOM evaluation, the study charge was understood as evaluating the initial implementation of PEPFAR 3 years after authorization to provide guidance for Congress in time for its consideration of the reauthorization of the program (IOM, 2005).

To plan, conduct, and report on this short-term implementation evaluation, the IOM empaneled an independent, expert committee. The scope of the evaluation was limited to the implementation of PEPFAR in the focus countries and did not include the U.S. contribution to the Global Fund, which is also overseen by the Coordinator. Although direct evaluation of the Leadership Act was beyond its scope, the IOM Committee for

[2]For purposes of this target, PEPFAR defines treatment narrowly as ART and categorizes other aspects of treatment—such as therapy for opportunistic infections or for pain management—under care.

the Evaluation of PEPFAR Implementation (the Committee) examined and drew conclusions about factors that appeared to be having a pronounced effect on implementation, some of which have their roots in the Leadership Act.

Evaluation Plan

The Committee began its study in January 2005 with a series of information-gathering and deliberative meetings, and in October 2005 published a letter report outlining its plan for the evaluation (IOM, 2005). Figure 1-1, from the letter report, summarizes the major foci and high-level questions of the evaluation plan (see Appendix C for the full letter report).

As Figure 1-1 illustrates, the Leadership Act is not the subject of the evaluation; rather, it is one of the major points of reference for evaluating PEPFAR implementation. Thus, the Committee did not examine the major features of the program that were determined by the legislation, such as its single-disease focus, the concentration of resources in specified countries, or the established targets and goals, but regarded them as the parameters within which the program was required to be implemented. However, the Committee did address the other major points of reference for evaluating PEPFAR shown in Figure 1-1: global consensus regarding the major components of an HIV/AIDS strategy and the evidence base for specific programs and activities. The Committee recognized that discordance was possible—both among elements of the legislation and between the legislation and other points of reference—and that such discordance could affect program implementation. In such instances, the Committee addressed aspects of the legislation that directly affect implementation and thereby the ability of the program to achieve the goals of the legislation.

Figure 1-1 also illustrates how the U.S. commitment to harmonization lies at the core of the complex structure and approach of PEPFAR, which involves numerous U.S. government agencies, is centrally coordinated by the Office of the U.S. Global AIDS Coordinator (OGAC), but is implemented by the U.S. teams in the focus countries (Country Teams) (UN, 2003a; The Rome Declaration, 2003; The Paris Declaration, 2005; OGAC, 2005). The central tenet of harmonization is that sustainable gains against the AIDS pandemic require that each country own and lead its response to its epidemic. The role of donors is to support and participate in three country-determined elements critical to an effective response—one national AIDS plan, one national AIDS coordinating mechanism, and one national AIDS monitoring and evaluation framework (UNAIDS, 2004b). Thus, the

Committee evaluated the implementation of PEPFAR primarily through the lens of harmonization and sought to determine how effectively the program is meeting its commitment to support the focus countries' responses to their HIV/AIDS epidemics (IOM, 2005). The evolution of harmonization and PEPFAR's participation in the process is discussed in detail in Chapter 2.

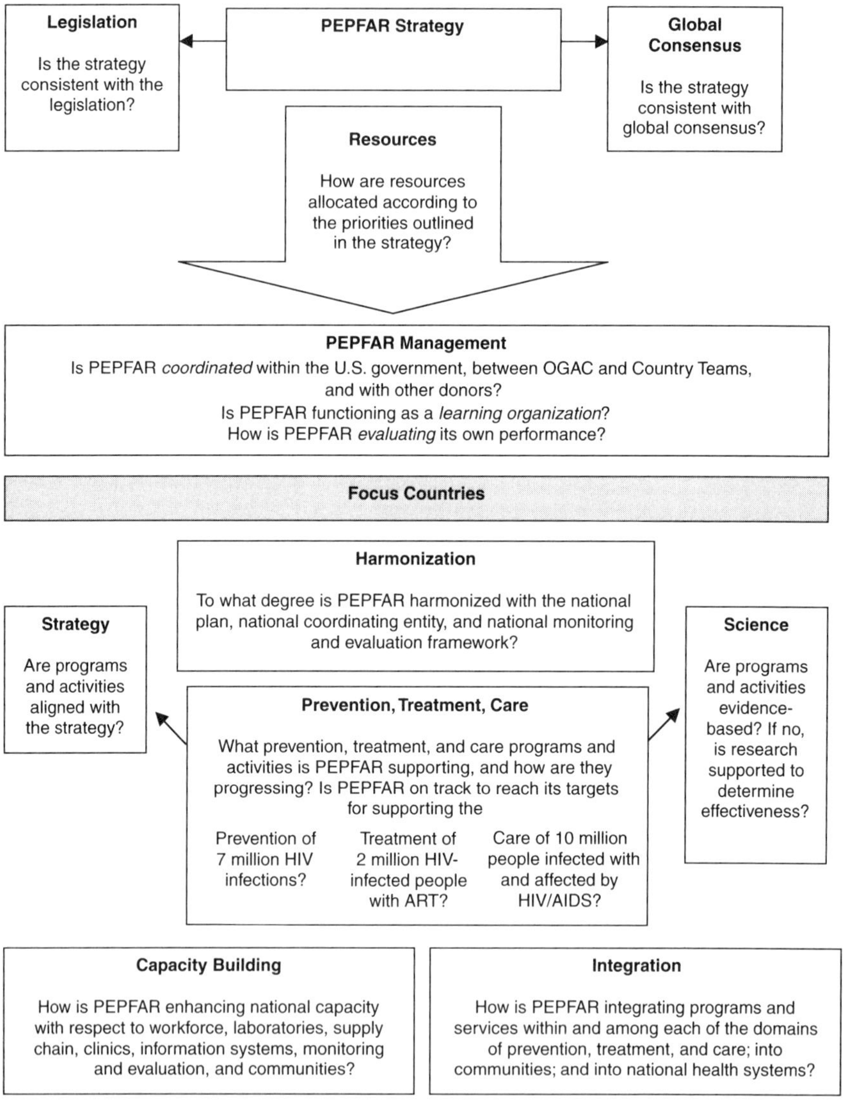

FIGURE 1-1 Short-term PEPFAR evaluation plan.

CONDUCT OF THE EVALUATION

In carrying out this evaluation, the Committee used several approaches to examine PEPFAR's strategic development and programmatic implementation, including review of the relevant literature and PEPFAR documentation, review and analysis of budgetary and programmatic data, information-gathering Committee meetings, discussions with relevant parties, and visits to the PEPFAR focus countries to observe activities directly and hold face-to-face discussions. The Committee endeavored to respect global efforts at harmonization of monitoring and evaluation—in which the United States was participating prior to PEPFAR (Rugg et al., 2004)—and relied on existing indicators and data sources to the extent possible. Beginning with its first meeting, the Committee reviewed global monitoring and evaluation efforts already under way, systems and processes already in place, and existing data (IOM, 2005).

In addition to the scientific literature, the Committee reviewed a wide range of documents, including PEPFAR's authorizing legislation, strategy, guidance, and reports; global consensus and guidance documents, such as those of the World Health Organization (WHO) and UNAIDS; national plans and other documents from the focus countries; and reports of other HIV/AIDS donors and PEPFAR partners. In addition to its three information-gathering meetings, the Committee held an extensive series of discussions with U.S. government officials at OGAC, at the implementing agencies, and on the Country Teams; focus country officials; partners; program officials; community groups; and officials from other donor organizations. To encourage the participants in these discussions to speak candidly, the Committee assured them that it would not attribute their statements to individuals by name, organization, or country. The Committee took this approach because consultation with a wide range of people and organizations during its development of the evaluation plan indicated that such an approach would be necessary to facilitate candid discussions (IOM, 2005). Appendix A lists the people and organizations with whom the Committee held discussions; Appendix B shows the generic agenda for the Committee's visits to the focus countries; and the letter report reprinted in Appendix C details the issues and questions covered in these discussions.

Focus Country Visits

From October 2005 through February 2006, small delegations from the Committee visited 13 of the 15 focus countries. Each visit lasted 1 week and included discussions with the U.S. Country Team, country government officials, officials from other donor groups working in the country, partners implementing PEPFAR programs, and representatives of groups of people living with HIV/AIDS. The Committee's delegations visited sites of all types conducting programs focused on prevention, treatment, care, the needs of orphans and vulnerable children, system strengthening, and training. The Committee's analysis of its country visits, as well as its synthesis of this information with that from other sources, is described in Appendix B. The visits were not designed or intended to allow the Committee to delve deeply into and reach definitive conclusions about any one focus country, program, or aspect of implementation, perhaps with the exception of PEPFAR's overall management, coordination, and harmonization. Thus, the Committee did not attempt to draw conclusions about specific countries or programs and did not base its conclusions about any aspect of PEPFAR solely on information obtained during the visits. However, the Committee believes that the cumulative information from all of the visits—effectively 13 weeks in PEPFAR focus countries, discussions with hundreds of people, and visits to dozens of sites—provided a comprehensive and detailed picture of PEPFAR implementation overall as viewed from the focus countries.

A great deal of information about the focus countries is a matter of public record—for example, information about the nature of their HIV/AIDS epidemics, their national AIDS strategies and sometimes their operational plans, and their PEPFAR Country Operational Plans. When discussing this kind of information in the report, the Committee identifies specific countries by name. When discussing information that is based on discussions held in the focus countries, however, the Committee avoids attribution of comments even by country.

The Committee provides examples of PEPFAR-supported programs throughout the report. These examples were selected from the Country Operational Plans simply to illustrate the types of programs and activities included in the various PEPFAR categories. The Committee did not visit or review the details of all of the programs described in the examples provided, nor did it evaluate any of these programs.

Budget and Performance Data

As suggested above, the Committee attempted to respect global efforts at harmonization of monitoring and evaluation by relying on existing data sources to the maximum extent possible. The Committee reviewed and analyzed all publicly available PEPFAR budget and performance data, as well as information about HIV/AIDS funding, epidemiology, and activities in the focus countries. The primary sources for PEPFAR data were Congressional Notifications, Country Operational Plans, annual reports and other interim reports, and analyses of the Country Operational Plan Reporting System provided by OGAC. The primary sources of data on the focus countries were their own websites and publications, OGAC, UNAIDS, WHO, the World Bank, and the Kaiser Family Foundation. The Committee did not audit or independently verify these data; however, it performed some checks for internal consistency, as well as for congruence with external sources. The Committee did not audit any aspect of the program and thus is unable to address such issues as contract compliance, diversion of funds, and corruption.

Appendix A acknowledges the many people and organizations who generously assisted the Committee with its study. Appendix B provides more detailed information about the Committee's methods.

Challenges for the Evaluation

In addition to the size and complexity of PEPFAR, two features made the Committee's task an especially challenging one: (1) PEPFAR is of necessity a dynamic, evolving program, and (2) it is still relatively early in its implementation.

The Coordinator has implemented PEPFAR on an emergency basis and, as acknowledged by the Leadership Act, has had to "maintain sufficient flexibility and remain responsive to the ever-changing nature of the HIV/AIDS pandemic" (P.L. 108-25, p. 718). Thus PEPFAR is a rapidly moving, continually evolving target for evaluation. The Committee was prepared to find considerable changes in PEPFAR throughout its evaluation, and attempted to develop an evaluation approach that would allow it to adapt not only to changes in PEPFAR implementation, but also to what the Committee learned as its work proceeded. PEPFAR indeed continued to evolve rapidly as the Committee conducted this study, and the Committee has attempted to remain current with these developments. Clearly, the Committee's findings and conclusions, particularly its observations of activities in the focus countries, are based on its examination of a particular period in PEPFAR's development. The Committee's main recommendations are for the future of the U.S. Global AIDS Initiative as a whole, and so are largely independent of ongoing changes in the management of PEPFAR. However, the Committee hopes that PEPFAR's dynamism will not diminish, and thus that parts of this report related to PEPFAR management may become outdated rather quickly.

EVALUATING THE SUCCESS OF PEPFAR

Ultimately the "success" of PEPFAR will be judged by whether it has achieved its targets of effectively supporting the prevention of 7 million HIV infections, treatment for 2 million people with HIV/AIDS with ART, and care for 10 million people living with and affected by HIV/AIDS, as well as its longer-term goal of achieving sustainable gains against the HIV/AIDS epidemics in the focus countries. However, although the Leadership Act was passed in May 2003, the initial funds for the program were not appropriated until January 2004, and the majority of the first year's funding was not obligated until September 2004. Thus at the close of the Committee's short-term evaluation, PEPFAR had been supporting the implementation of programs for prevention, treatment, care, and orphans and vulnerable children in the focus countries for less than 2 years—less time, perhaps, than Congress had envisioned when it wrote the mandate for this study. The Committee recognized that it would not be reasonable or feasible to judge PEPFAR's success solely against the above targets and goal this early in the program's implementation, and therefore planned instead in this short-term evaluation to examine how well PEPFAR has been establishing the foundation for and making reasonable progress toward achieving and measuring these targets and this goal. In so doing, the Committee aimed to make constructive suggestions for improvement to ensure that the program ultimately meets the targets and goal. The Committee recognized that it was too early in the program for this short-term evaluation to provide the information necessary to judge true success, that is, to adequately measure what matters most—the program's impact on the lives of the people whom the Leadership Act sought to serve. The Committee urges that a long-term evaluation be conducted to determine whether the U.S. Global AIDS Initiative has ultimately succeeded in improving the lives of people in the focus countries by preventing infections, treating patients, and caring for people. To this end, the Committee is planning to conduct a workshop to encourage collaboration among evaluators, and to discuss and develop considerations for designing an evaluation of PEPFAR's impact on the focus countries, their HIV/AIDS epidemics, and, most important, their people.

ORGANIZATION OF THE REPORT

This report is organized into three main parts (see Box 1-1). Part I describes the nature and object of the study—the U.S. Global AIDS Initiative—and its context. Following this introductory chapter, Chapter 2 briefly describes the HIV/AIDS pandemic that the Leadership Act was designed to address, as well as the global context for the U.S. Global AIDS Initiative, briefly highlighting the challenges for the implementation of PEPFAR, and indeed any such donor program. Chapter 2 also provides background on the U.S. Global AIDS Initiative, beginning with the historic legislation that enabled it and concluding with the current structure for implementing the first 5-year strategy of the initiative—PEPFAR. Part II describes the progress of PEPFAR to date; its structure is aligned with how the Coordinator reports to Congress. Chapter 3 presents the Committee's assessment of the Coordinator's management of the U.S. Global AIDS Initiative, including

BOX 1-1
Report Structure

development of the strategy required by the Leadership Act. Chapters 4 through 7 provide progress reports on the implementation of the strategy according to its four major categories of activities and programs—prevention, treatment, care, and orphans and vulnerable children—and suggest how the Coordinator could improve programming in each of these categories. Part III looks to the future—both the immediate future of the remaining years of the PEPFAR 5-year strategy and the longer-term future of the U.S. Global AIDS Initiative. The one chapter in this section, Chapter 8, focuses on the common themes that emerged when the Committee considered PEPFAR as a whole, that is, without being bound by the program's four categories. This final chapter draws on what the Committee learned from the implementation of PEPFAR thus far to suggest how the U.S. Global AIDS Initiative could advance most effectively toward achieving the primary goal of its landmark enabling legislation—U.S. leadership to address the HIV/AIDS pandemic.

REFERENCES

CSIS (Center for Strategic and International Studies). 2005. *More than humanitarianism: A strategic U.S. approach toward Africa.* Washington, DC: CSIS.

IOM (Institute of Medicine). 2005. *Plan for a short-term evaluation of PEPFAR implementation.* Washington, DC: The National Academies Press.

Kates, J., and E. Lief. 2006. *International assistance for HIV/AIDS in the developing world: Taking stock of the G8, other donor governments and the European Commission.* Washington, DC: Kaiser Family Foundation.

OGAC (Office of the U.S. Global AIDS Coordinator). 2004. *The President's Emergency Plan for AIDS Relief: U.S. five-year global HIV/AIDS strategy.* Washington, DC: OGAC.

OGAC. 2005. *The President's Emergency Plan for AIDS Relief: Defining U.S. support for national strategies* (PowerPoint Presentation, July 2005). Washington, DC: OGAC. http://www.pepfar.gov (accessed July 19, 2005).

The Paris Declaration on aid effectiveness: Ownership, harmonisation, alignment, results and mutual accountability. 2005. High level forum on harmonization, February 28–March 2, 2005, Paris, France. http://www.aidharmonization.org (accessed November 10, 2006).

The Rome Declaration on harmonization. 2003. High level forum on harmonization, February 24–25, 2003, Rome, Italy. http://www.aidharmonization.org (accessed November 10, 2006).

Rice, S. 2006. *Global poverty, weak states, and insecurity.* The Brookings Blum Roundtable. Washington, DC: The Brookings Institution.

Rugg, D., G. Peersman, and M. Carael. 2004. *Global advances in HIV/AIDS monitoring and evaluation.* Minneapolis, MN: Wiley Periodicals, Inc.

UN (United Nations). 2003a. *Monterrey Consensus of the International Conference on Financing for Development: The final text of agreements and commitments adopted at the International Conference on Financing for Development, Monterrey, Mexico, 18–22 March 2002.* Geneva, Switzerland: UN.

UN. 2003b. *Organizing the UN response to the triple threat of food insecurity, weakened capacity for governance and AIDS, particularly in southern and eastern Africa. Document discussed at the UN high-level committee on programmes, 6th Session, Rome, Italy, September 18–19, 2003.* Geneva, Switzerland: UN.

UNAIDS (Joint United Nations Programme on HIV/AIDS). 2004a. *2004 report on the global AIDS epidemic: 4th global report.* Geneva, Switzerland: UNAIDS.

UNAIDS. 2004b. *"Three ones" key principles.* Conference paper 1, Washington consultation of April 4, 2004. Geneva, Switzerland: UNAIDS. http://www.unaids.org/NetTools/Misc/DocInfo.aspx?LANG=en&href=http://gva-doc-owl/WEBcontent/Documents/pub/UNA-docs/Three-Ones_KeyPrinciples_en.pdf (accessed September 20, 2006).

UNAIDS. 2006. *2006 report on the global AIDS epidemic.* Geneva, Switzerland: UNAIDS.

UNICEF (United Nations Children's Fund). 2006. *Africa's orphaned and vulnerable generations: Children affected by AIDS.* New York: UNICEF.

2

The U.S. Global AIDS Initiative: Context and Background

Summary of Key Points

- PEPFAR, the largest bilateral initiative for HIV/AIDS funding, is one of many efforts taking concerted action against the pandemic. Multiple donor efforts eventually led the Joint United Nations Programme on HIV/AIDS (UNAIDS) to propose a framework and set forth principles for supporting countries' ownership of their responses to their epidemics and harmonizing national HIV/AIDS responses.
- The development, implementation, monitoring, and evaluation of global HIV/AIDS programming are complicated by contextual challenges, such as concurrent public health epidemics; poor nutrition; poverty; capacity constraints with respect to human, fiscal, technical, and infrastructure/system resources; and sociocultural challenges of stigma and discrimination, and the vulnerable status of women, girls, orphans, and other children in many of the focus countries.
- PEPFAR's landmark authorizing legislation prescribes many aspects of the program, including development of a comprehensive global strategy for programming based on sound science and available best practices, budgetary allocations for categories of programmatic activities, creation of the oversight position of the U.S. Global AIDS Coordinator, expectations for unprecedented coordination among U.S. government agencies and international stakeholders, assignment of responsibilities to involved U.S. government agencies and programs, and identification of the priority countries for action.
- The U.S. Global AIDS Coordinator is charged with coordinating all U.S. international activities to combat HIV/AIDS. The Office of the U.S. Global AIDS Coordinator (OGAC) is the central headquarters for the initiative. It consists of a small staff of experts in areas critical to headquarters-level coordination of the different agencies involved, as well as the development of policy and programmatic guidance for the field. Program implementation is accomplished primarily by teams in the focus countries. These Country Teams are based in the embassy and led by the ambassador, and are supported by core teams and technical working groups based at OGAC.

2

The U.S. Global AIDS Initiative: Context and Background

The first half of this chapter provides a brief overview of the HIV/AIDS pandemic; identifies some of the key partners responding to the pandemic; and explores the global context for implementing HIV/AIDS programs, including challenges faced by all donor programs. The second half provides an introduction to the President's Emergency Plan for AIDS Relief (PEPFAR) focus countries and describes the legislation that created the program.

THE HIV/AIDS PANDEMIC

The HIV/AIDS pandemic has already claimed more than 25 million lives. Cases have been reported in all regions of the world, but most people living with HIV/AIDS (95 percent) reside in low- and middle-income countries, where most new HIV infections and AIDS-related deaths occur.

The year 2006 marks the twenty-fifth anniversary of the description of acquired immunodeficiency syndrome (AIDS). AIDS was first recognized among gay men in the United States. By 1983, the etiological agent of the disease, the human immunodeficiency virus (HIV), had been identified. By 1985, at least one case of HIV infection had been reported in each region of the world (UNAIDS, 2006). The 1980s also marked the pandemic status of HIV/AIDS, which has been increasing in incidence and prevalence globally ever since. The nature of the virus is such that without intervention, only a minuscule proportion of HIV-positive individuals will not progress to AIDS, and predictably to death from AIDS and its complications. The twenty-fifth anniversary of the identification of AIDS was marked by numerous histories, perspective reviews, and publications. Appendix D provides a short list of sources offering more detailed global overviews.

Figure 2-1 shows a global view of the prevalence of HIV/AIDS, with the majority of cases occurring in low- and middle-income countries (UNAIDS, 2006; WHO, 2006a). The nations of sub-Saharan Africa are the hardest hit, but concern is increasing about the next wave of the pandemic that is emerging in parts of Eastern Europe and Asia. AIDS is the leading cause of death worldwide among those aged 15 to 59 (UNAIDS, 2006). The pandemic is also considered a threat to the economic well-being and social and political stability of many nations (UN, 2003b; CSIS, 2005; Rice, 2006). The stark facts are these (UNAIDS, 2006):

- More than 39 million people are living with HIV/AIDS worldwide, twice the number in 1995.
- During 2006, more than 4 million people became infected with HIV, including more than half a million children.
- Nearly 3 million people died of AIDS-related illnesses in 2006.
- Worldwide, most people living with HIV are unaware that they are infected.
- At any given time, many more people are infected—are HIV-positive—than are clinically ill with AIDS.

Although undeniably pandemic, HIV/AIDS can best be addressed if it is viewed as many separate epidemics with distinct origins and characteristics of spread. The epidemics can be described in terms of geography or of subpopulations affected within larger populations, and involve different transmission patterns that result from varying patterns of behaviors conducive to spread of the virus. The main methods of transmission are sexual contact, blood exposure from injecting drug use involving shared needles, and transmission from mother to child before or during childbirth. Other methods of transmission that may be especially important focally are blood transfusions from people who are HIV-positive, medical accidents, and unsafe medical injection practices. It is estimated that in sub-Saharan Africa, transmission through sexual contact, from mother to child, and via health care procedures (including blood transfusions and medical injections) account for 80–90 percent, 5–35 percent, and 5–10 percent of new infections, respectively, with regional variation (NAS, 1994; Quinn et al., 1994; Quinn, 1996, 2001; WHO, 2002b; Askew and Berer, 2003; Bertozzi et al., 2006).

Bertozzi and colleagues (2006) classified country-level AIDS epidemics into three states: low, concentrated, and generalized, with numeric indicators for HIV prevalence among populations (see Table 2-1). In the low state, HIV infection has not spread to significant levels in any subpopulation and

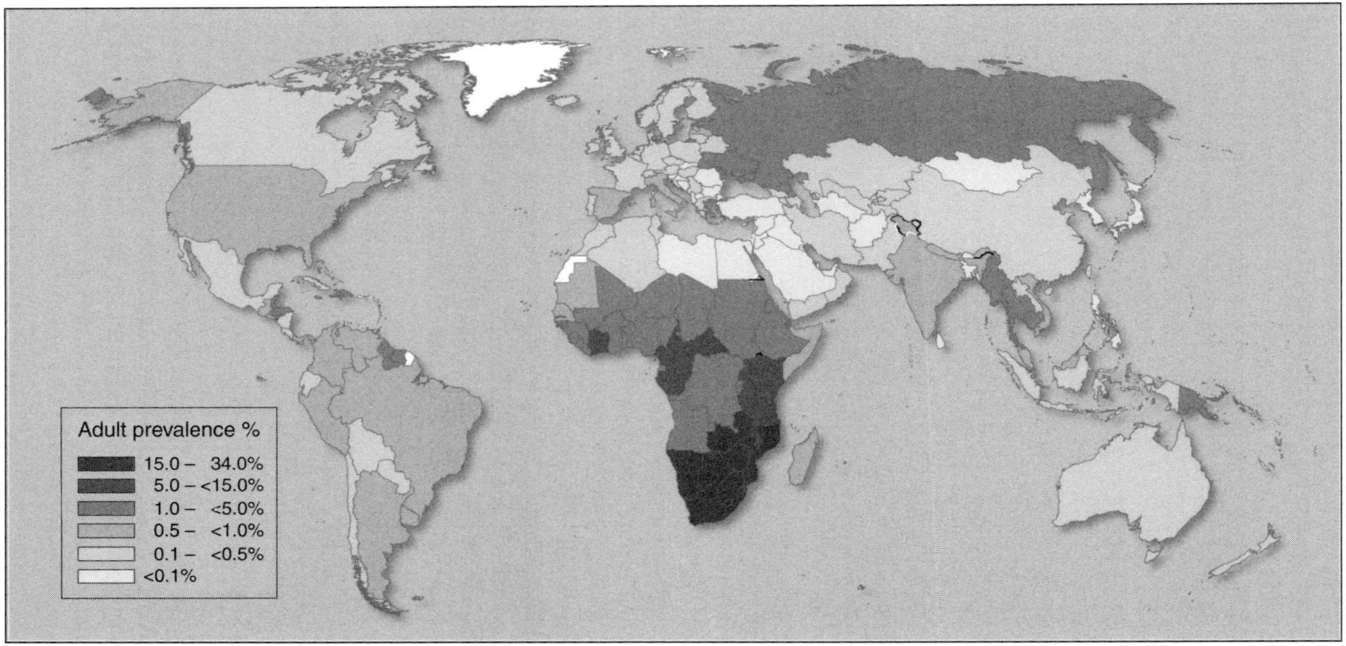

FIGURE 2-1 Global view of the prevalence of HIV/AIDS.
SOURCE: Reprinted with the kind permission of UNAIDS, 2006.

TABLE 2-1 Classification of Country-Level AIDS Epidemics

Extent of HIV Infection	Highest Prevalence in a Key Population (percentage)*	Prevalence in the General Population (percentage)
Low	<5	<1
Concentrated	>5	<1
Generalized Low	≥5	1–10
Generalized High	≥5	≥10

*Key populations include sex workers, men who have sex with men, and people who use injecting drugs.

SOURCE: Bertozzi et al., 2006.

is largely confined to individuals with higher-risk behaviors, such as sex workers, people who use injecting drugs, and men who have sex with other men. This epidemic state suggests that networks of those at high risk are diffuse (that is, low levels of partner exchange or sharing of drug-injecting equipment) or that the virus has been introduced relatively recently. No focus country epidemic is characterized by this state.

In the concentrated state, HIV has spread rapidly in a defined subpopulation but is not well established in the general population. This state suggests active networks of risk within the subpopulation, and the future course of the epidemic is determined by the frequency and nature of links between the highly infected subpopulation and the general population.

In the generalized state, HIV is firmly established in the general population. Although subpopulations at high risk may continue to contribute disproportionately to the spread of HIV, sexual networking in the general population is sufficient to sustain an epidemic independent of subpopulations at higher risk of infection. Low and high subcategories of the generalized epidemic are recognized.

THE GLOBAL RESPONSE TO HIV/AIDS IN THE DEVELOPING WORLD

Major Funding Sources for HIV/AIDS Assistance

In response to the intensifying global HIV/AIDS crisis, international funding for HIV/AIDS programs has increased steadily since 2001. In 2005, commitments from donor governments to respond to HIV/AIDS rose to $4.3 billion, up from $3.6 billion in the previous year (Kates and Lief, 2006).

U.S. funding to combat global HIV/AIDS has steadily increased since 2001 (see Table 2-2). In 2006 PEPFAR contributed 26 percent of official

TABLE 2-2 Total U.S. Funding for Global HIV/AIDS for Fiscal Years 2001–2007 (in millions of U.S. dollars)

2001	2002	2003	2004	2005	2006	2007	2008*
785	1,083	1,540	2,311	2,719	3,290	4,556	5,400

*Proposed.

SOURCE: OGAC, 2007a.

development assistance[1] from donor governments for programs to address global HIV/AIDS (OGAC, 2005b, 2006a; Kates and Lief, 2006).

The U.S. Global AIDS Initiative is one of several significant sources of international HIV/AIDS assistance. Multilateral organizations—such as the Global Fund to Fight AIDS, Tuberculosis and Malaria (the Global Fund); the World Bank; and UNAIDS, which coordinates the various United Nations (UN) agencies[2]—are also primary providers of international HIV/AIDS funding (UNAIDS, 2005b). These key global partners for the U.S. Global AIDS Initiative are briefly described in Box 2-1.

Governments of affected countries have also increased their spending, with amounts depending on, among other factors, gross national income, national debt, political stability, and the status of the working class (Kates and Lief, 2006). The private sector (including foundations, corporations, international nongovernmental organizations, and individuals) represent another vital funding stream for responses to HIV/AIDS. U.S.-based philanthropies committed an estimated $395 million in 2003 to HIV/AIDS activities in the United States and internationally, with the Bill and Melinda Gates Foundation making the greatest contribution. International development banks, including the Inter-American Development Bank, the Asian Development Bank, and the African Development Bank, play contributory roles as well (Kates and Lief, 2006). The Joint United Nations Programme

[1]Official development assistance is defined as those flows to developing countries and to multilateral institutions for developing countries (1) which are provided by official agencies, including state and local governments, or by their executing agencies; and (2) each transaction of which (a) is administered with the promotion of the economic development and welfare of developing countries as its main objective, and (b) is concessional in character and conveys a grant element of at least 25 percent (OECD, 2006).

[2]The agencies coordinated by UNAIDS are the United Nations Refugee Agency; United Nation's Children Fund; World Food Programme; United Nations Development Programme; United Nations Population Fund; United Nations Office on Drugs and Crime; International Labour Organization; United Nations Educational, Scientific, and Cultural Organization; World Health Organization; and World Bank.

BOX 2-1
Multilateral Organizations Contributing to Responses to Global HIV/AIDS

The Global Fund was created in 2001 as an independent public–private partnership with the intent of providing grants to countries to finance programs targeting AIDS, tuberculosis, and malaria. As of July 2006, about $9 billion had been pledged to the Global Fund from all sources, and $5.5 billion had been committed to 132 countries. Fifty-seven percent of the funds had been allocated to HIV/AIDS (Global Fund, 2005, 2006).

The World Bank began supporting HIV/AIDS programming in 1986, and has since launched major efforts in Africa (2000) and the Caribbean (2001) through its Multi-Country AIDS Program. The World Bank also offers financial assistance for HIV/AIDS programs through the International Development Association, which provides grants and interest-free loans to the world's poorest countries, and through the International Bank for Reconstruction and Development, which offers nonconcessional loans to countries able to repay them. The majority of funds are derived directly from member country contributions, primarily from the G8. As of April 2006, the World Bank had committed a total of $2.6 billion to combat HIV/AIDS, approximately $1.9 billion of which was distributed through the International Development Association (Kates and Lief, 2006).

UNAIDS, the Joint United Nations Programme on HIV/AIDS, brings together the efforts and resources of 10 UN agencies to help the world prevent new HIV infections, care for those already infected, and mitigate the impact of the pandemic. UNAIDS is based in Geneva and works on the ground in more than 75 countries. Established in 1994 by a resolution of the UN Economic and Social Council and launched in January 1996, the organization is guided by a Programme Coordinating Board including representatives of 22 governments from all geographic regions; the UNAIDS Cosponsors; and five representatives of nongovernmental organizations, including associations of people living with HIV (UNAIDS, 2007). HIV/AIDS funding from the UN increased from $1.3 billion for 2004–2005 to $2.6 billion for the 2006–2007 budget (UNAIDS, 2003, 2005c).

on HIV/AIDS (UNAIDS) estimates spending from all of these sources at approximately $2.1 billion for 2005.

Despite the large sums of money available, funding is far below what is needed (UNAIDS, 2006). A publication from the Henry J. Kaiser Family Foundation entitled *International Assistance for HIV/AIDS in the Developing World: Taking Stock of the G8, Other Donor Governments and the European Commission*, available at http://www.kff.org, provides an in-depth review of international donor assistance for HIV/AIDS efforts.

Global Efforts to Improve Coordination Among Donors

The scope and size of the U.S. Global AIDS Initiative are closer to the scale of a multilateral than a bilateral effort, and while the United States is not the only donor of funding for HIV/AIDS programs, in some countries its magnitude makes it a dominant source and thus influential in policy and program development. In 2005, the UNAIDS Secretariat convened leaders from governments and the civil sector, UN agencies, and other multinational and international organizations to review the global response to HIV/AIDS. Issues such as the absorptive capacity of developing countries, duplication of effort among donors, gaps in funding, and the burden on countries for reporting results and administering the funds were examined. The magnitude of PEPFAR and its contributions to the increase in funding were also recognized and considered. These examinations prompted the formation of the Global Task Team, whose primary purpose was to improve HIV/AIDS coordination among multilateral institutions and international donors. The ultimate goal was to accelerate global action to achieve significant progress toward international goals for the delivery of services to people affected by the epidemics in low- and middle-income countries by making recommendations for addressing the above issues (UNAIDS, 2005a). The Global Task Team comprised representatives from 24 countries and institutions, and its work was facilitated by three working groups. Officials from the Office of the U.S. Global AIDS Coordinator (OGAC) participated in the working group on harmonization of monitoring and evaluation, which made recommendations for improving policies, systems, and practices of multilateral institutions, as well as global initiatives to coordinate and improve monitoring and evaluation systems (UNAIDS, 2005a). The expectation for aligning the work of the Global Task Team with the Three Ones principles of harmonization (discussed further later in this chapter) was expressed early in the process (UNAIDS, 2005a).

To implement the recommendations of the Global Task Team, the Global Implementation Support Team was formed in July 2005. By November 2006, the Global Implementation Support Team had expanded and included additional representatives from the civil sector and bilateral donors, including the U.S. Global AIDS Initiative. The Global Implementation Support Team "centers on country-driven problem solving to unblock obstacles to accelerated grant implementation . . . [with] members meeting on a monthly basis to review immediate and medium-term technical support needs, make decisions on joint and coordinated technical support to be provided, evaluate progress and assess performance of such support, and look at ways to improve interaction between Global Implementation Support Team member organizations and countries" (GIST, 2006, p. 1).

HARMONIZATION IN THE GLOBAL RESPONSE TO HIV/AIDS

Evolution of the Three Ones Principles of Harmonization

Significant global events and economic development agreements were the precursors to the formal drafting of and commitment to what would become known as the Three Ones principles of harmonization (see Box 2-2). These principles were "specifically developed to cope with the urgency and need to ensure effective and efficient use of resources and focus on delivering results—in ways that will also enhance national capacity to deal with the AIDS crisis long-term" (UNAIDS, 2004b, p. 1). Though developed to foster improved coordination of HIV/AIDS responses, the principles were designed to be fully compatible with the guidelines of the Organisation for Economic Co-operation and Development's Development Assistance Committee for "Harmonising Donor Practices for Effective Aid Delivery" and the February 2003 "The Rome Declaration on Harmonisation" by "accommodating different aid modalities while ensuring effective management procedures and reducing transaction costs for countries" (OECD, 2003; The Rome Declaration, 2003; UNAIDS, 2004b, p. 1), as well as with the concept of national ownership described in the "Monterrey Consensus," which provides the framework for national ownership of social and economic development (UN, 2003a).

In April 2004, UNAIDS, the United Kingdom, and the United States co-hosted a high-level meeting at which all major donors and programs (including PEPFAR) formally endorsed the Three Ones principles of harmonization (UNAIDS, 2004a). A primary intent of harmonization is to reinforce the consistency and simplification of policies, practices, and procedures among donors (UNAIDS, 2004b).

BOX 2-2
The Three Ones Principles for the Harmonization of National HIV/AIDS Responses

- One agreed HIV/AIDS Action Framework that provides the basis for coordinating the work of all partners
- One National HIV/AIDS Coordinating Authority, with a broad-based multisectoral mandate
- One agreed HIV/AIDS country-level Monitoring and Evaluation System

SOURCE: UNAIDS, 2004a.

One HIV/AIDS Action Framework

The first principle of harmonization requires broad participation in the development, review, and periodic update of the national framework for HIV/AIDS response, as well as in its successful implementation. Broad participation of key stakeholders in the governmental, private, civil, and international sectors is also expected to contribute to the quality and comprehensiveness of the framework (UNAIDS, 2005d). Stakeholder participation applies not only to implementation and innovation, but also to public policy, advocacy, and oversight functions such as monitoring and evaluation (UNAIDS, 2004b). National ownership of participatory planning and execution, which is becoming increasingly common, is critical. National ownership has many elements, but key is both the respect and continued support of donors for national governments, as well as strong leadership, governance, communication, and transparency on the part of both national entities and donors (UNAIDS, 2004a, 2005d). National frameworks require work plans and budgets that can be tracked, especially to coordinate the support of donors and other stakeholders (UNAIDS, 2005d). Frameworks that have these plans and budgets are often characterized as being prioritized and costed.

One National HIV/AIDS Coordinating Authority

UNAIDS has stated that developing, reviewing, and updating national plans requires human resource capacity for coordination and calls for strong leadership and commitment, which are ideally provided by the highest level of government. This highest level of government is also expected to delegate its authority to a national AIDS authority, which may include a governing council and a secretariat, that also has a mandate to broadly recruit other national, local, and international stakeholders from all sectors into the collaborative process and to coordinate all action related to that process. The complex dynamics seen in several countries among the various stakeholders have demonstrated the need for effective leadership and coordination to maximize the contributions made by all (UNAIDS, 2005d).

One Monitoring and Evaluation System

Monitoring and evaluation of activities can facilitate the allocation of limited resources to the best advantage and provide information needed for a country and its partners to respond to emerging trends in the epidemic in a timely manner. UNAIDS recommends that monitoring and evaluation occur in the context of a unified national strategic plan for these activities, with the country adopting a single set of standardized indicators endorsed by all stakeholders and using a national information system that ensures the effective flow of information at all levels (UNAIDS, 2005d).

While they are essential activities, monitoring and evaluation pose a tremendous challenge. UNAIDS has described three directions of accountability—upward to donors of all types, downward to people directly affected by HIV/AIDS, and horizontally within and across partnerships and to the civil sector to encourage mutual accountability (UNAIDS, 2004b). According to UNAIDS, "a central focus for accountability in this situation is to strengthen partner countries' capacity to manage and monitor so that reporting can be country-led and country-owned and reporting and monitoring should support the partner countries' own needs. Credible monitoring and evaluation must serve two essential functions: to improve programme implementation, while also allowing donor sources to ensure that their funding is effectively spent" (UNAIDS, 2004b, p. 3). Follow-up to the United Nations General Assembly Special Session on HIV/AIDS has shown that among the challenges faced by countries and their partners are weak collaboration among stakeholders; shortages of monitoring and evaluation skills; insufficient resources to support the activities; and a lack of the strategic information systems needed to collect, analyze, and report the data (UNAIDS, 2005d).

Strategic Planning and Major Elements of HIV/AIDS Programs at the Country Level

As early as 1998, UNAIDS published a guide for countries to assist them in developing national strategic plans for their response to HIV/AIDS. The guidelines offer practical assistance for planning at the national, district, and community levels by governments, nongovernmental organizations, donors, and other agencies (UNAIDS, 1998). The major steps or strategic planning at the country level as outlined by UNAIDS are listed in Box 2-3.

Strategic planning may result in different priorities in different countries, but the major elements of all HIV/AIDS programs are similar (see Box 2-4). Interventions and services involve both help for those living with HIV/AIDS or otherwise affected by the epidemic (for example, children orphaned because of AIDS and family members of people who are HIV-positive) and efforts to curtail the spread of the virus through a variety of measures.

A Family-Centered and Community-Based Approach to HIV/AIDS

Programs can be offered in a variety of settings, but UNAIDS has urged that services be available in the communities where those affected live and

BOX 2-3
UNAIDS Guidelines on Major Steps of Strategic Planning at the Country Level

1. A situational analysis to look at situations that may be relevant to HIV, factors that favor or impede its spread, and factors that improve or impede the best possible quality of life for people living with HIV and for their families.
2. A response analysis, in which relevant initiatives in priority areas are examined, including those that augment or supplement "official national programs," including activities organized by the community, the private sector, civil society, academic organizations, and nongovernmental organizations.
3. The formulation of a strategic plan through a process that addresses how a country responds to its epidemic currently and in the future. This plan should include detailed strategies for changing the current situation and successive intermediate steps necessary to achieve the stated objectives.
4. Acquisition of the resources needed to carry out the activities, as well as identification of currently available resources (and how they are being used) and how additional resources and partners can be identified and accessed.

SOURCE: UNAIDS, 1998.

to families, which are the main source of support and care for people with HIV/AIDS. With a few exceptions, however, community-based primary health care services are fragmented, have inadequate resources, and place "little emphasis on health promotion, prevention, and systematic screening and referrals" (WHO, 2002a, p. 1). Remedying this situation means supporting and strengthening local capacity to provide all necessary services (UNAIDS, 2001).

A healthy community has been described as "one that is continually creating and improving physical and social environments and expanding those community resources which enable people to mutually support each other in performing all the functions of life and developing to their maximum potential." An empowered community must have both a system to provide help, including both formal and informal elements, and an empowered and mobilized citizenry (Kaye and Wolff, 2002, pp. 1–2). Local communities, even when composed mainly of people who are illiterate, have the capacity to work as partners with governments, with health and development agencies, and with nongovernmental organizations in identifying local priorities and implementing appropriate strategies (WHO, 2002a). These issues are discussed further in Chapter 6.

BOX 2-4
Major Elements of HIV/AIDS Programs Identified by UNAIDS

- **Prevention interventions and programs,** including use of mass media, testing and counseling, and social marketing of condoms to reduce risk behaviors by vulnerable populations (such as people who use injecting drugs, sex workers and their clients, youths in and out of school, men having sex with men, and people living with HIV infection). In the general population, interventions include preventing transmission from mother to child; management and treatment of sexually transmitted infections; preventing transmission in the workplace; and improving safety in health facilities through the use of universal precautions and of postexposure prophylaxis to reduce the risks of occupational exposure, and improved blood and medical injection safety (see Chapter 4 for discussion of PEPFAR's prevention programs). Coverage for the greatest impact will vary depending on how the country's epidemic is defined by prevalence (see Table 2-1).
- **Treatment and care interventions** to provide access to antiretroviral and other medications, palliative care, provider-initiated HIV testing, management and treatment of opportunistic infections, nutritional support, and laboratory support (see Chapters 5 and 6, respectively, for discussion of PEPFAR treatment and care programs).
- **Support for all orphans and vulnerable children,** including those made vulnerable and orphaned by HIV/AIDS. This support includes primary and secondary education for children and skills training for out-of-school youths; routine and specific health care, including sexual and reproductive health for older children; family and home support, including income generation or support; community support, including training and support of full-time community workers and child care; and administrative costs for birth certificates, as well as for other administrative and institutional arrangements necessary for the implementation for child care (see Chapter 7 for discussion of PEPFAR's programs for orphans and vulnerable children).
- **Significant investment in human resources,** including the training of clinicians, as well as strengthening cadres of community health workers. Analyses should also be conducted to assess the costs for additional tiers of health workers, such as nurse practitioners, clinical officers, and laboratory technicians (see Chapter 8 for discussion of PEPFAR's workforce programs).
- **Management and infrastructure** for AIDS programs, monitoring and evaluation, advocacy, and facility upgrading through purchases of telecommunications and laboratory equipment (see Chapters 5 and 8 for discussion of PEPFAR's infrastructure programs).

SOURCE: UNAIDS, 2005b.

CHALLENGES TO HIV/AIDS PROGRAMS

Even assuming harmonization among stakeholders, countries and their assistance partners are faced with myriad challenges to successful implementation of HIV/AIDS programs. These challenges include economic and social conditions; the capacity of health care systems; the capacity of the health care workforce; competing health priorities, the increasing burden of HIV/AIDS on women and girls; growing numbers of orphans and other vulnerable children; the increasing need for children and grandmothers to serve as caregivers; stigma and discrimination; and gaps in the current evidence base for the prevention, care, and treatment of people with HIV/AIDS. These challenges are highlighted briefly here and discussed further in the subsequent chapters. With the levels of aid being provided and the infusion of commodities, the potential for corruption is another challenge countries face (Lyman, 2005). However, an examination of the kind necessary to detect corruption was beyond the scope of this study (see Chapter 1 and Appendix B for discussion of data and methods).

Economic and Social Conditions

The countries hardest hit by HIV/AIDS are among the poorest in the world. AIDS has been identified as a serious challenge to development, with both short- and long-term economic effects (UNAIDS, 2006). Because HIV/AIDS often hits working-age populations hardest, the workforces of many nations have been affected by the loss of skilled workers to the epidemic. This loss of skilled workers in turn affects nations' ability to respond to their epidemics. (The special case of the health care workforce is discussed below.)

The education sector in many countries has been severely affected. A growing number of studies have been examining the impact of HIV/AIDS on education, including supply, demand, and quality. As early as December 1999, the United Nations Children's Fund (UNICEF) reported that the "educational systems of much of Eastern and Southern Africa were experiencing problems due to absenteeism and the loss of teachers, education officers, inspectors, and planning and management personnel" (Africa Renewal, 1999, p. 1). In some severely affected countries in Africa, the number of teachers dying of AIDS-related complications is higher than the number of new graduates produced by teacher-training colleges (Africa Renewal, 2007).

The demographic effects of the epidemic are significant, as it alters the population structure of hard-hit countries, affecting population growth and mortality rates and ultimately age and sex distributions. People die prematurely, during their most productive and reproductive years. One consequence of this is that fewer working-age people must support children and the elderly. In parts of the world where women are disproportionately affected, HIV has changed the ratio of caregivers (mainly women) to those needing care.

Especially in sub-Saharan Africa, HIV is only one of several ongoing health crises, the most pressing being malaria, tuberculosis, pneumonia, and diseases of poor nutrition. These challenges are interrelated with HIV/AIDS, each intensifying and complicating the effects of the other. Abu-Raddad and colleagues (2006) found that repeated and transient increases in HIV viral load resulting from coinfection with malaria can amplify HIV prevalence, suggesting that malaria may be an important factor in the rapid spread of HIV infection in sub-Saharan Africa (see Chapter 6 for further discussion of this issue).

Poverty exacerbates all efforts to improve the well-being of populations, especially health. Often, there is a constellation of diseases that occur more consistently among the poor than among the more affluent. When health is viewed from a multiple-determinant model, such as that proposed by Evans and colleagues (Evans et al., 1994), it is clear that socioeconomic and physical environmental factors—including nutrition; housing; air, food, and water quality; waste disposal; injury control; infectious disease management; workplace and road safety; and issues concerning energy sources and use—play critical contributory roles in determining individual and population health outcomes, particularly in developing countries (Kindig, 1997). Poverty and environmental degradation are intricately linked, and their mutual reinforcement can have consequences that directly impact a country's ability to meet the basic human needs (food, health, and education) of its population (UN, 2003b; Rice, 2006).

Capacity of Health Care Systems

An adequate health care infrastructure is critical to implementing efficient and effective HIV/AIDS prevention, treatment, and care programs. While this section focuses on the health sector, the Committee acknowledges that many other sectors, including education, agriculture, and transportation, also play a critical role in comprehensively addressing each country's epidemic. Increasing demand for health care services is overwhelming the public health infrastructure in many developing countries. The health care system is central to surveillance, prevention, diagnosis, and treatment of HIV/AIDS and related conditions. Some efforts have been made to build the capacity of health systems in developing countries, but donor support has not kept pace with the increasing demand for scale-up of the delivery of HIV/AIDS services (World Bank, 2006). Physical infrastructure, clinics, laboratories, the supply chain, and information systems all are stretched thin by the implementation of a national HIV/AIDS program.

On an operational level, the ability to implement programs effectively is often contingent on physical infrastructure, such as transportation routes, water and sanitation, schools, and other social resources. These elements of the health infrastructure are weakest in rural areas, where most people in the focus countries reside. Only about one-third of the population of the focus countries live in urban areas, although this varies widely among countries (U.S. DOS, 2006). Of the focus countries, Botswana and South Africa have the largest urban populations, documented at 54 percent and 53 percent, respectively; whereas Ethiopia and Uganda have the smallest—less than 15 percent in urban areas in both countries (UNAIDS, 2006).

The ability to procure HIV/AIDS drugs and supplies also affects the overall success of programs. Despite donor support, some existing procurement systems are fragile, lacking trained personnel, handicapped by antiquated technology, and limited in their forecasting ability. The capacity of smaller countries to negotiate successfully with manufacturers is also limited. Various procurement methods, including multicountry purchasing through organizations such as UNICEF, are currently in use. Group purchasing mechanisms are available through international partners, which supply many of the focus countries.

Capacity of the Health Care Workforce

Stephen Lewis, the UN Special Envoy for AIDS in Africa, remarked at the close of the 16th International AIDS Conference in 2006:

> What has clearly emerged as the most difficult of issues, almost everywhere, certainly in Africa, is the loss of human capacity. In country after country, the response to the pandemic is sabotaged by the paucity of doctors, nurses, clinicians and community health workers. The shortages are overwhelming. Everyone is struggling. Most of the shortage stems from death and illness; some stems from brain-drain and poaching. But whatever the source, we have a problem of staggering dimensions.

The Institute of Medicine has previously reported that human resource capacity is very weak in resource-constrained settings, especially sub-Saharan Africa. Such limited capabilities pose a critical obstacle to providing access to antiretroviral therapy and prevention of mother-to-child transmission, particularly in rural settings (IOM, 2005). Policy makers and field staff in some of the most affected countries have identified the lack of human resources for health as the single most serious obstacle to scaling up treatment. The HIV/AIDS pandemic has exacerbated workforce shortages, as many countries lose large numbers of health care workers to AIDS. In some African countries, AIDS may be responsible for half of all deaths among employees in the public health sector.

Increasing Burden of HIV/AIDS on Women and Girls

As of 2006, almost half of all people living worldwide with HIV/AIDS were women (UNAIDS, 2006). In sub-Saharan Africa, however, women now represent 59 percent of all people living with HIV/AIDS, and the proportion is growing (see Figure 2-2) (UNAIDS, 2006). Today's statistics are the product of a trend toward increasing rates of infection among women, given that the pandemic started in men. The reasons underlying this trend include the inferior social and economic status of women in many countries, which affects their chances of gaining access to either means for prevention of or treatment for HIV/AIDS and related complications; violence against women and girls, including domestic, sexual, and war-related violence; and biological factors that increase the susceptibility of women to infection. UNAIDS has expressed concern about gender-based inequalities in access to treatment, with some evidence of women paying more for services and being hospitalized less frequently when clinically appropriate (UNAIDS, 2004b).

Teens and young adults (aged 15 to 24) continue to be at the center of the epidemic with heavy concentrations among those newly infected, accounting for more than 40 percent of new adult HIV infections in 2000. In sub-Saharan Africa, three young women are infected for every young man in this age group. The situation is similar in the Caribbean, where young women are about twice as likely as men their age to be infected with HIV (UNAIDS, 2006).

Biological characteristics place women at greater risk than men of contracting the virus from engaging in unprotected sex, but gender disparities

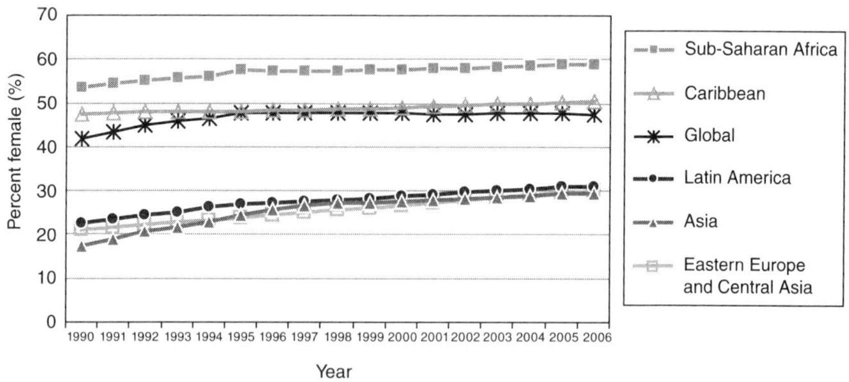

FIGURE 2-2 Percent of adults living with HIV who are female, 1990–2006.
SOURCE: Reprinted with the kind permission of UNAIDS, 2006.

and inequity are probably more responsible for rising infection rates in women. Even in the case of women who are married and engaging in intercourse only with their husbands, if their husbands have other sexual contacts, they are at increased risk of infection. For the past 5 years, HIV incidence has increased among married women and girls globally. In South Africa, infection rates have risen to more than 35 percent among pregnant women aged 25 to 29, and remain at more than 30 percent among pregnant women aged 30 to 34. At least in some places, women are aware of their vulnerability. In a 1999 national reproductive and child health survey in Tanzania, 62 percent of married women reported that they perceived the greatest risk factor for HIV infection to be their partners having other sexual contacts (National Bureau of Statistics Dar es Salaam, Tanzania and Macro International, 2000).

Most evidence suggests that women are at higher risk of infection from an infected male partner than vice versa. Although not entirely consistent, recent studies support an estimate that HIV is two to four times more transmissible to women than to men (NWHRC, 2006). Young girls whose reproductive systems are not fully developed are at even greater risk because of a higher propensity to develop microlesions and vaginal tearing, particularly in cases of sexual coercion (NWHRC, 2006). Women suffer from the same complications of AIDS that afflict men, but they also experience gender-specific manifestations of HIV infection that occur with less frequency or severity in HIV-negative women. These manifestations include recurrent vaginal yeast infections; severe pelvic inflammatory disease; and an increased risk of precancerous cervical lesions, which may indicate an increased risk of cervical cancer (NIAID/NIH, 2006).

Women are particularly vulnerable to HIV infection through heterosexual transmission because of substantial mucosal exposure to seminal fluids. This major biological factor of women's susceptibility may be increased by the symptoms of sexually transmitted infections, especially those causing ulcerations of the vagina, such as genital herpes, syphilis, and chancroid, which increase the risk of transmission of HIV through sexual intercourse by two- to tenfold (Johns Hopkins School of Public Health, 2000; NIAID/NIH, 2006; NWHRC, 2006). Other infections can also increase a woman's risk of contracting HIV. For example, although the specific bacteria involved have not been identified, bacterial vaginosis, the most prevalent vaginal infection in women of childbearing age, may double a woman's susceptibility to HIV infection (Myer et al., 2005). The strategy of identifying and treating bacterial vaginosis has been proposed as a means of HIV prevention; however, the practicality of such an approach has yet to be demonstrated (Schwebke, 2005).

As the pandemic continues to take its toll on families and communities, the growing burden of caring for the sick, the dying, and those left behind falls to women and girls. According to UNAIDS, most of the care for people living with HIV in the hardest-hit countries occurs at home, with up to 90 percent of such care being provided by women and girls (UNAIDS, 2006). According to UNAIDS, special attention should be paid to the difficulties women and children face as caregivers, including economic vulnerability due to widowhood and the lack of developmentally appropriate income-generating skills in the young, exacerbated by discrimination in property inheritance and employment. While they are caring for the sick and dying, they are also coping with the loss of their parents, siblings, other relatives, or adult children (UNAIDS, 2006). Elderly caregivers shoulder the additional concern of what will happen to the children for whom they are providing care when they themselves die. (See also the discussion of children and elderly women as caregivers below.)

Growing Numbers of Orphans and Other Vulnerable Children

The rising human cost of the pandemic can be measured not only by the rising toll of people losing their lives to the disease, but also by the escalating numbers of orphans and other vulnerable children. UNAIDS estimates that globally, more than 20 million children having lost at least one parent, will have been orphaned as a result of HIV/AIDS by 2010. This estimate does not include children who will have died (UNAIDS et al., 2002). In the 15 focus countries, the number of orphans due to all causes ranges from 33,000 in Guyana to an estimated 7 million in Nigeria (U.S. DOS, 2006). In 12 of the 15 focus countries, orphan populations due to all causes exceeding 500,000 have been reported (UNICEF, 2006a). Kenya, South Africa, Tanzania, and Uganda each have more than 1 million children orphaned because of AIDS. Namibia has reported the smallest population of children orphaned by AIDS in Africa, estimated at 85,000, which is slightly more than 4 percent of its total population of approximately 2 million people. No data are currently available for orphans due to AIDS for Ethiopia, Guyana, Haiti, and Vietnam (UNICEF, 2006a) (see Chapter 7). Estimates for children living with HIV/AIDS at the end of 2005 ranged from fewer than 1,000 in Guyana to 240,000 in both Nigeria and South Africa. Seven of the focus countries have reported more than 100,000 children living with HIV/AIDS (UNAIDS, 2006).

Attention to the needs of orphans and other vulnerable children is a critical element of a long-term HIV/AIDS strategy. While estimates of numbers of orphans do not include children made vulnerable by HIV/AIDS or any other health or social condition, they may well be the proverbial tip of the iceberg in terms of the visibility and extensive needs of children in these countries. These children become vulnerable not only to the risk of HIV infection, but also to a host of social and economic ills. Academic performance may suffer or schooling may end prematurely because they must be caregivers or because family finances no longer allow them to be in school. The cascading effects of academic vulnerability often lead to economic vulnerability, including loss of income and/or property and lack of adequate shelter and food, which in turn may lead to increased risk of HIV exposure and infection through transactional or transgenerational sex in exchange for food, money, shelter, and other basic needs. Psychosocial vulnerability may develop from the need for emotional support due to HIV/AIDS from the individual child as well as the family and the burden of caregiving and guardianship for younger siblings. Survivor vulnerability may lead to poor nutrition, poor health, and lack of resources for basic care to meet the developmental needs of children. Finally, these children are vulnerable to exploitation and abuse when they have lost the protection of parents and the community (UNAIDS et al., 2004).

Children and Elderly Grandmothers as Caregivers

When young children (of any age up to 18) or elderly grandmothers are forced to head households, they face many challenges in terms of not only their ability to generate income, but also their own health and social service needs. Grandmothers are typically of the age at which physical labor, such as farming for subsistence or income generation, is difficult for them. They often need assistance themselves, even for chores such as carrying water and firewood. Many elderly grandmothers are concerned about what will happen to their grandchildren and other wards when they die. Succession planning and issues related to inheritance and property rights are crucial not only when the grandmothers die, but also during their caretaking years to ensure that there is a stable and physical environment in which the children can be raised and then assume caretaking responsibilities if they have no other extended family. Children whose parents have died or are too busy caring for a dying spouse or partner to pass on essential knowledge and skills (e.g., farming) are left behind their peers in preparing for adulthood (UNICEF, 2006b).

Elderly grandmothers and children are often framed as victims of the pandemic, but they appear to be forgotten in terms of their need for HIV/AIDS prevention information and education. Grandmothers are too often and incorrectly assumed to be sexually inactive, and children are not expected to engage in sex. If household and community safety nets fail, children are at risk for sexual and labor exploitation to meet their basic needs and thus are at risk for exposure to HIV. Children also have basic age-specific health needs for other common conditions (such as malaria and pneumonia), vaccinations against childhood diseases, and maintenance of hygienic conditions to prevent exposure to parasitic and other infections.

Children who are HIV-positive need a range of prevention, care, and treatment services (UNICEF, 2006b).

Stigma and Discrimination

Stigma and discrimination pose obstacles to responses to HIV/AIDS epidemics, but programs increasingly are addressing these issues and the challenges they present. Weiss and Ramakrishna (2001) make the point that for targeted strategies against stigma to be developed, the phenomenon needs to be better understood and measured. There is a need to understand the sociocultural context of stigma and its effects, to document its impact, to develop strategies needed to measure it, and to track its impact over time. While programs are focusing efforts on understanding and addressing stigma as well as monitoring these efforts, much of what has been reported about the effects of stigma and discrimination is anecdotal. That the effects are significant, however, particularly in sub-Saharan Africa, is not doubted.

Stigma has been categorized for study as perceived, experienced, and internalized; and according to several domains—fear of casual transmission, values (shame, blame, and judgment), enacted stigma (discrimination), and disclosure (USAID, 2005). Common manifestations of stigma include social isolation or distancing in the community; family rejection; loss of respect; physical or verbal abuse or violence; expressed fear of casual transmission; feelings of shame and worthlessness for those infected with HIV and their family members; the experience of being blamed for contracting HIV; and denial of rights, education, employment, and health services. Moreover, health care workers may be stigmatized because they care for HIV patients (Project Siyam'kela, 2003; USAID, 2005). High levels of stigma have been associated with less willingness to care for a family member with HIV/AIDS (Letamo, 2003).

It has been reported that the availability of antiretroviral therapy has reduced the prevalence of AIDS-related stigma and resulted in increases in voluntary testing and counseling (Castro and Farmer, 2005); however, this phenomenon is not well documented. According to UNAIDS, reports from more than 30 countries indicate that stigma and discrimination against people with HIV remain pervasive (UNAIDS, 2006). Other researchers have reported that stigma has emerged as a major limiting factor in primary and secondary HIV/AIDS prevention and care by discouraging voluntary testing and counseling and care seeking, thus increasing suffering and shortening life (Weiss and Ramakrishna, 2001; Newman et al., 2002).

Few tested and validated indicators exist with which to measure stigma and efforts to reduce it (USAID, 2005). Stigma and its effects affect even the ability to gather HIV-related data. For example, individuals may misreport (either way, in different circumstances) whether they have been tested (OGAC, 2005c) and certainly, if known, their HIV status. According to the U.S. Agency for International Development (USAID), "current measures of stigma focusing on HIV/AIDS knowledge, fear of casual transmission, and social distancing often suffer from ambiguity and the inability to specify the underlying cause (motive) for the action" and are often presented with respect to hypothetical situations that may not accurately reflect people's responses and actions in given situations (USAID, 2005, p. 5). Other difficulties associated with the study of stigma include very small samples that are not representative of the community or general population or large samples with few, ambiguous questions. One final challenge to understanding the complexity of stigma is the need to understand the motivation for such behavior in order to develop targeted interventions at the population level, including those to address "compound stigma," defined as "HIV stigma that is layered on top of pre-existing stigmas, frequently toward homosexuals, commercial sex workers, injecting drug users, women, and youth" (USAID, 2005, p. 6).

Gaps in the Evidence Base

Planning and implementation of an integrated national HIV/AIDS program requires a reasonable base of evidence on the effectiveness and other characteristics of particular interventions and programs as applied in specific cultural, economic, and social contexts. However, significant gaps exist in understanding of the epidemic, how to best address it, and how to expand what is working. These gaps relate to every aspect of implementing an HIV/AIDS program, from precisely how HIV infections are spreading to how to assess clinical status without the capacity to measure viral load or CD4 (Bertozzi et al., 2006). As increasing amounts of HIV/AIDS funding are spent in the countries hardest hit by the pandemic, these gaps in the knowledge base will increasingly impair the ability of host countries and donors to achieve their HIV/AIDS control targets. Without this information, allocating the finite resources available is an even more difficult task (Grassly et al., 2001; Bollinger et al., 2004; Bertozzi et al., 2006).

A major research challenge in all areas is how to adapt strategies that originate mainly in wealthy countries to low-income, low-technology settings with low human resource capacity. As programs have been implemented, host countries, donors, and international organizations have been working to increase what is known about implementing a comprehensive HIV/AIDS program in a developing country (see, for example, the World Health Organization's guidelines for antiretroviral therapy in resource-limited settings). But gaps in knowledge remain, and, as more is learned about combating HIV/AIDS in these settings, questions continue to arise.

THE PEPFAR FOCUS COUNTRIES

Funds from PEPFAR support HIV/AIDS relief in more than 120 countries, but two-thirds of the funds—$10 billion out of $15 billion over 5 years—is to be spent on the development of comprehensive and integrated prevention, treatment, and care programs in the 15 focus countries (OGAC, 2004, 2005b). PEPFAR has established 5-year targets for its prevention, treatment, and care programs in these countries to support prevention of 7 million new HIV infections; treatment of 2 million HIV-infected people with antiretroviral therapy; and care for 10 million people infected and affected by HIV/AIDS, including orphans and other vulnerable children.[3]

Among the 12 PEPFAR focus countries in sub-Saharan Africa, the adequacy of the health workforce varies considerably. For example, the average doctor-to-population ratio is 22 per 100,000 among the focus countries. Only South Africa and Vietnam report more than 50 doctors per 100,000; Ethiopia, Mozambique, Rwanda, Tanzania, and Uganda report 5 or fewer. (By comparison, the United States has 256 physicians per 100,000 population.) Similar disparities exist for other types of health care workers (see Table 2-3).

The focus countries are among those nations with the lowest per capita incomes in the world, but important variations exist in their gross domestic product and unemployment rates (see Table 2-4). The average gross domestic product per capita for the 15 focus countries at the end of 2005 was approximately US$3,003 (UNAIDS, 2006). Among the focus countries, Botswana, Namibia, and South Africa have gross domestic products per capita greater than US$5,000. At US$10,960, South Africa has the highest per capita gross domestic product (CIA, 2006) At the other end of the spectrum, Ethiopia, Nigeria, Tanzania, and Zambia have gross domestic products per capita of less than US$1,000. Tanzania has the lowest of all, at US$660 (UNAIDS, 2006). The World Bank has classified 9 of the focus countries—Ethiopia, Guyana, Mozambique, Rwanda, Tanzania, Uganda, Zambia, Côte d'Ivoire, and Haiti—as "heavily indebted poor countries." In 3 focus countries, half of the population lives on less than US$1 per day; in Nigeria, the proportion is 70 percent (UNDP, 2005). Unemployment rates in the focus countries are highly variable. Five have unemployment rates below 10 percent, with Nigeria having the lowest at 3 percent (World Bank, 2006). In contrast, Kenya, Namibia, South Africa, and Zambia all report unemployment rates higher than 25 percent. Zambia's is highest, at 50 percent (World Bank, 2006).

The focus countries all are generally experiencing devastating HIV/

---

[3]For purposes of this goal, PEPFAR defines "treatment" narrowly as antiretroviral therapy (ART) and categorizes other types of treatment—such as therapy for opportunistic infections or for pain management—under "care."

TABLE 2-3 Density of Selected Health Care Workers in the PEPFAR Focus Countries

Country (year represented by data)	Health Care Workers (Total)[a]	Physicians		Nurses		Midwives		Other Health Workers		Medical Assistants	Community Health Workers	
		Total	Density Per 1000	Total	Density Per 1000	Total	Density Per 1000	Total	Density Per 1000	(Total)[c]	Total	Density Per 1000
United States (2002)	15,959,391	730,801	2.56	2,669,603	9.37	N/A	N/A	4,177,609	14.66	N/A	N/A	N/A
Botswana (2004)	7,117	715	0.40	4,753	2.65	N/A	N/A	829	N/A	N/A	N/A	N/A
Côte d'Ivoire (2004)	17,214	2,081	0.12	7,773	0.60	2,407	N/A	147	0.01	25	N/A	N/A
Ethiopia (2003)	48,972	1,936	0.03	14,270	0.21	1,274	0.01	43	0.10	7,311	13,433	0.26
Guyana (2000)	2,134	366	0.48	1,738	2.29	N/A	N/A	N/A	N/A	N/A	N/A	N/A
Haiti (1998)	2,877	1,949	0.25	834	0.11	N/A	N/A	N/A	N/A	N/A	N/A	N/A
Kenya (2002/04)	66,956	4,506[b]	0.14	37,113[b]	1.14	N/A	N/A	5,610	0.17	N/A	N/A	N/A
Mozambique (2004)	20,129	514	0.03	3,947	0.21	2,236	0.12	1,225	0.09	434	N/A	N/A
Namibia (2004)	16,244	598	0.30	6,145	3.06	N/A	N/A	597	0.30	N/A	N/A	N/A
Nigeria (2003/04)	371,726	34,923[b]	0.28	127,580[b]	1.70	82,726[b]	N/A	1,220	0.01	N/A	115,761	0.91

continued

TABLE 2-3 Continued

Country (year represented by data)	Health Care Workers (Total)[a]	Physicians		Nurses		Midwives		Other Health Workers		Medical Assistants	Community Health Workers	
		Total	Density Per 1000	Total	Density Per 1000	Total	Density Per 1000	Total	Density Per 1000	(Total)[c]	Total	Density Per 1000
Rwanda (2004)	18,427	401	0.05	3,570	0.42	77	0.01	446	0.06	75	12,557	1.41
South Africa (2004)	319,992	34,829	0.77	184,459	4.08	N/A	N/A	40,479	0.90	13	14,306	0.20
Tanzania (2002)	48,508	822	0.02	13,292	0.37	N/A	N/A	3,755	0.82	25,967	N/A	N/A
Uganda (2004)	35,445	2,209	0.08	15,161	0.61	4,164	0.12	3,772	0.14	N/A	N/A	N/A
Vietnam (2001)	107,505	42,327	0.53	44,539	0.56	14,662	0.19	N/A	N/A	N/A	N/A	N/A
Zambia (2004)	41,429	1,264	0.12	16,990	1.74	5,020	0.27	3,330	0.30	N/A	N/A	N/A

NOTE: N/A = Data not available.

[a]Estimated number of total health care workers in each country including physicians, nurses, midwives, dentists, pharmacists, public and environmental health workers, community health workers, laboratory technicians, other health care workers, and health management and support workers.

[b]The data provided is only for the year 2004.

[c]The numbers provided for Medical Assistants are the total of assistants in each country. No density rates are available for this category of worker.

SOURCE: Compiled from data from WHO, 2006b.

TABLE 2-4 Selected Economic and Health-Related Indicators of the PEPFAR Focus Countries

Country	Population[a]	Income Status[b]	GDP per Capita (US$)[a]	Life Expectancy[c]	Adult HIV/AIDS Prevalence [Range] (ages 15–49)[a]	Infant Mortality Rate (deaths/1,000 live births)[d]
Botswana	1,765,000	Upper middle	8,920	35	24.1 [23.0–32.0]	54.58
Côte D'Ivoire	18,154,000	Low	1,390	47	7.1 [4.3–9.7]	90.83
Ethiopia	77,431,000	Low	810	48	[0.9–3.5]	95.32
Guyana	751,000	Lower middle	4,110	63	2.4 [1.0–4.9]	33.26
Haiti	8,528,000	Low	1,680	52	3.8 [2.2–5.4]	73.45
Kenya	34,256,000	Low	1,050	47	6.1 [5.2–7.0]	61.47
Mozambique	19,792,000	Low	1,160	42	16.1 [12.5–20.0]	130.79
Namibia	2,031,000	Lower middle	6,960	46	19.6 [8.6–31.7]	48.98
Nigeria	131,530,000	Low	930	44	3.9 [2.3–5.6]	98.80
Rwanda	9,038,000	Low	1,300	44	3.1 [2.9–3.2]	91.23
South Africa	47,432,000	Upper middle	10,960	52	18.8 [16.8–20.7]	61.81
Tanzania	38,329,000	Low	660	44	6.5 [5.8–7.2]	98.54
Uganda	28,816,000	Low	1,520	48	6.7 [5.7–7.6]	67.83
Vietnam	84,238,000	Low	2,700	72	0.5 [0.3–0.9]	25.95
Zambia	11,668,000	Low	890	37	17.0 [15.9–18.1]	88.29

NOTE: GDP = gross domestic product.

[a]UNAIDS, 2006.

[b]World Bank, 2006.

[c]PRB, 2005.

[d]CIA, 2006.

SOURCE: Compiled from data from CIA, 2006; PRB, 2005; UNAIDS, 2006; World Bank, 2006.

AIDS epidemics, but the specifics vary considerably by country. With reference to the classification of country-level epidemics in Table 2-1, except for Vietnam, the HIV/AIDS epidemic is generalized in all of the focus countries, with unprotected heterosexual intercourse remaining the most prevalent mode of HIV transmission and people at risk spanning all age groups and both sexes (UNAIDS, 2006). Adult prevalence is above 5 percent in Botswana, Côte d'Ivoire, Kenya, Mozambique, Namibia, South Africa, Tanzania, Uganda, and Zambia (UNAIDS, 2006). Adult prevalence is below 5 percent in Ethiopia, Guyana, Haiti, Nigeria, Rwanda, and Vietnam (UNAIDS, 2006). Vietnam is the only PEPFAR focus country whose epidemic is characterized as concentrated, with the lowest reported adult HIV prevalence rate of the focus countries at 0.5 percent (UNAIDS, 2006).

Underlying the common classification of generalized epidemic are 14 distinct epidemics occurring in 14 unique contexts. PEPFAR will succeed in reaching its stated targets only if programs are tailored to differences in the state of the epidemics, demographics, political and economic situations, health systems, and social structure (specifically regarding gender and equality). For example, differences in infrastructure affect drug delivery, a critical component of PEPFAR's treatment arm. Each country has a different array of internal systems and external partners, which require coordination and communication. Physical infrastructure and human resource capacity also vary from country to country.

PEPFAR'S AUTHORIZING LEGISLATION: THE LEADERSHIP ACT

In early 2001, at the start of the 107th session of the U.S. Congress, two seminal bills were introduced in the Senate. The first, known as the International Infectious Diseases Control Act of 2001 (S.1032), called for an increase in funding of $200 million for the prevention of HIV transmission from mother to child (along with other provisions) through the establishment of a Global Fund to Fight Against HIV/AIDS, Malaria and Tuberculosis.[4] The second was the Kerry-Frist Global AIDS bill (S.15), formally known as the U.S. Leadership against HIV/AIDS, TB and Malaria Act of 2002. This latter bill was the first coordinated effort by U.S. leadership to respond to the global AIDS pandemic.[5] Although neither of these bills was

[4] S.1032IS, International Infectious Diseases Control Act of 2002, accessed from http://thomas.loc.gov on September 11, 2006.

[5] Presentations by Allen Moore (former deputy chief of staff and policy director for Senator Bill Frist) and Dr. Nancy Stetson (senior foreign policy advisor to Senator John Kerry) to the Institute of Medicine's PEPFAR Evaluation Committee's Open Meeting, September 15, 2005, in Washington, DC.

passed, elements of both were incorporated into what would become the Leadership Act that authorized PEPFAR.[6]

On January 28, 2003, President Bush delivered his State of the Union address, in which he proposed a 5-year, $15 billion initiative to treat and prevent HIV/AIDS in some of the world's most affected countries. Legislation to enact this initiative was introduced in the House of Representatives on March 17, 2003, and in the Senate on May 7, 2003. Many amendments were introduced and debated, a few of which, related mainly to the focus countries, substantively changed the legislation. One amendment established priorities for the "distribution of resources based on factors such as the size and demographic characteristics of populations affected by HIV/AIDS, TB, and malaria; the needs of that population; and the existing infrastructure or funding levels to cure, treat, and prevent HIV/AIDS, TB, and malaria" (P.L. 108-25, §101). A further provision called for "[the Centers for Disease Control and Prevention] in coordination with the Global [AIDS] Coordinator, [the National Institutes of Health, the World Health Organization], UNICEF, and national governments to develop and implement effective strategies to improve injection safety, including eliminating unnecessary injections, promoting sterile injection practices and technologies, strengthening the procedures for proper needle and syringe disposal, and improving the education and information provided to the public and to health professionals" (P.L. 108-25, §306).

Another amendment required "assistance for the purpose of encouraging men to be responsible in their sexual behavior, child rearing, and to respect women" (P.L. 108-25, §301, §104(d)(1)(c)). The next created a pilot program of assistance for children and families affected by HIV/AIDS to "ensure the importance of inheritance rights of women, particularly women in African countries, due to the exponential growth in the number of young widows, orphaned girls, and grandmothers becoming heads of households as a result of the HIV/AIDS pandemic" (P.L. 108-25, §314(b)(4)). An additional amendment required not less than 10 percent of appropriated PEPFAR funds to be allocated to programs that would serve orphans and other vulnerable children affected by HIV/AIDS, at least half of this 10 percent allotment being provided through nonprofit, nongovernmental organizations, including faith-based organizations, that would implement programs on the community level (P.L. 108-25, § 403(b)).

Several amendments added features to the legislation that have been the subject of ongoing debate. For example, the Leadership Act underscores the importance of involving faith-based organizations in the initiative and also exempts them from participating in activities to which they hold

[6]S.1099, United States Emergency Plan for AIDS Relief Act of 2003 and HR 1298, United States Emergency Plan for AIDS Relief Act of 2003, accessed from http://thomas.loc.gov on September 11, 2006.

religious or moral objection. The legislation states that "an organization that is otherwise eligible to receive assistance . . . to prevent, treat, or monitor HIV/AIDS shall not be required, as a condition of receiving the assistance, to endorse or utilize a multisectoral approach to combating HIV/AIDS, or to endorse, utilize, or participate in a prevention method or treatment program to which the organization has a religious or moral objection" (P.L. 108-25, p. 733). Further, the legislation states that "no funds made available to carry out this Act, or any amendment made by this Act, may be used to promote or advocate the legalization or practice of prostitution or sex trafficking. Nothing in the preceding sentence shall be construed to preclude the provision to individuals of palliative care, treatment, or post-exposure pharmaceutical prophylaxis, and necessary pharmaceuticals and commodities, including test kits, condoms, and, when proven effective, microbicides. No funds made available to carry out this Act, or any amendment made by the Act, may be used to provide assistance to any group or organization that does not have a policy explicitly opposing prostitution and sex trafficking" (P.L. 108-25, pp. 733–734). Finally, the legislation required that of the amounts appropriated, "an effective distribution of such amounts would be 20 percent of such amounts for HIV/AIDS prevention . . . of which such amount at least 33 percent should be expended for abstinence-until-marriage programs" (P.L. 108-25, p. 746).

Congress passed the Leadership Act, and on May 27, 2003, the President signed it to become P.L. 108-25, The United States Leadership against HIV/AIDS, Tuberculosis, and Malaria Act of 2003. The Leadership Act called for bold leadership by the United States in international HIV/AIDS programs; however, it stressed the overarching need to coordinate with local, national, and international partners. In particular, the act recognized that the new resources being provided could not meet all needs, and it sought to complement existing programs that might already be meeting some needs. The legislation stated that the Global AIDS Coordinator would collaborate and coordinate with civil sector organizations to plan, fund, implement, monitor, and evaluate all programs addressing HIV/AIDS.

Requirement for a Comprehensive 5-Year Strategy

The Leadership Act directed the President to submit a strategy meeting specified objectives (see Box 2-5) to the Committee on Foreign Relations of the Senate and the Committee on International Relations of the House of Representatives, the committees with jurisdiction over the legislation.

Specification of Focus Countries

The PEPFAR legislation named 14 focus countries, which at the time accounted for more than half of the world's HIV/AIDS cases. These 14

BOX 2-5
Central Objectives of P.L. 108-25 for Strategy Development

- Include specific objectives, designed to develop and implement national and community-based multisectoral approaches, and specific strategies to treat individuals infected with HIV/AIDS and to prevent the further spread of HIV infections, with a particular focus on the needs of families with children (including the prevention of mother-to-child transmission), women, young people, and children (such as unaccompanied minor children and orphans) [that will enhance leadership capacity, particularly at the community level].
- Implement a tiered approach to direct delivery of care and treatment through a system based on central facilities augmented by expanding circles of local delivery of care and treatment through local systems and capacity.
- Assign priorities for relevant executive branch agencies primarily in those areas where the agency has the greatest expertise, technical capabilities, and potential for success.
- Provide that the reduction of HIV/AIDS behavioral risks shall be a priority of all prevention efforts in terms of funding, educational messages, and activities by promoting abstinence from sexual activity and substance abuse, encouraging monogamy and faithfulness, promoting the effective use of condoms, and eradicating prostitution, the sex trade, rape, sexual assault, and sexual exploitation of women and children [with specific strategies to target the unique economic and social needs of women, young people, and children (and keeping families intact) that make them vulnerable to infection].
- [Provide a description of the mechanisms to] improve coordination and reduce duplication among relevant executive branch agencies, foreign governments, and international organizations [as well as heightening the engagement of member states of the G-8 and strengthening key financial and coordination mechanisms such as the Global Fund and UNAIDS].
- Project general levels of resources needed to achieve the stated objectives.
- Expand public–private partnerships and the leveraging of resources.
- Maximize U.S. capabilities in the areas of technical assistance and training and research, including vaccine research.
- Establish priorities for the distribution of resources based on factors such as the size and demographics of the population with HIV/AIDS, tuberculosis, and malaria and the needs of that population and the existing infrastructure or funding levels that may exist to cure, treat, and prevent HIV/AIDS, tuberculosis, and malaria.
- Include initiatives describing how the President will maximize the leverage of private-sector dollars in reduction and treatment of HIV/AIDS, tuberculosis, and malaria.

SOURCE: P.L. 108-25.

countries—12 in Africa and 2 in the Caribbean—had been named by President Bush in his 2003 State of the Union address. The law gave the President the authority to add focus countries, which he did, adding a 15th—Vietnam—in June 2004. The focus countries are the Republic of Botswana (Botswana), the Republic of Côte d'Ivoire (Côte d'Ivoire), the Federal Democratic Republic of Ethiopia (Ethiopia), the Cooperative Republic of Guyana (Guyana), the Republic of Haiti (Haiti), the Republic of Kenya (Kenya), the Republic of Mozambique (Mozambique), the Republic of Namibia (Namibia), the Federal Republic of Nigeria (Nigeria), the Republic of Rwanda (Rwanda), the Republic of South Africa (South Africa), the United Republic of Tanzania (Tanzania), the Republic of Uganda (Uganda), the Socialist Republic of Vietnam (Vietnam), and the Republic of Zambia (Zambia). The goal of concentrating the majority of the PEPFAR funds in selected focus countries is to scale up rapidly to have impact on their epidemics at the national level.

The U.S. Global AIDS Coordinator

The legislation established the position of a U.S. Global AIDS Coordinator to be appointed by the President, with the advice and consent of the Senate. The Office of the U.S. Global AIDS Coordinator (OGAC) was established within the Department of State. The Coordinator, who reports directly to the Secretary of State, has primary responsibility for oversight and coordination of all resources for the U.S. government's international activities to combat the HIV/AIDS pandemic.

Reporting Requirements

In addition to other reports, the Leadership Act required the President to deliver annual reports to the committees with jurisdiction to describe progress, in particular to assess the impact of the program in reducing the spread of HIV/AIDS (particularly among women and girls and through mother-to-child transmission) and in

- Providing treatment for HIV/AIDS
- Improving health delivery systems
- Treating and curing people with tuberculosis and malaria

As required, three annual reports have been submitted to date. The first, entitled *Engendering Bold Leadership*; the second, entitled *Action Today: A Foundation for Tomorrow*; and the third, entitled *The Power of Partnerships*; covered fiscal years 2004, 2005, and 2006, respectively (OGAC, 2005b, 2006a, 2007b). Many other reports have been submitted in response to requests on specific topics. In 2006, for example, OGAC submitted reports on workforce capacity, food and nutrition, supplying antiretrovirals, primary and secondary education for children, and refugees and internally displaced persons (OGAC, 2006b–f).

Performance Targets

The Leadership Act did not provide a rationale for the derivation of the performance targets for prevention, treatment, and care. However, the Committee did learn at one of its public meetings that the prevention target represented roughly half of the expected new infections in the focus countries (Dybul, 2005). The Committee also learned that a group of economists with UNAIDS was consulted to help derive the targets (personal communication, Stefano Bertozzi).

Budget Allocations

The Leadership Act specified several budget allocations that were originally intended as guidance for the first 2 years of the legislation, but many became mandatory beginning in fiscal year 2006. They include the following:

- 55 percent for "therapeutic medical care of individuals infected with HIV, of which such amount at least 75 percent should be expended for the purchase and distribution of antiretroviral pharmaceuticals and at least 25 percent should be expended for related care"
- 20 percent for "HIV/AIDS prevention, of which such amount at least 33 percent should be expended for abstinence-until-marriage programs"
- 15 percent for "palliative care of individuals with HIV/AIDS"
- Not less than 10 percent for "assistance for orphans and vulnerable children affected by HIV/AIDS, of which such amount at least 50 percent shall be provided through non-profit, nongovernmental organizations, including faith-based organizations, that implement programs on the community level"

THE 5-YEAR STRATEGY: THE PRESIDENT'S EMERGENCY PLAN FOR AIDS RELIEF

The Leadership Act required development of a comprehensive 5-year strategy, guided by the legislation (Box 2-3). The strategy (which includes elements cited in Box 2-4) was developed and presented to Congress by Ambassador Tobias, the U.S. Global AIDS Coordinator, on February 23, 2004, 9 months after the act had been signed into law. The Ambassador stressed that the strategy should be viewed as a "work in progress," something that could change in response to changes in the HIV/AIDS pandemic and the knowledge and tools available. The strategy has four main emphases: (1) rapidly expanding services, building on existing successful programs; (2) identifying new partners and building capacity for sustainable, effective, and widespread HIV/AIDS responses; (3) encouraging bold leadership and fostering a sound enabling policy environment for combating HIV/AIDS and mitigating its consequences; and (4) implementing strong strategic information systems that will contribute to continued learning and identification of best practices.

The strategy also stresses collaboration and coordination with a wide range of partners, including relevant parts of the U.S. government, nongovernmental organizations of all types, the private sector, and international organizations. Responsiveness to local needs as well as to national priorities and strategies is also key (OGAC, 2004).

As required, the strategy assigns priorities for and allocates resources to relevant executive branch agencies, including the Departments of State, Defense, Commerce, Labor, Health and Human Services (specifically, the Centers for Disease Control and Prevention, National Institutes of Health, U.S. Food and Drug Administration, and Health Resources Services Administration), the U.S. Agency for International Development, and the Peace Corps. Most of these agencies were already involved in global HIV/AIDS efforts prior to PEPFAR (OGAC, 2004) (see Box 2-6).

The PEPFAR strategy is responsive to legislative imperatives while containing the major elements of an HIV/AIDS strategy recommended by normative entities such as the World Health Organization and UNAIDS.

The Network Model

PEPFAR's 5-year strategy describes a network model developed to deliver prevention, treatment, and care services for HIV/AIDS, consistent with the priorities and requirements of the Leadership Act. The basic design, adopted from a successfully implemented model in Uganda, relies on centralized, core facilities (staffed by different practitioners of varying skill) from which technical support and products flow to facilities in the periphery, especially to rural and underserved areas. In turn, facilities and staff at different points in the network identify and refer people needing more complex care to the more advanced central facilities (OGAC, 2004) (see Figure 2-3).

The model relies on existing medical facilities, such as district-level hospitals and local health clinics, for basic services. Private—often faith-based—medical facilities are relied upon to rapidly scale up existing palliative care services for adults and children with AIDS, with the aim of ensuring long-term sustainability. Finally, information systems are to be set

BOX 2-6
HIV/AIDS Activities of U.S. Government Agencies Implementing PEPFAR

Department of State:

- HIV/AIDS prevention activities and small-scale programs in 162 countries through U.S. embassies in those countries
- Diplomatic exchanges to generate more resources for HIV/AIDS
- Exchange programs and community involvement
- Support for the Office of the U.S. Global AIDS Coordinator in coordinating global HIV/AIDS efforts

Department of Health and Human Services:

- Centers for Disease Control and Prevention: Prevention, surveillance, infrastructure development, care, and field activities through its Global AIDS Program; field staff work with the Global Fund's Country Coordinating Mechanisms
- National Institutes of Health: Basic, clinical, and behavioral research on HIV, opportunistic infections, and other HIV-associated conditions; development of therapies, vaccines, and microbicides
- Health Resources and Services Administration: Training, technical assistance, twinning, and palliative care programs
- U.S. Food and Drug Administration: Advisory resource on HIV/AIDS drug quality, safety, and efficacy, and conduct of related HIV/AIDS activities

Department of Defense:

- Military-to-military HIV/AIDS awareness and prevention education
- Policy development for HIV/AIDS issues in military settings
- Construction of facilities used for HIV/AIDS activities

Department of Labor:

- Workplace HIV/AIDS prevention education and stigma reduction
- Technical assistance to governments, employees, and labor leaders
- Capacity building to improve worker access to testing, counseling, and other support services
- Multilateral programs targeting HIV-infected children forced to work and child prostitution
- Cross-sector collaboration
- Reduction of trade barriers to facilitate delivery systems for health care products

U.S. Agency for International Development:

- Bilateral programs in 50 countries; regional programs including 48 countries
- Expertise in pharmaceutical logistics management
- Operational and biomedical research
- Health care system strengthening in host countries
- Coordination with other development programs

Peace Corps:

- 3,000+ volunteers working on HIV/AIDS (PEPFAR commits 1,000 more)
- Training of African volunteers as HIV/AIDS educators and advocates
- Building of community-level capacity
- Short-term Crisis Corps that can be harnessed to address HIV/AIDS

SOURCE: OGAC, 2004.

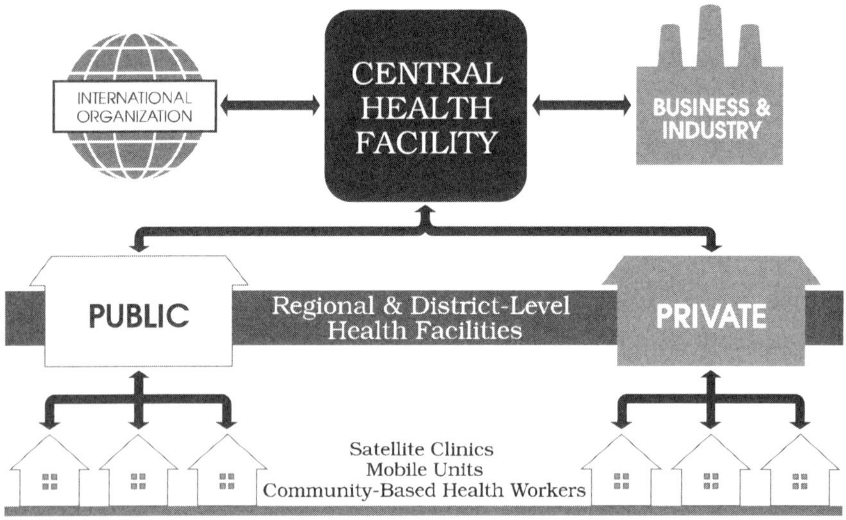

FIGURE 2-3 PEPFAR's network model.
SOURCE: OGAC, 2004.

up to monitor progress and ensure that programs comply with PEPFAR's stated policies and strategies (OGAC, 2004, 2006g). The network model envisions information systems in facilities at all levels, with links and regular feedback loops to provide information to health providers and policy makers (OGAC, 2006g). Recognizing the severe shortages of health care personnel in focus countries, the model includes training for community health workers to deliver routine care, manage symptoms, and monitor for treatment adherence.

The description of the network model focuses on medical services, with less attention to social services. The model states the intent to use and strengthen linkages among the levels of support, but does not explain how this will be accomplished. Home-based services, largely for palliative care, are acknowledged as important and cost-effective, but are otherwise not elaborated upon.

Organizational Structure

The U.S. Global AIDS Coordinator

The first U.S. Global AIDS Coordinator, Randall Tobias, was sworn in with the rank of Ambassador on October 6, 2003; on February 23, 2004, he presented to Congress the U.S. 5-year global HIV/AIDS strategy. The Coordinator's office, OGAC, is responsible for maintaining the focus of

PEPFAR by leading policy development, program oversight, and coordination both among U.S. government departments and agencies and with other donors and governments (Box 2-5). The Coordinator is responsible for the allocation of funds that are distributed through the U.S. government departments and agencies cited earlier.

Coordination and Support Within the Office of the U.S. Global AIDS Coordinator

Within OGAC, staff are organized into several groups, all of which include OGAC staff and representatives from the other U.S. government departments and agencies coordinated by OGAC (Table 2-5). These groups include the Policy Group, incorporating representation from the U.S. Agency for International Development, the Department of Health and Human Services, the White House, and the National Security Council; the Deputy Principals Group, handling program management and logistics, with representation from the majority of the government department and agencies cited above; and a Scientific Steering Committee, consisting of representatives from the two largest of the above implementing departments and agencies and the Department of Defense (Moloney-Kitts, 2005). Finally, Core and Technical Teams, which draw members from a wide range of U.S. government agencies, are responsible for supporting programs in PEPFAR countries in addressing specific technical and implementation issues.

PEPFAR Focus Country Teams

Each focus country has a U.S. Government Country Team that is responsible for coordinating PEPFAR-sponsored programs in the country. The Country Team is led by the U.S. ambassador to the country and includes representatives from all of the implementing departments and agencies. The staff of Country Teams serve in foreign-service posts. The Committee observed that the teams varied in size, expertise, and length of time served in the country.

The Country Team is supported by a core team at OGAC headquarters. Often, an ambassadorial steering committee works with the in-country team and the minister of health on HIV/AIDS efforts (in some countries this committee also serves as the Country Coordinating Mechanism for the Global Fund) (OGAC, 2005a).

Funding

The Leadership Act authorized $15 billion, including about $10 billion in new resources, for efforts to combat global HIV/AIDS. The majority of the funding is intended to be concentrated in the 15 focus countries.

TABLE 2-5 Structure for Coordination and Support Within the Office of the U.S. Global AIDS Coordinator

Group	Responsibility	Involved Agencies
Ambassador	*Leadership of Initiative* • Ensure policy and program coordination at the highest levels • Holds strong mandate for accountability	U.S. Global AIDS Coordinator, Ambassadors
Agency Principals	*Policy*	Office of the U.S. Global AIDS Coordinator, U.S. Agency for International Development, Department of Health and Human Services, National Security Council, White House
Deputy Principals	*Management/Programs* • Addresses how to operationalize programs • Can move policy issues up to agency principals	Office of the U.S. Global AIDS Coordinator, U.S. Agency for International Development, Department of Health and Human Services, Peace Corps, Department of Defense, Department of Labor
Scientific Steering Committee	*Scientific Integrity* • Assesses evidence base for policies and programs • Can be involved in evaluation and monitoring	Office of the U.S. Global AIDS Coordinator, U.S. Agency for International Development, National Institutes of Health, Department of Health and Human Services, Department of Defense
Core Teams	*General Field Support* • Channels information • Addresses problems • Leverages technical support as needed by the field	Office of the U.S. Global AIDS Coordinator, U.S. Agency for International Development, Department of Health and Human Services, Peace Corps, Department of Defense, Department of State
Technical Working Groups	*Technical Assistance and Review to Support the Field* • Addresses specific program components (e.g., care, prevention, food, orphans and vulnerable children)	Office of the U.S. Global AIDS Coordinator, U.S. Agency for International Development, Department of Health and Human Services, Peace Corps, Department of Defense, National Institutes of Health, U.S. Department of Agriculture

SOURCE: Moloney-Kitts, 2005.

PEPFAR funds are appropriated through several agencies, with the bulk of the funding appropriated through the State Department's Global HIV/AIDS Initiative account. Foreign operations (such as the Peace Corps) are funded by the Global HIV/AIDS Initiative account, but are not generally under the PEPFAR umbrella.

As noted, the Leadership Act directs most PEPFAR funding to the focus countries. The roughly $10 billion that is intended for the focus countries is directed primarily either centrally from OGAC or locally from the Country Teams, with a 7 percent cap for OGAC and the Country Teams for operating costs (P.L. 108-25). Most focus country funding comes from the State Department's Global HIV/AIDS Initiative account. Funding concentrated in the focus countries in the first 3 years totaled over $3.4 billion (see Table 2-2). This total includes funding to the Country Teams, centrally funded programs, strategic information activities, and technical management and oversight funding for the U.S. agencies involved in the program's implementation. As the program scaled up, the annual funding directed to the focus countries increased from $470 million in fiscal year 2004 to more than $1.6 billion in fiscal year 2006. The remaining $5 billion is intended for other bilateral activities, including the Global Fund and activities in non-focus countries. Chapter 3 provides greater detail about PEPFAR funding.

REFERENCES

Abu-Raddad, L. J., P. Patnaik, and J. Kublin. 2006. Dual infection with HIV and malaria fuels the spread of both diseases in sub-Saharan Africa. *Science* 314:1603–1606.

Africa Renewal (formerly Africa Recovery). 1999 (December). *AIDS saps Africa's educational system.* http://www.un.org/ecosocdev/geninfo/afrec/ (accessed January 3, 2007).

Africa Renewal (formerly Africa Recovery). 2007. Education in Africa: Africa Recovery special report. *Schools struggling with crises: Financial constraints hamper expansion of primary education in Africa.* http://www.un.org/ecosocdev/geninfo/afrec/ (accessed January 3, 2007).

Askew, I., and M. Berer. 2003. The contribution of sexual and reproductive health services to the fight against HIV/AIDS: A review. *Reproductive Health Matters* 11(22):51–73.

Bertozzi, S., P. Padian, J. Wegbreit, L. M. DeMaria, B. Feldman, H. Gayle, J. Gold, R. Grant, and M. T. Isbell. 2006. HIV/AIDS prevention and treatment. In *Disease control priorities in developing countries.* 2nd ed., edited by D. T. Jamison, J. G. Breman, A. R. Measham, G. Alleyne, M. Claeson, D. B. Evans, P. Jha, A. Mills, and P. Musgrove. New York and Washington, DC: Oxford University Press and World Bank.

Bollinger, L., K. Cooper-Arnold, and J. Stover. 2004. Where are the gaps? The effect of HIV-prevention interventions on behavior change. *Studies in Family Planning* 35(1):27–38.

Castro, A., and P. Farmer. 2005. Understanding and addressing AIDS-related stigma: From anthropological theory to clinical practice in Haiti. *American Journal of Public Health* 95(1):53–59.

CIA (Central Intelligence Agency). 2006. *CIA World Factbook.* http://www.cia.gov/cia/publications/factbook/index.html (accessed June 10, 2006).

CSIS (Center for Strategic and International Studies). 2005. *More than humanitarianism: A strategic U.S. approach toward Africa.* Washington, DC: CSIS.

Dybul, M. 2005 (April 21). *Remarks at the second meeting of the Institute of Medicine Committee for the Evaluation of PEPFAR Implementation, Washington, DC.*

Evans, R., M. Barer., and T. Marmor. 1994. *Why are some people healthy and others not? The determinants of health populations.* New York: Aldine de Gruyter.

GIST (Global Implementation Support Team). 2006. *Fact sheet: The Global Implementation Support Team: Coordinating UN action and provision of technical support for accelerating HIV/AIDS responses in countries.* http://data.unaids.org/pub/BrochurePamphlet/2006/2006_gist_en.pdf (accessed January 12, 2007).

Global Fund. 2005. *Global Fund ARV fact sheet: 1st December, 2005.* Geneva, Switzerland: Global Fund. http://www.theglobalfund.org/en/files/publications/factsheets/aids/ARV_Factsheet_2006.pdf (accessed November 3, 2006).

Global Fund. 2006. *Distribution of funding after 5 rounds.* Geneva, Switzerland: Global Fund. http://www.theglobalfund.org/en/funds%5Fraised/distribution/ (accessed November 3, 2006).

Grassly, N., G. Garnett, B. Schwartlander, S. Gregson, and R. Anderson. 2001. The effectiveness of HIV prevention and the epidemiological context. *Bulletin of the World Health Organization* 79:1121–1132.

IOM (Institute of Medicine). 2005. *Scaling up treatment for the global AIDS pandemic: Challenges and opportunities.* Washington, DC: The National Academies Press.

Johns Hopkins School of Public Health. 2000. *Population reports: Series A, number 9 oral contraceptives.* Baltimore, MD: Johns Hopkins University. http://www.infoforhealth.org/pr/a9/a9chap5_3.shtml (accessed January 31, 2007).

Kates, J., and E. Lief. 2006. *International assistance for HIV/AIDS in the developing world: Taking stock of the G8, other donor governments and the European Commission.* Washington, DC: Kaiser Family Foundation.

Kaye, G., and T. Wolff. 2002. *From the ground up! A workbook on coalition building and community development.* Amherst, MA: AHEC/Community Partners.

Kindig, D. 1997. *Purchasing population health: Paying for results.* Ann Arbor, MI: University of Michigan Press.

Letamo, G. 2003. Prevalence of, and factors associated with, HIV/AIDS-related stigma and discriminatory attitudes in Botswana. *Journal of Health, Population, and Nutrition* 21(4):347–357.

Lyman, P. 2005. *Remarks at the second meeting of the Institute of Medicine Committee for the Evaluation of PEPFAR Implementation, Washington, DC.*

Moloney-Kitts, M. 2005 (April 19). *Office of the Global AIDS Coordinator.* Presentation at the second meeting of the Institute of Medicine Committee for the Evaluation of PEPFAR Implementation, Washington, DC.

Myer, L., L. Denny, R. Telerant, M. Souza, T. C. Wright, Jr., and L. Kuhn. 2005. Bacterial vaginosis and susceptibility to HIV infection in South African women: A nested case-control study. *The Journal of Infectious Diseases* 192(8):1372–1380.

NAS (National Academy of Sciences). 1994. Population migration and the spread of types 1 and 2 human immunodeficiency viruses. *Proceedings of the National Academy of Sciences (USA)* 91(7):2407–2414.

National Bureau of Statistics Dar es Salaam, Tanzania and Macro International, Inc. 2000. *Tanzania 1999 reproductive and child health survey.* Calverton, MD: Macro International, Inc.

Newman, P., O. Grusky, S. J. Roberts, and I. Rivkin. 2002. *Organizational factors in the early detection of HIV.* Presentation provided at the XIV International AIDS Conference, Barcelona, Spain.

NIAID/NIH (National Institute of Allergy and Infectious Diseases/National Institutes of Health). 2006. *HIV infection in women.* Rockville, MD: NIAID/NIH. http://www.niaid.nih.gov/factsheets/womenhiv.htm (accessed January 12, 2007).

NWHRC (National Women's Health Resource Center). 2006. *National women's health report: Women & HIV.* Red Bank, NJ: NWHRC.

OGAC (Office of the U.S. Global AIDS Coordinator). 2004. *The President's Emergency Plan for AIDS Relief: U.S. five-year global HIV/AIDS strategy.* Washington, DC: OGAC.

OGAC. 2005a. *The President's Emergency Plan for AIDS Relief: Compassionate action provides hope through treatment success.* Washington, DC: OGAC.

OGAC. 2005b. *PEPFAR first annual report to Congress.* Washington, DC: OGAC.

OGAC. 2005c. *The President's Emergency Plan for AIDS Relief: Indicators, reporting requirements, and guidelines for focus countries* (revised for FY2006 reporting). Washington, DC: OGAC.

OGAC. 2006a. *PEPFAR second annual report to Congress.* Washington, DC: OGAC.

OGAC. 2006b. *PEPFAR report on food and nutrition for people living with HIV/AIDS.* Washington, DC: OGAC.

OGAC. 2006c. *PEPFAR report on work force capacity and HIV/AIDS.* Washington, DC: OGAC.

OGAC. 2006d. *Bringing hope: Supplying antiretroviral drugs for HIV/AIDS treatment: The President's Emergency Plan for AIDS Relief report on antiretroviral drugs for HIV/AIDS treatment.* Washington, DC: OGAC.

OGAC. 2006e. *Report on education: The President's Emergency Plan for AIDS Relief.* Washington, DC: OGAC.

OGAC. 2006f. *Report on refugees and internally displaced persons: The President's Emergency Plan for AIDS Relief.* Washington, DC: OGAC.

OGAC. 2006g. *HIV/AIDS palliative care guidance #1: An overview of comprehensive HIV/AIDS care services in the President's Emergency Plan for AIDS Relief.* Washington, DC: OGAC.

OGAC. 2007a. Office of the Global AIDS Coordinator's Suggested Factual Changes to the PEPFAR Implementation: Progress and Promise Report. Email communication to IOM staff on March 29, 2007.

OGAC. 2007b. *PEPFAR third annual report to Congress.* Washington, DC: OGAC.

OECD (Organisation for Economic Co-operation and Development). 2003. *Harmonising donor practices for effective aid delivery good practice papers: A DAC reference document.* Paris, France: OECD.

OECD. 2006. *Aid activities: CRS user's guide: Basic concepts—official development assistance, official aid.* http://www.oecd.org/document/28/0,2340,en_2649_34469_15070940_1_1_1_1,00.html (accessed November 1, 2006).

PRB (Population Reference Bureau). 2005. *2005 world population data sheet.* Washington, DC: PRB. http://www.prb.org/pdf05/05WorldDataSheet_Eng.pdf (accessed May 25, 2006).

Project Siyam'kela. 2003. *Siyam'kela: A report on the fieldwork leading to the development of HIV/AIDS stigma indicators and guidelines.* http://www.poplicyproject.com/siyamkela.cfm (accessed November 1, 2006).

Quinn, T. C. 1996. Global burden of the HIV pandemic. *The Lancet* 348:99–106.

Quinn, T. C. 2001. *AIDS in Africa: A retrospective.* Bulletin of the World Health Organization. Geneva, Switzerland: World Health Organization.

Quinn, T. C., A. Ruff, and N. Halsey. 1994. Special considerations for developing nations. In *Pediatric AIDS: The challenge of HIV infection in infants, children, and adolescents.* Edited by P. A. Pizzo and C. M. Wilfert. Baltimore, MD: Williams & Wilkins. Pp. 31–49.

Rice, S. 2006. *Global poverty, weak states and insecurity; The Brookings Blum Roundtable.* Washington, DC: The Brookings Institution.

Schwebke, J. R. 2005. Abnormal vaginal flora as a biological risk factor for acquisition of HIV infection and sexually transmitted diseases. *The Journal of Infectious Diseases* 192(8):1315–1317.

The Rome Declaration on harmonization. 2003. High level forum on harmonization, February 24–25, 2003, Rome, Italy. http://www.aidharmonization.org (accessed November 10, 2006).

UN (United Nations). 2003a. *Monterrey Consensus of the International Conference on Financing for Development: The final text of agreements and commitments adopted at the International Conference on Financing for Development, Monterrey, Mexico, 18–22 March 2002.* Geneva, Switzerland: UN.

UN. 2003b. *Organizing the UN response to the triple threat of food insecurity, weakened capacity for governance and AIDS, particularly in southern and eastern Africa. Document discussed at the UN High-Level Committee on Programmes, 6th session, Rome, Italy, 18–19 September 2003.* Geneva, Switzerland: UN.

UNAIDS (Joint United Nations Programme on HIV/AIDS). 1998. *UNAIDS best practice collection: Guide to the strategic planning process for a national response to HIV/AIDS, modules 1–4.* Geneva, Switzerland: UNAIDS.

UNAIDS. 2001. *The global strategy framework on HIV/AIDS.* Geneva, Switzerland: UNAIDS.

UNAIDS. 2003 (April 29). *Unified budget and workplan 2004–2005, UNAIDS/PCB(14)/03.3.* Geneva, Switzerland: UNAIDS.

UNAIDS. 2004a. *"Three ones" key principles.* Conference paper 1, Washington consultation of April 4, 2004. Geneva, Switzerland: UNAIDS. http://www.unaids.org/NetTools/Misc/DocInfo.aspx?LANG=en&href=http://gva-doc-owl/WEBcontent/Documents/pub/UNA-docs/Three-Ones_KeyPrinciples_en.pdf (accessed September 20, 2006).

UNAIDS. 2004b. *Clearing the common ground for the "three ones": Report of a consultation process.* Conference paper 2, Washington consultation of April 25, 2004. Geneva Switzerland: UNAIDS. http://data.unaids.org/UNA-docs/Three-Ones_ConsultationReport_en.pdf (accessed September 20, 2006).

UNAIDS. 2005a. *Global task team on improving AIDS coordination among multilateral institutions and international donors.* Geneva, Switzerland: UNAIDS.

UNAIDS. 2005b. *Resource needs for an expanded response to AIDS in low- and middle-income countries.* Geneva, Switzerland: UNAIDS.

UNAIDS. 2005c (June 27–29). *Unified budget and workplan 2006–2007, UNAIDS/PCB(17)/05.4.* Geneva, Switzerland: UNAIDS.

UNAIDS. 2005d. *The "three ones" in action: Where we are and where we go from here.* Geneva, Switzerland: UNAIDS.

UNAIDS. 2006. *2006 report on the global AIDS epidemic.* Geneva, Switzerland: UNAIDS.

UNAIDS. 2007. *About UNAIDS.* Geneva, Switzerland: UNAIDS. http://www.unaids.org (accessed January 10, 2007).

UNAIDS, UNICEF, USAID (Joint United Nations Programme on HIV/AIDS, United Nations Children's Fund, U.S. Agency for International Development). 2002. *Children on the brink: A joint report on orphan estimates and program strategies.* Washington, DC: TVT Associates.

UNAIDS, UNICEF, USAID. 2004. *Children on the brink: A joint report on new orphans estimates and a framework for action.* New York: UNICEF.

UNDP (United Nations Development Programme). 2005. *Human development report 2005.* http://hdr.undp.org/reports/global/2005/pdf/HDR05_complete.pdf (accessed May 25, 2006).

UNICEF (United Nations Children's Fund). 2006a. *Information by country (Côte d'Ivoire, Ethiopia, Haiti, Kenya, Mozambique, Nigeria, Rwanda, South Africa, Tanzania, Uganda, Vietnam, and Zambia).* http://www.unicef.com (accessed June 10, 2006).

UNICEF. 2006b. *Africa's orphaned and vulnerable generations: Children affected by AIDS.* New York: UNICEF.

U.S. DOS (U.S. Department of State). 2006. *Office of the Global AIDS Coordinator: Focus countries.* Washington, DC: U.S. DOS. http://www.state.gov/s/gac/countries/fc/index.htm (accessed May 25, 2006).

USAID (U.S. Agency for International Development). 2005. *Working report: Measuring HIV stigma: Results of a field test in Tanzania.* Washington, DC: USAID.

Weiss, M. G., and J. Ramakrishna. 2001. Conference examines need for more study of AIDS stigma. *AIDS Policy Law* 16(18):4.

WHO (World Health Organization). 2002a. *Perth framework for age-friendly community-based primary health care.* http://www.who.int/ageing/projects/perth/en/ (accessed January 13, 2007).

WHO. 2002b. *Blood safety: Aide-memoire for national blood programmes.* Geneva, Switzerland: WHO.

WHO. 2006a. *Fact sheet: Progress in scaling up access to HIV treatment in low- and middle-income countries.* Geneva, Switzerland: WHO.

WHO. 2006b. *WHO global health atlas.* http://www.who.int/globalatlas/DataQuery/default.asp (accessed August 1, 2006).

World Bank. 2006. *2006 world development indicators.* Washington, DC: World Bank. http://devdata.worldbank.org/wdi2006/contents/index2.htm (accessed November 1, 2006).

Part II

Progress on the First 5-Year Strategy—PEPFAR

3

PEPFAR's Management

Summary of Key Findings

- The Office of the U.S. Global AIDS Coordinator (OGAC) is committed to learning by doing and contributing to the evidence base for how to combat global HIV/AIDS most effectively. PEPFAR's virtual organization, composed of OGAC, numerous other implementing agencies, and the Country Teams, has demonstrated an increasing capacity for responding to and sharing knowledge acquired over the course of the program's implementation.
- PEPFAR's accomplishments include the ongoing development, revision, and dissemination of program policies and procedures, as well as dissemination of evidence on how to provide and scale up quality services to those affected by HIV/AIDS in resource-constrained settings. Mechanisms for planning and reporting, coordination, and knowledge sharing at all levels have also been developed. Going forward, OGAC needs to increase its emphasis on operations research and develop an overall plan for the collection and management of strategic information.
- PEPFAR policies demonstrate a commitment to supporting host countries' leadership and ownership of their responses to their HIV/AIDS epidemics. Country Teams have endeavored to work closely with host country governments and coordinating bodies, as well as other donors, to carry out PEPFAR activities within the framework of harmonization. PEPFAR has been increasingly successful in this regard, but concerns about the transparency of the planning process remain. Moreover, congressional budget allocations have created a substantial administrative burden, hampering harmonization and requiring that considerable local effort be expended on new planning, budgeting, and reporting mechanisms.
- PEPFAR's initial decision to jump-start the program by relying heavily on central programming and using experienced nongovernmental organizations for implementation has had mixed results. Although some of the disadvantages of this approach are still evident, OGAC has shifted greater control of centrally funded grants to Country Teams to facilitate integration of these activities within the larger PEPFAR portfolios in the focus countries.
- PEPFAR and other donors plan to rely on national data from the focus countries to determine the program's impact in the long term. Thus, strong support for creating, implementing, and strengthening a unified and coherent monitoring and evaluation system at the country level continues to be critical.

Recommendations Discussed in This Chapter

Recommendation 3-1: To support country leadership, the U.S. Global AIDS Coordinator should seek to identify and remove barriers to coordination with partner governments and other donors, with a particular focus on promoting transparency and participation throughout the annual planning process.

Recommendation 3-2: *The commitment of the U.S. Global AIDS Initiative to work toward reducing stigma and discrimination against people living with HIV/AIDS requires that marginalized and difficult-to-reach groups receive prevention, treatment, and care services. These groups include sex workers, prisoners, those who use injecting drugs, and men who have sex with men—groups that not only are characterized by their high-risk behavior, but also tend to be stigmatized and subject to discrimination.* The U.S. Global AIDS Coordinator should document how these groups are included in the program planning, implementation, and evaluation of PEPFAR activities.

Recommendation 3-3: *Although they may have been helpful initially in ensuring a balance of attention to activities within the four categories of prevention, treatment, care, and orphans and vulnerable children, the Committee concludes that rigid congressional budget allocations among categories, and even more so within categories, have also limited PEPFAR's ability to tailor its activities in each country to the local epidemic and to coordinate with the level of activities in the countries' national plans.* Congress should remove the budget allocations and replace them with more appropriate mechanisms that ensure accountability for results from Country Teams to the U.S. Global AIDS Coordinator and to Congress. These mechanisms should also ensure that spending is directly linked to and commensurate with necessary efforts to achieve both country and overall performance targets for prevention, treatment, care, and orphans and other vulnerable children.

3

PEPFAR's Management

The Office of the U.S. Global AIDS Coordinator (OGAC) has created a virtual organization that, as mandated by the Leadership Act, coordinates among many different entities both within and outside of the U.S. government and between the central and country levels. In contrast to recent reorganizations of other government entities, OGAC has deliberately been kept small, with use being made of temporary assignments and coordinating bodies rather than a large, entirely new structure being created. This chapter reviews key aspects of the management of this virtual organization: (1) coordination, (2) harmonization, (3) policy guidance, (4) planning and reporting, (5) technical working groups, (6) functioning as a learning organization, (7) budget allocations, (8) targets, and (9) resource allocation.

COORDINATION

This section reviews coordination among the U.S. implementing agencies under the auspices of OGAC both at the headquarters and country levels, between OGAC and other international HIV/AIDS donors, and between OGAC and the U.S. teams working in the focus countries (Country Teams). Coordination of the Country Teams with partner governments and other donors working at the country level is addressed in the next section in the discussion of the Second One of harmonization—One National HIV/AIDS Coordinating Authority.

The Leadership Act called for the newly established U.S. Global AIDS Coordinator (the Coordinator) to coordinate

- Programs and policies of designated executive branch agencies and nongovernmental organizations.
- Resolution of policy, program, and funding discrepancies among these organizations.
- Field activities of the designated executive branch agencies.
- Related assistance by other countries and international organizations.

The President's Emergency Plan for AIDS Relief (PEPFAR) strategy was to identify the existing capacity of the implementing agencies and harness and expand their comparative strengths into one synergistic U.S. government response coordinated by OGAC (OGAC, 2004).

Central Coordination: The Office of the U.S. Global AIDS Coordinator

Unification of all U.S. international HIV/AIDS activities and coordination of PEPFAR implementation are the responsibility of OGAC, a relatively small central office staffed largely by people detailed from the implementing agencies and supplemented by positions created and staffed on an as-needed basis. OGAC officials reported that the office has also relied heavily on numerous interagency coordinating committees, task forces, and working groups to address the challenge of bringing together the many disparate implementing agencies. To ensure coordination among participating agencies at the central headquarters level, OGAC created the Deputy Principals Group, which handles program management and logistics and includes high-level representation from all of the implementing agencies (see Chapter 2).

Interagency Coordination

The two principal implementing agencies—the U.S. Agency for International Development (USAID) and the Centers for Disease Control and Prevention (CDC)—have different systems and structures for operating, different established budget cycles, and even different salary scales.[1] For purposes of PEPFAR, all agencies are expected to collaborate in program funding that was previously managed separately by each agency. Prior to PEPFAR, USAID and CDC had limited funds available to prepare for scale-up of antiretroviral therapy (ART). USAID's HIV/AIDS programs had

[1]Some CDC employees are part of the Public Health Service Corps; this option is not available in USAID.

previously been focused primarily on prevention, including prevention of mother-to-child transmission. CDC's HIV/AIDS programs also provided support for prevention of mother-to-child transmission. CDC staff worked with ministries of health in various technical areas, such as surveillance, and on the development of national AIDS plans.

OGAC and agency officials believe that previous joint monitoring and evaluation activities provided a foundation for improving collaboration between CDC and USAID. The agencies had engaged in an ongoing coordination process that included agency visits, biweekly conference calls, quarterly meetings, review of agency-specific guidance, and cosigned letters of concurrence on major issues (Rugg et al., 2004). The agencies had also jointly organized and conducted monitoring and evaluation workshops and training courses and collaborated to develop core indicators. In addition, they had been collaborating on monitoring and evaluation with global partners, such as UNAIDS, the World Health Organization (WHO), the United Nations Children's Fund (UNICEF), the World Bank, and the Global Fund to Fight AIDS, Tuberculosis and Malaria (Global Fund). The people involved reported that this foundation for interagency collaboration on monitoring and evaluation did not develop easily and required significant ongoing effort, as well as "setting realistic expectations and seeing a balance between what is contributed and what is gained from the partnership" (Rugg et al., 2004, p. 74).

All donors, large and small, are attempting to improve their coordination with one another so as to minimize the transactional burden—the difficulties governments experience in handling the demands of multiple donors, such as attendance at meetings and reporting requirements—associated with the influx of large amounts of funding in the focus countries (UNAIDS, 2005b; Shakow, 2006). Considerable evidence shows that uncoordinated donor actions can result in pressures on country systems that weaken, rather than strengthen, the partner government's ability to manage its own programs (OECD, 2003; The Rome Declaration, 2003; UNAIDS, 2005a,b).

As the largest single bilateral donor, PEPFAR can lead the way in furthering such efforts. Effective coordination will mean that both U.S. dollars and money from other donors will be spent effectively, minimizing the potential for waste arising from poorly coordinated independent funding streams.

Field Coordination: The Country Teams

In the focus countries, PEPFAR Country Teams are coordinated through the U.S. embassy and thus led by the U.S. ambassador. All agencies working in a country on HIV/AIDS—such as the Department of Defense, the Peace Corps, the National Institutes of Health, USAID, and CDC—are part of the

Country Team, and each team has a designated leader (OGAC, 2004). The typical coordinating mechanism is a regular meeting chaired by the ambassador or his/her most senior staff member. OGAC intends this structure to ensure coordination among all agencies, and to provide a single voice speaking for the entire Country Team in interactions with partner governments and other donors.

In its visits to the focus countries, the Committee observed that Country Teams were generally collaborating effectively, although a few examples of rivalry and poor communication persist. In addition, further efforts could be made to coordinate planning and contracting cycles and requirements among the implementing agencies, particularly CDC and USAID. The Committee was told that timing discrepancies between agencies had in some cases resulted in funding gaps and resource shortages; that confusion existed around the management of certain programs, resulting in a lack of clear accountability for those programs; and that coordination at the country level continued to be complicated by the presence of numerous, large, centrally-managed contractors.

Coordination Among International Donors

OGAC recently (January 2006) met with representatives from the Global Fund and the World Bank to discuss program implementation and ways of improving donor coordination (OGAC et al., 2006). The three partners have agreed to work together, particularly on coordinating procurement, organizing annual implementation reviews, improving communication, and supporting country strategies and action plans. The role of donors in the country planning process is addressed below in the discussion of the First One of harmonization—One HIV/AIDS Action Framework.

Communications

Communication is a central element of PEPFAR's coordination strategy. OGAC has worked to develop a number of mechanisms for communicating not only across agencies, but also between Country Teams and central staff (OGAC, 2004, 2005a, 2006a).

According to OGAC, weekly teleconferences are held between each Country Team and the Washington-based interagency core team, which includes a coordinator within OGAC. The core team is expected to be aware of both OGAC policy and country programs so it can support the Country Teams in a variety of ways, from program management to identification of areas in which technical assistance may be needed (Moloney-Kitts, 2005) (see the discussion of Technical Working Groups later in the chapter).

To enhance communication, the PEPFAR Extranet was created in 2006.

Currently limited to internal use, the Extranet offers access to archived *News to the Field* weekly newsletters, public affairs/public diplomacy resources, PEPFAR policies and guidance, presentations, budget figures and country data, and U.S. agency directories. Additionally, the Extranet is intended to give Country Teams the opportunity to collaborate and share information with their colleagues around the world. Available information includes lessons learned, best practices, national polices and guidelines, technical articles, presentations, and resources such as curricula and toolkits.

According to OGAC, the primary reason the Extranet was created was to help manage the volume of information needed to run a program as technically complex as PEPFAR and make this information available to those overseeing the program's implementation in the field. OGAC plans to allow implementing partners outside of the U.S. government access to the Extranet at some point in the near future; implementing partners have told the Committee that they eagerly await this change.

HARMONIZATION

PEPFAR, along with all other major donors, is committed to supporting the focus countries' ownership of their response to their AIDS epidemics. Country Teams work closely with partner governments, as well as other donors, to implement harmonized HIV/AIDS plans (OGAC, 2005a, 2006a,b,c). To this end, PEPFAR has committed to implementing its program within the Three Ones framework of harmonization agreed upon at a meeting with the United Kingdom and UNAIDS in April 2004: One agreed HIV/AIDS Action Framework, One National AIDS Coordinating Authority, and One agreed country-level Monitoring and Evaluation System (see Chapter 2) (UNAIDS, 2004a; OGAC, 2005b).

First One: One Action Framework

All of the focus countries have a national strategic plan to fight AIDS; most also have a national operational plan. The latter plans vary widely in detail and quality, particularly with regard to the specific steps to be taken and the associated costs. Responding to a call by UNAIDS, PEPFAR and other major donors are currently working with the host countries to help develop operational plans that are costed, evidence-based, and prioritized, and thus will provide the specificity necessary for funding and program development purposes for both the country itself and all donors (UNAIDS, 2004a; OGAC, 2005b).

OGAC has directed Country Teams to develop both a U.S. 5-year strategic country plan and an annual Country Operational Plan that are harmonized with the existing plans of the focus countries (OGAC, 2004,

2005d, 2006b,c,f). The U.S. plans are expected to reflect the priorities and interests of the partner government, as well as to identify strategic information, activities, and priorities for the coming year (OGAC, 2006a).

During the Committee's country visits, representatives of partner governments generally expressed their satisfaction with the level of harmonization achieved. To complement these reports, the Committee reviewed PEPFAR's annual Country Operational Plans against the plans of the focus countries and found them to be generally congruent. In most cases, however, the Committee was able to compare only the highly specific PEPFAR Country Operational Plans for fiscal years 2005 and 2006 with the much more general national strategic plans. Because the national strategic plans typically are not prioritized, the Committee could not determine how well PEPFAR support is aligned with national priorities. In most cases, for example, it is not possible to determine how PEPFAR allocations by the categories of prevention, treatment, care, and orphans and other vulnerable children compare with proposed national spending.

During its country visits, the Committee also heard reports of disharmony arising from constraints imposed by U.S. laws that prohibit or appear to prohibit or restrict the use of some of the means of prevention that are viewed by those in the field as important and potentially successful. These include restrictions on teaching young teens about the full scope of HIV prevention methods, the Leadership Act requirement for organizations to certify that they have a "policy explicitly opposing prostitution and sex trafficking" (P.L. 108-25, p. 734) in order to receive funding, and the prohibition against support for clean needles to combat the spread of HIV among people who use injection drugs. The Committee was told of examples of innovative programs that PEPFAR was unable to support, such as those that integrate messages about HIV prevention into traditional teaching at the time of sexual initiation, those organized by sex workers to conduct peer counseling, and those that provide clean needles in communities where injecting drug use is a major source of spread of HIV infection.

By far the most often-cited obstacle to harmonization, however, is the requirement that U.S. funds be used only for medications that have received approval from the U.S. Food and Drug Administration. Country Teams, host country officials, and implementing partners all agreed that, although workaround arrangements had been developed to deal with this requirement, such arrangements were awkward, costly, and difficult to administer, reducing the ability of PEPFAR and the host countries to use funds in the most cost-effective manner possible. This issue and the Committee's related recommendation are discussed in greater detail in Chapter 5 in the overall context of treatment.

Coordination is also crucial to the development of a unified action framework. As noted earlier, failure of bilateral donors to coordinate with one another can lead to duplication and conflict in the delivery of needed services (OECD, 2003; The Rome Declaration, 2003; UNAIDS, 2005a,b). A number of countries have more or less formal donor groups that enable donors to speak to the government, to the extent possible, with a single voice. OGAC officials stressed that a significant amount of time is dedicated to working with other international donors, and the Country Teams confirmed this. Of particular importance is for all donors to know what the others are planning so they can ensure that their money is being spent in the most effective way, whether or not they participate in basket funding. Full transparency of U.S. plans is therefore particularly important.

One complaint voiced by both donors and Country Teams during the Committee's visits was that because the Country Operational Plans are procurement sensitive, they cannot be fully shared with other donors. The Country Teams share the Country Operational Plans with the partner governments before completion, and are required to obtain approval from the partner governments before submitting the plans to OGAC (OGAC, 2006c). Subsequent to the Committee's visits, OGAC made nonsensitive versions of the Country Operational Plans available on the PEPFAR website, and OGAC officials reported that they have taken additional steps to encourage Country Teams to share as much information as appropriate with their counterparts from other donors working in a country. However, the Committee was unable to confirm with other donors at the country level whether the situation has improved in their view. Since the preparation of the Country Operational Plans is such a prominent part of the Country Teams' work, the inability to disclose their content to other donors represents an impediment to harmonization; resolution of any remaining issues would therefore be an important improvement.

Recommendation 3-1: To support country leadership, the U.S. Global AIDS Coordinator should seek to identify and remove barriers to coordination with partner governments and other donors, with a particular focus on promoting transparency and participation throughout the annual planning process.

Second One: One National Coordination Authority

The Second One essentially challenges each country to create a single coordinating authority to develop, implement, and monitor its plans for supporting its response to its HIV/AIDS epidemic, and calls for donors to participate in that authority (UNAIDS, 2004a). Unfortunately, the Global Fund's required Country Coordinating Mechanisms were not fully congruent with the existing National HIV/AIDS Coordinating Authorities already in place in most countries (UNAIDS, 2005a). Although some countries have successfully combined the two, in many cases there are still two coordinating bodies, sometimes with conflicting and confusing mandates. Recent work by the Global Fund and the World Bank promises to help ameliorate this problem (OGAC et al., 2006; Shakow, 2006).

National HIV/AIDS Coordinating Authorities vary in their capacity to oversee the approach to the epidemic; an important donor task is to continue supporting and strengthening these bodies. As one step to that end, OGAC encourages Country Teams to sign a memorandum of understanding with the Global Fund so the PEPFAR planning process can be fully integrated under the Country Coordinating Mechanism. The Committee was told of some successful early examples of this arrangement already in place.

During its visits to the focus countries, the Committee was told by all parties involved—partner governments, Country Teams, and other donors—that they recognize the importance of a unified, country-led coordinating authority but find this challenging to achieve. The Committee heard some concern expressed, particularly by other donors, about PEPFAR's domination of the agenda by virtue of its large size. Overall, however, the view from the focus countries of PEPFAR's support of and participation in the Second One was largely positive.

Third One: One National Monitoring and Evaluation System

The importance of creating, implementing, and strengthening a single, unified, and coherent monitoring and evaluation system at the country level cannot be overemphasized (UNAIDS, 2004a; OGAC, 2005b). A strong unified monitoring and evaluation system ensures that (1) relevant, timely, and accurate data are made available to program leaders and managers at each level of the program and health care system; (2) selected quality data can be reported to national program leaders; and (3) the national program is able to meet donor and international reporting requirements under a unified global effort to contain the HIV/AIDS pandemic (UNAIDS, 2004b).

In its first year, PEPFAR proceeded simultaneously with program implementation and the development of monitoring and evaluation systems. Since then, PEPFAR has worked with countries to develop and strengthen monitoring and evaluation plans and systems. PEPFAR, like other donors, is largely dependent on a country's capacity to provide the data needed for monitoring and evaluation of its own programs. Thus, PEPFAR's own monitoring and evaluation capabilities are improved by its support for the building of local capacity to collect, synthesize, and disseminate information on the HIV/AIDS programs in the host countries through technical assistance, the development of health management information systems, efforts to improve data standards, and training of personnel at all levels of the health system (OGAC, 2005a, 2006a).

During its visits, the Committee found that at the country level, there is agreement with the Third One in principle, but there is frustration with the lack of progress toward achieving the aim of a single monitoring and evaluation system. A major difficulty cited by many was that of conducting joint planning for the collection of data needed immediately while concurrently building the necessary infrastructure. PEPFAR's need to collect U.S.-specific information to report to Congress is another cited barrier to the Third One. PEPFAR's monitoring and evaluation requirements and how they compare with those of other global donors are discussed in Chapter 8.

OGAC reported that it is currently developing guidelines for building an intermediate information system that can become part of a larger national system designed to facilitate data flow and communication. Recently, OGAC participated in global monitoring and evaluation training in collaboration with the Global Fund and WHO (OGAC, 2005d, 2006f). Despite these efforts, however, achievement of the Third One is far from a reality and will require continued support from and effort by PEPFAR and other donor programs.

Challenges of Harmonization

Harmonization does not mean simply passively accepting policies developed by partner governments. In the developing world, governments are dependent on a variety of sources for the formulation of scientific policy: faculty of their own universities; resident technical advisors funded by donors; and short-term consultants and the permanent staff of donors, both bilateral and multilateral. Outside advisors who reside in the country, speak the local language, and understand local politics are particularly valuable to government experts (UNAIDS, 2004a). The United States has the advantage of maintaining a relatively large and highly skilled staff in the countries; these individuals are often actively involved in supporting, and at times urging, efforts by the partner government to incorporate in their plans new scientific advances and lessons learned in the field. In so doing, Country Teams need to be able to collaborate with other donors and the partner government in policy development, as well as to be patient when new technology is not adopted as quickly as might appear desirable. As a recent study conducted for the Gates Foundation notes, the country must take the lead in determining the "timing, pace and scale of new technology and policies" if their implementation is to be sustainable (McKinsey and Company, 2005, p. 1).

Another challenge to harmonization is the development of equitable programs that ensure access for the most vulnerable members of the population. The Joint United Nations Programme on HIV/AIDS (UNAIDS) recently published a document entitled *Considerations for Countries to Set Their Own Targets for AIDS Prevention, Treatment, and Care* (UNAIDS, 2006). The Global Steering Committee on Scaling Up Towards Universal Access recommended that national governments set a small number of their own targets in approaching universal access, rather than having UNAIDS or WHO attempt to establish global targets (UNAIDS et al., 2006). Among the principles recommended in the UNAIDS document are the following: "The movement to scale up towards universal access should address needs and rights in terms of health, nondiscrimination and gender equality"; and "The goal of moving towards universal access is only meaningful to the extent to which access is measured across different populations—ensuring that access to prevention, treatment and care is available for those least advantaged and socially marginalized" (UNAIDS, 2006, pp. 5–6).

In countries where certain marginalized groups are, in the view of donors, receiving insufficient attention in scale-up plans, PEPFAR and other donors may need to serve as advocates for those groups. Striking a balance between respecting local decisions and speaking effectively for those who do not have their own local voice is a core challenge to harmonization.

> **Recommendation 3-2:** ***The commitment of the U.S. Global AIDS Initiative to work toward reducing stigma and discrimination against people living with HIV/AIDS requires that marginalized and difficult-to-reach groups receive prevention, treatment, and care services. These groups include sex workers, prisoners, those who use injection drugs, and men who have sex with men—groups that not only are characterized by their high-risk behavior, but also tend to be stigmatized and subject to discrimination.*** **The U.S. Global AIDS Coordinator should document how these groups are included in the program planning, implementation, and evaluation of PEPFAR activities.**

POLICY GUIDANCE

Given the rapid implementation of PEPFAR and the formal process involved in developing official guidance documents, such documents for PEPFAR activities have been slow in coming. To date, OGAC has issued relatively few official policy documents; however, it has issued numerous less formal reports that provide information to guide program implementation. Nonetheless, during its country visits, the Committee heard that the lack of clear guidance in certain areas had caused many programs to self-censor and in some instances not to support particular services even though they are allowed. The absence of clear policy direction was confirmed by the fact that Country Teams in different countries sometimes described very different "official policy" under which they were working. For example, nutritional support in the early phase of treatment was variously described as encouraged, permitted but not encouraged, and prohibited. OGAC officials reported that they are working both to provide official guidance in a timelier manner and to continue to provide information in other forms to guide program implementation. The schedule of new materials coming from the Technical Working Groups supports this assertion.

PLANNING AND REPORTING

Country Operational Plans are used as planning tools for the Country Teams and allow for the aggregation of data across funding sources. They enable the consolidation of all relevant information, such as that related to budgeting, reporting, reviewing, and data analysis. The agencies that make up a Country Team are also required to work together to submit one strategic information plan as part of the Country Operational Plan (OGAC, 2006a).

OGAC officials described how a 2004 discussion between PEPFAR's central office and the Country Teams led to the development and implementation of a fully web-based system for developing and managing the Country Operational Plans—the Country Operational Plan and Reporting System (COPRS). COPRS is also used for collecting and reporting information on the progress of PEPFAR—for example, progress toward the prevention, treatment, and care targets. To this end, it includes mechanisms for and warehouses data from semiannual and annual reports by the Country Teams. According to OGAC, COPRS was designed to allow the Country Teams to meet individual agency reporting requirements in addition to OGAC requirements.

OGAC and Country Teams informed the Committee that the process of developing and implementing the Country Operational Plans and managing COPRS strained the resources of the Country Teams, particularly in the first year. The process reportedly has improved over time, however, as the planning and reporting cycle has become more regular, the system has been streamlined and made more user-friendly, and the Country Teams have received more support and become more experienced.

At the same time, Country Teams and implementing partners described a number of remaining planning challenges. The fact that the Country Operational Plan planning cycle spans only 1 year makes it difficult for Country Teams to manage their own time and develop mid- and long-term programs. The 1-year planning cycle also takes time away from implementation and monitoring and evaluation efforts. The inability to make midcourse changes to programming decisions because of contractual obligations and the rigidity of plans makes it difficult to improve programs during the year. In response to these concerns, OGAC announced at its 2006 annual meeting that it was considering moving to a 2-year Country Operational Plan cycle beginning with fiscal year 2008.

TECHNICAL WORKING GROUPS

Interagency Technical Working Groups are PEPFAR's principal mechanism for providing technical support to Country Teams for the implementation of program activities (see Chapter 2). These groups, which include members from all agencies, both headquarters and Country Teams, are charged with drafting program guidance and making and implementing evidence-based recommendations regarding changes in current and future programming. The work of these groups is supplemented by consultations with outside experts, such as one on substance abuse and HIV/AIDS in 2005 and one on gender and HIV/AIDS in 2006. OGAC views the Technical Working Groups as an effective way to tap the scientific and technical resources of the U.S. government to ensure that guidance issued by PEPFAR is of the highest quality (OGAC, 2005a, 2006a–c). The development of indicators has been an important focus of the Technical Working Groups. According to OGAC, all PEPFAR programs, regardless of implementing agency, were reporting on the same indicators by June 2006.

A major charge to the Technical Working Groups is providing several types of technical assistance to the Country Teams, including program design and/or reviews, direct assistance to implementing partners, training sessions, and assistance with the development of Country Operational Plans (OGAC, 2006b,c). To support the development of the Country Operational Plans, the Technical Working Groups prepare Technical Considerations documents for their respective areas. These documents serve as sources of available evidence, as well as guides to the recommendations of global normative bodies, such as UNAIDS and WHO. They also include PEPFAR priorities for country-funded targeted evaluations (OGAC, 2006b,c). The Technical Working Groups are intended to support OGAC's goal of reducing duplicative and/or conflicting directives from different agencies by planning and providing technical assistance as a U.S. government–wide effort.

FUNCTIONING AS A LEARNING ORGANIZATION

Over the course of this study, the Committee observed a number of examples of OGAC's commitment to learning from experience and contributing to the evidence base on how to combat HIV/AIDS most effectively. This adaptability was necessary given the emergency nature of PEPFAR's response to the pandemic and its consequent lack of time to develop policies and procedures prior to program implementation.

Garvin defines a learning organization as ". . . skilled at creating, acquiring, and transferring knowledge, and at modifying its behavior to reflect new knowledge and insights" (Garvin, 2000, p. 11). This definition emphasizes a systematic, ongoing commitment to the strategic collection, communication, analysis, and use of knowledge gained through experience. In attempting to determine how well PEPFAR is functioning as a learning organization, the Committee looked for evidence of transparent structures and processes, the allocation of time and resources to support learning, and changes over time showing that the organization can learn from both its mistakes and its successes.

A number of examples of PEPFAR's willingness to learn and adapt have already been described. Further examples are presented below.

Research

When PEPFAR was initiated, the Country Teams perceived a "ban" on using PEPFAR funds other than those flowing through the National Institutes of Health for research (OGAC, 2004), and the Committee was told that this inhibited them from supporting even operations research that was an integral part of program implementation. Over time, however, OGAC has recognized the need to clarify the policy and to encourage Country Teams to support operations research. The intent of such research is both to evaluate currently funded programs and to develop information that can answer important questions about how best to respond to the pandemic (OGAC, 2006g).

OGAC is currently providing about $22 million for targeted evaluations, primarily in the focus countries (OGAC, 2005c, 2006d,e). These evaluations cover a wide range of topics related to the program categories of prevention, treatment, care, and orphans and other vulnerable children. OGAC recently published a PEPFAR strategy for targeted evaluation to ensure the best use of these funds, and a list of priorities for such evaluations was included among the materials distributed to support the development of fiscal year 2007 Country Operational Plans (OGAC, 2006b). The strategy lays out a process for the review and approval of targeted evaluations. OGAC intends this process to support the systematic collection of information, as well as a mechanism for sharing that information both across the PEPFAR program and with partners. Additional discussion of PEPFAR's targeted evaluations appears in Chapter 8.

Quality Improvement

One important element of learning by doing is the use of modern quality improvement techniques to permit practitioners to continuously measure and improve their work. USAID's Quality Assurance Project applies these techniques in developing countries and is now in its third 5-year funding phase (USAID, 2006b). The project's objectives are to "build capacity in countries to develop and sustain quality assurance and workforce improvement activities; assist countries to achieve demonstrable results in quality of care and outcomes; strengthen USAID programming under its Global Health Strategic Objective programs through quality assurance approaches, methods, and tools; carry out research to develop and test new quality assurance and workforce development approaches and methods; and provide leadership in the technical development of the quality improvement field and in advocacy of the essential goal of high quality of care worldwide" (USAID, 2006a, p. 1). PEPFAR is supporting these activities in several of the focus countries, including Rwanda, South Africa, Tanzania, and Uganda.

PEPFAR is also supporting the updating and dissemination of two HIV clinical care data management software programs that enhance the ability of practitioners to improve their results. CAREWare, originally developed by the Health Resources and Services Administration within the Department of Health and Human Services for use in the United States, promotes quality care by providing a customizable and confidential platform for entering, collecting, and reporting demographic, service, and clinical information. An international version has been developed and implemented with PEPFAR support in Uganda, Zambia, Kenya, Tanzania, and Nigeria, with plans for adoption in Vietnam and Thailand (USAID, 2006a). PEPFAR is also supporting some focus countries' use of the HIVQUAL software program, an HIV-specific data system designed to enhance quality improvement activities. HIVQUAL helps participants measure key quality indicators and use these measurements to benchmark and make progress toward objectives (USAID, 2006a). PEPFAR support for HIVQUAL, which was piloted in Thailand, has expanded to include Uganda, Nigeria, and Mozambique (USAID, 2006a).

PEPFAR's Annual Meetings as a Learning Model

PEPFAR's annual meetings have evolved to provide an opportunity for PEPFAR staff and implementing partners to discuss issues, exchange information on program and management successes and challenges, and share lessons learned. OGAC officials reported that at the first meeting, held in South Africa, there were approximately 100 invitees, including ambassadors, Country Team directors, and chargés d'affaires. The focus of the meeting, which took place less than 6 months after PEPFAR funding was available, was the management and structure of the new program. Topics discussed included policies, procedures, staffing issues, and the development of Country Operational Plans. OGAC officials said that based on the results of these discussions, they decided there was a need to open future meetings to partners so that PEPFAR policies could be as widely understood as possible.

The second PEPFAR annual meeting was held in Addis Ababa, Ethiopia, in 2005. The number of invitees increased to approximately 450, including U.S. implementing partners. The press and representatives of the Committee were also invited. Country poster presentations were encouraged with no review other than a limit on the total number that each country could present. The entire meeting was a plenary session, with a scientific focus. OGAC officials believe that positive programmatic changes took place in the countries after information was shared at this meeting. After the meeting, OGAC developed a task force to address reporting burden, a commonly shared challenge in the field that was communicated during the meeting. OGAC officials and Country Teams reported that since then, the task force and its recommendations have contributed to progress in streamlining reporting requirements.

The third annual meeting was held in Durban, South Africa, in June 2006. An application process was instituted instead of invitations; the sole criterion for acceptance of an application was whether the person was involved in program implementation. Approximately 1,000 people from 50 countries attended; 500 presentations were made (Dybul, 2006). New features included an abstract-driven program and the use of an International Program Committee for planning and review of abstracts. The International Program Committee also selected the topics and plenary speakers. While the Committee did not seek access to the formal evaluation of this meeting, it heard from a number of individual participants who praised the "by implementers, for implementers" approach.

OGAC reported that the fourth annual meeting, to be held in 2007, would be cosponsored by the World Bank, the Global Fund, and UNAIDS and that it expected 1,500–2,000 people to attend.

Communications

Initially, PEPFAR created ill will in some countries and among other donors because successes were attributed only to the United States in official statements and speeches. The U.S. Global AIDS Coordinator responded by changing this language to communicate the fact that PEPFAR is a partner, not a solo actor. The Coordinator has also worked closely with the Global Fund to derive jointly their estimates of the numbers of people being served by each program.

Changes have been initiated as well to respond to the focus countries' call for more communication from headquarters on matters of policy and implementation. Weekly email "Notes to the Field" disseminate the most recent news and guidance from OGAC headquarters and address issues raised in the field.

Institutionalizing the Learning Organization Concept

PEPFAR would benefit from developing a detailed, overall strategy for institutionalizing the concept of being a learning organization, including how it is going to track and report on its progress in this regard. Such a strategy would include the following:

- Articulation of the learning agenda of PEPFAR programs, including a strategy for the conduct and use of results of operations, behavioral, and epidemiological research and implementation studies.
- Continued support for targeted evaluation efforts.
- Specification of how PEPFAR structures and processes will be modified to ensure ongoing communication and access to information and lessons learned at the country and cross-country levels and among others in the global HIV/AIDS community.
- Definition of the indicators by which PEPFAR will track its progress toward becoming a learning organization and how those indicators will be measured.

An annual report, or a specific section in the overall program's annual report, on these issues would highlight the importance of this area and enhance its visibility.

BUDGET ALLOCATIONS

PEPFAR is accountable to Congress for implementing a relatively large set of specific budget allocations (see Chapter 2). These allocations derived from Congress' desire to articulate and enforce certain priorities, in particular to ensure that the scale-up of ART would be the centerpiece of the program. At the time the legislation was passed, the international community, including CDC and USAID, was still debating whether treatment on this scale could be achieved. Relatively little information existed with which to determine precisely how resources should be allocated to achieve the performance targets in the focus countries; thus the budget allocations could not be fully evidence-based. Even in instances where the available information allowed reasonable estimates, the situation has since changed so rapidly that those estimates are no longer accurate. For example, when the Leadership Act was drafted, Congress estimated that antiretroviral medications (ARVs) would account for 75 percent of the cost of providing

ART—hence the 75 percent suballocation for ARVs within the 55 percent allocation for treatment. According to some current estimates, however, ARVs now account for a relatively small and declining proportion of the total cost of ART (Martinson, 2006), while increases in the number of children being treated, as well as in the number of individuals on second-line medications, are likely to shift cost patterns once again.

The lack of an evidence base for the budget allocations and a rationale linking the allocations to performance targets and goals has adversely affected implementation in a number of ways described by the Country Teams and others. First, the budget allocations limit the Country Teams' ability to harmonize PEPFAR's activities with those of the partner government and other donors. Although OGAC requires each Country Team to meet the same allocations, national plans and epidemiologic data suggest that the relative allocations among categories would appropriately vary by country. For example, approximately 10 percent of all children under age 17 are estimated to be orphans in Nigeria, whereas the proportion in Botswana is 20 percent (USAID et al., 2004).

Second, PEPFAR's categories of prevention, treatment, and care and the subcategories within them fragment the natural continuum of needs and services, often in ways that do not correspond to global standards, do not align with an individual focus country's perspective, and do not permit optimal management of patients and their families. ART programs (categorized as treatment) and counseling and testing programs (categorized as care) need to be closely linked so that HIV-positive people can be quickly referred from counseling and testing sites for evaluation for treatment, and the partners and families of patients can receive counseling and testing promptly. Separate funding can serve to sever these linkages.

There has also been some misalignment of activities across the program categories of prevention, treatment, and care. The result has been a lack of emphasis on some crucial activities. For example, voluntary counseling and testing is included in the care category (mainly for HIV case finding) rather than under prevention, although it has long been considered an important element of prevention approaches. Consequently, there has been insufficient emphasis on quality counseling and testing as a prevention tool. Likewise, treatment is narrowly defined as ART, but a comprehensive basic treatment package includes elements categorized as both prevention (for example, services addressing sexually transmitted infections) and care (for example, treatment of opportunistic infections and pain management) (OGAC, 2004). Care, which is the fundamental organizing principle for the full spectrum of HIV/AIDS interventions and typically includes both preventive care and ART, is instead a catch-all for what does not fit easily within the prevention and treatment categories and budget allocations. To achieve longer-term targets and the ultimate goals of the Leadership Act—

improvements in survival and reversal of the epidemic—it will be necessary to eliminate the fragmentation introduced by the PEPFAR categories and budget allocations and better capitalize on the synergy that results from effective integration.

The suballocations and corresponding subcategories that OGAC has developed to manage them have also been problematic within categories. According to many of the Country Teams, the abstinence-until-marriage allocation within the prevention category has been the most difficult to manage. The adverse effect of this budget allocation on prevention programming that is responsive to and harmonized with host country plans was also found in a recent Government Accountability Office study (GAO, 2006) that examined countries in addition to the focus countries. By requiring the Country Teams to isolate funding for these activities, this budget allocation has undermined the teams' ability to integrate prevention programming.

The abstinence-until-marriage budget allocation in particular has fueled a divisive U.S. debate over the ABC concept. It is important to understand that ABC represents neither a program nor a strategy, but a goal of changing key behaviors. There is good evidence that behavior changes such as delaying sexual activity (A), reducing the number of sexual partners (B), and using condoms correctly and consistently (C), reduce the risk of transmitting HIV/AIDS (Stanton et al., 1998; Furguson et al., 2004; Bunnell et al., 2006; Riedner et al., 2006). While no one argued during the Committee's visits that funding for ABC should exclude activities focused on changing abstinence behaviors, the Committee has been unable to find evidence for the position that abstinence can stand alone or that 33 percent is the appropriate allocation for such activities even within integrated programs.

The ABC debate has also served to obscure the importance of other behaviors that put people at high risk of contracting HIV/AIDS, such as alcohol use and violence toward women. Since programs aimed at reducing alcohol dependence or empowering women are not officially ABC activities, they are less likely to be funded.

Finally, the budget allocations do not allow program implementers sufficient flexibility to respond to change. Moreover, the Leadership Act stipulated that the budget allocations were recommended for the first 2 years of the program and many would be required beginning in 2006. Thus the allocations were set to become more, rather than less, restrictive as the program evolved and attempted to adapt to changes in science, country epidemics, and circumstances. OGAC's management of the allocations for the first 3 years of funding are shown later in the chapter in Table 3-3.

The difficulties posed by budget allocations will become more pronounced as the HIV/AIDS pandemic and the science of controlling it evolve. For example, several new approaches to prevention are currently being investigated, including male circumcision, microbicides, and vaccines. These new approaches will change the appropriate mix and costs of prevention services in unforeseen ways. Without greater flexibility, the ability of the U.S. Global AIDS Initiative to lead the way in utilizing such new techniques when proven effective will be greatly reduced.

> **Recommendation 3-3:** ***Although they may have been helpful initially in ensuring a balance of attention to activities within the four categories of prevention, treatment, care, and orphans and vulnerable children, the Committee concludes that rigid congressional budget allocations among categories, and even more so within categories, have also limited PEPFAR's ability to tailor its activities in each country to the local epidemic and to coordinate with the level of activities in the countries' national plans.*** **Congress should remove the budget allocations and replace them with more appropriate mechanisms that ensure accountability for results from Country Teams to the U.S. Global AIDS Coordinator and to Congress. These mechanisms should also ensure that spending is directly linked to and commensurate with necessary efforts to achieve both country and overall performance targets for prevention, treatment, care, and orphans and other vulnerable children.**

TARGETS

Some of the indicators being collected by PEPFAR do not yet provide appropriate information on the progress being made toward the ultimate goal of controlling the epidemic. As is appropriate for a program this early in its implementation, most results reported to date are for targets that can be measured in the short term; thus they reveal more about the process of implementation than the impact of the program. PEPFAR plans to measure more meaningful mid- and long-term results, and the program is supporting countries in developing the measures and skills needed to evaluate the impact of initiatives at the country level.

One issue related to targets concerns requiring that results be specifically and uniquely attributed to the U.S. initiative. Such a requirement creates disincentives for international coordination among donors and harmonization at the country level, and can work against the use of U.S. funds to leverage other donors' interests in a particular area. The most important result is impact on a country's epidemic, and that impact can best be attributed to collective actions taken in partnership with all donors and, most critically, the host country. PEPFAR would do well to consider a step taken by some other large donors: evaluating Country Teams on how well they cooperate with the partner government and the donor group as a whole and how effective they are at leveraging a successful package of services.

Finally, targets that are defined in terms of whether programs meet the full spectrum of needs of an individual person across his or her lifespan, of all members of the family or household, and of communities as a whole would create improved incentives for programming that is comprehensive, integrated, and accountable to those being served. At present, however, PEPFAR is not reporting referral or linkage indicators in its annual report, and few such indicators are required to be reported to OGAC across the four program categories. Over the course of the program, OGAC has increased its emphasis on integration in guidance provided to the focus countries (Dybul, 2005). Integration was included in the fiscal year 2005 guidance in a general manner; by fiscal year 2007, that guidance was expanded, outlining points of possible integration for all program activities, including voluntary counseling and testing, ART, diagnosis and treatment of sexually transmitted infections, and services for orphans and other vulnerable children (OGAC, 2006b,c). OGAC has also provided Country Teams with additional information on integrated services and activities required to address the needs of key populations, such as people living with HIV/AIDS (OGAC, 2006b,c). This improved guidance can have greater impact if it is enhanced by tracking of the results of integration.

RESOURCE ALLOCATION

Financial Management

Over the course of the program, there have been a number of changes in the way funding is managed, as well as in the interactions between the Country Operational Plans and funding decisions. Country Teams originally developed Country Operational Plans under the assumption that they would have the available minimum level of funding OGAC had assigned to them. If, as happened in fiscal year 2006, more money was appropriated after the plans had been approved, new versions of the plans had to be developed that described how the additional funds would be spent. These new plans, called "plus-up plans," were then reviewed through the usual mechanisms. OGAC was dissatisfied with the quality of the plus-up plans, and the Country Teams were unhappy about writing and reviewing planning documents twice in one year. As a result, for fiscal year 2007, the interagency Deputy Principals Group assumed the highest possible level of potential funding when developing the country planning budgets and requested that Country Teams formulate a short statement indicating how spending would be prioritized if funding were decreased by 5–10 percent.

Since its inception, PEPFAR has undergone one evaluation by the Office of Management and Budget. The Office of Management and Budget developed the Program Assessment Rating Tool to assess and drive the improved performance of U.S. government programs by examining all factors that affect and reflect program performance, such as program purpose and design, performance measurement, evaluations, strategic planning, program management, and results (OMB, 2007a). Programs that are categorized as performing (versus nonperforming) receive ratings from effective (highest rating) to adequate (lowest rating). All U.S. government agencies involved in PEPFAR are rated in a single assessment, and the program received an overall rating of moderately effective when assessed in 2005. Specifically for fiscal accountability, however, the assessment found that "the implementing agencies' mechanisms for financial accountability and control did not yet meet the standards for strong financial management practices." In addition, audits conducted by USAID's Inspector General in 2005 and 2006 found financial management problems in PEPFAR programs implemented by USAID in some of the focus countries (USAID, 2005, 2006c).

OGAC's response to its assessment was that it was establishing and implementing a new system to capture program expenditures by country and undertaking an internal review of budget allocations to focus countries based on performance data and pipeline capacity (OMB, 2007b). Additionally, a new financial management system has been implemented at CDC and at USAID for both headquarters and Country Team management.

OGAC officials also explained to the Committee that they are funding a number of new projects aimed at improving PEPFAR's financial management. These include the following:

- Development of a country-level portfolio review process. This process is intended to improve program management and evaluate funding pipelines by partner and activity type.
- A pipeline analysis to determine whether improvements can be made in how funds move from congressional appropriation to the end user.
- An addition, on the part of the Office of Management and Budget, OGAC, and the PEPFAR implementing agencies, of an annual outlays report to the current quarterly obligations and outlays reports. According to OGAC, this new approach will serve to provide greater detail and transparency.
- A joint effort with State Department information technology experts to develop a budget interface system that will be flexible and web-based. In related activities, OGAC is working with a contractor to improve COPRS reports.

PEPFAR Focus Country Funding by Agency Account

A 357 percent increase in focus country funding from the State Department Global HIV/AIDS Initiative account from fiscal year 2004 to fiscal year 2006 resulted from both an increase in new monies for HIV/AIDS and the shifting of funding from other agency accounts, such as CDC's Global AIDS Program account and the Department of Defense's Prevention account. The AIDS budgets of USAID and the Department of Defense were shifted in their entirety to the State Department account, as was a large proportion of the budget of the Department of Health and Human Services for the CDC Global AIDS and Prevention of Mother-to-Child Transmission programs (see Table 3-1).

PEPFAR Central and Focus Country Funding

PEPFAR activities are funded either centrally—through OGAC or one of the implementing agencies—or through the Country Teams. The majority of PEPFAR funds (84 percent), totaling almost $3 billion over the first 3 years of the program, has been planned and granted by the Country Teams. The proportion of country funds implemented through central programs has decreased by almost half—from 24 percent in fiscal year 2004 to 13 percent in fiscal year 2006 (see Table 3-2) (OGAC, 2005a, 2006a). PEPFAR's initial rounds of funding were intended to capitalize

TABLE 3-1 Focus Country–Implemented Funding by Agency for Fiscal Years 2004–2006 (in millions of U.S. dollars)

	Fiscal Year 2004		Fiscal Year 2005		Fiscal Year 2006		Total Fiscal Year 2004–2006	
Agency	Funding	Percent	Funding	Percent	Funding	Percent	Funding	Percent
USAID	194	34	0	0	0	0	194	6
Department of Health and Human Services (CDC)	84	15	59	6	59	4	202	7
Department of Defense	0.4	<1	0	0	0	0	0.4	<1
State Department	292	51	969	94	1,336	96	2,597	87
Total	$570	100	$1,028	100	$1,395	100	$2,993	100

SOURCE: OGAC, 2005d, 2006f.

TABLE 3-2 PEPFAR Focus Country–Implemented and Central-Implemented Funding for Fiscal Years 2004–2006 (in billions of U.S. dollars)

	Focus Country		Central		Total Focus Country and Central
Fiscal Year	Funding	Percent	Funding	Percent	Funding
2004	.57	76	.18	24	.75
2005	1.03	84	.19	16	1.22
2006	1.39	87	.21	13	1.60
Total 2004–2006*	$2.99	84	$.58	16	$3.58

*Numbers may not sum to the totals shown because of rounding.

SOURCE: OGAC, 2005d, 2006f.

on the existing operations of both international and country-based non-governmental organizations to allow for rapid scale-up. Contracts with international organizations—which were required to be already operating in at least four of the focus countries—were centrally managed, while contracts with country-based organizations were managed by the Country Teams. During the Committee's country visits, Country Teams described the challenges of managing a comprehensive HIV/AIDS program when as much as a third (on average 16 percent) of the country's PEPFAR funding was centrally managed.

While OGAC has worked to facilitate linkages between the Country Teams and centrally funded grantees, issues remain. Centrally funded programs were selected at the headquarters level, and Country Teams had little or no control over the types of activities funded, the size of the contracts, or the evaluation of performance. Although the initial centrally managed contracts were seen by OGAC as a way to get the funding on the ground as quickly as possible, Country Teams regarded them as a circumvention of country planning and Country Team funding decisions. This situation raised concerns, some of which persist, regarding PEPFAR's ability to comply with the tenets of harmonization. Moreover, the performance of centrally funded contracts appears to be quite variable, with some being singled out for praise in terms of country knowledge and integration with country policies and others being criticized for a lack of those characteristics.

In addition, OGAC has taken several steps to shift control of centrally funded grants to Country Teams so they can better integrate the activities with the larger PEPFAR portfolio in the focus country. Central funding for these contracts has been held constant, and the organizations involved have been required to negotiate increases with the Country Teams. Two examples of this shift in management of central programs are the Partnership for Supply Chain Management and the New Partners Initiative. The Partnership for Supply Chain Management is a program involving a technically skilled central structure from which Country Teams are able to buy specific commodities and services that address each country's specific needs (OGAC, 2006b,c). Since 2004, OGAC has requested approximately $36 million in central funds for the program, used for operations and management, but the bulk of the program's funding is expected to come from focus country budgets. The Quality Assurance Program of USAID, described previously, is managed in a similar style (USAID, 2006b).

The New Partners Initiative is a central grant-making mechanism focused on increasing the number of new partners. Initiated in 2005, it has received $35 million in central funding to date. There was concern that New Partners Initiative grants would be made with little input from the Country Teams. However, OGAC reported that it has been working with Country Teams to apply lessons learned about centrally managed programs to inform New Partners Initiative policies. Specifically, grantees are required to have Country Team approval to work in that country (OGAC, 2006a).

Both of these programs were established after the Committee made its visits to the focus countries. Thus the Committee was unable to obtain the perspective of the Country Teams on whether the implementation of these centrally managed programs represents an improvement.

PEPFAR Funding by Program Category

Of the approximately $3.6 billion allocated for the focus countries during the first 3 years of funding, the treatment category has accounted for approximately $1.4 billion (40 percent), while prevention and care have each accounted for about $.81 billion (23 percent) (see Table 3-3). The remaining $.51 billion (14 percent) has gone to other costs, such as strategic information activities, policy analysis and system strengthening, and management and staffing of the Country Teams.

With respect to the budget allocations, the proportion of funds allocated by OGAC for treatment has increased from 34 to 45 percent. The proportion for care has stayed constant at about 23 percent, while the proportion allocated for prevention has declined by about 9 percentage points. Since the program's inception, about 28 percent of the funds allocated to care and 6 percent of overall funding has been allocated for the orphans and other vulnerable children category (OGAC, 2006a).

As reported by OGAC to the Committee, it has a method to attribute the same "other" costs described above to their corresponding program categories for each fiscal year (OGAC, 2007). When this method is used, the totals for the full dollar amounts appropriated each year for the focus

TABLE 3-3 PEPFAR Funding by Program Category for Fiscal Years 2004–2006 (in billions of U.S. dollars)

	2004		2005		2006		Total 2004–2006	
Category	Funding	Percent	Funding	Percent	Funding	Percent	Funding	Percent
Prevention	.21	28	.29	24	.31	19	.81	23
Care	.16	23	.27	22	.37	23	.81	23
Treatment	.25	34	.48	39	.72	45	1.45	40
Other Costs	.13	17	.18	15	.20	13	.51	14
Total	$.75	100	$1.22	100	$1.60	100	$3.58	100

NOTE: Numbers may not add due to rounding.
SOURCE: OGAC, 2005d, 2006f.

countries (including central support) and the percentages of funding for each program area change from the data in Table 3-3 (see Table 3-4).

Focus Country Funding

Between $53 million (Guyana) and $459 million (South Africa) has been allocated for each of the 15 focus countries since fiscal year 2004, totaling a combined $3.6 billion (see Table 3-5). PEPFAR support for the focus countries collectively has increased by 113 percent, and each of the countries has seen at least an 80 percent increase in funds since the first year of the program. Botswana, Ethiopia, Haiti, Kenya, Mozambique, Namibia, Nigeria, South Africa, and Vietnam have all seen their support increase by more than 100 percent.

One of the major concerns of the Country Teams has been the relationship between their budgets and targets for prevention, treatment, and care. For many of the focus countries, the proportions of the prevention,

TABLE 3-4 PEPFAR Funding by Program Category for Fiscal Years 2004–2006 (in billions of U.S. dollars) with Distribution of Other Costs by OGAC Method

	2004		2005		2006		Total 2004–2006	
Category	Funding	Percent	Funding	Percent	Funding	Percent	Funding	Percent
Prevention	.28	33	.38	27	.40	23	1.06	27
Care	.24	28	.39	28	.54	31	1.17	29
Treatment	.32	38	.62	44	.82	47	1.76	44
Total	$.83	100	$1.40	100	$1.76	100	$3.99	100

NOTE: Data presented as received from OGAC.
SOURCE: OGAC, 2007.

TABLE 3-5 PEPFAR Funding by Focus Country for Fiscal Years 2004–2006 (in millions of U.S. Dollars)

Country	2004	2005	2006	Percent Increase 2004–2006	Total Funding 2004–2006
Botswana	24	52	55	129	131
Côte d'Ivoire	24	44	47	96	115
Ethiopia	48	84	123	156	255
Guyana	12	19	22	83	53
Haiti	28	52	56	100	135
Kenya	92	143	208	126	444
Mozambique	37	60	94	154	192
Namibia	24	43	57	138	124
Nigeria	71	110	164	131	345
Rwanda	39	57	72	85	168
South Africa	89	147	222	149	459
Tanzania	71	109	130	83	309
Uganda	91	147	170	87	409
Vietnam	17	27	34	100	79
Zambia	82	130	149	82	361
Total	$751	$1,223	$1,602	113	$3,580

NOTE: Numbers may not sum to the totals shown because of rounding. Some sources of central support for focus countries are not reflected in the table above.
SOURCE: OGAC, 2005d, 2006f.

treatment, and care targets they are responsible for achieving are close to the respective proportions of their funding. For 9 of the 15 focus countries, the target and funding proportions are within 3 percentage points of one another across the three program categories with targets. However, South Africa, which is responsible for approximately 25 percent of the targets in all three categories, is receiving between 11 and 14 percent of funding, depending on the program area. In contrast, Uganda is responsible for 2 to 3 percent of the targets and receives 10 to 15 percent of the funding. On the other hand, these figures do not take into account a number of factors that could impact the level of funding, such as existing infrastructure, other funding sources (e.g., the host country and other donors), human resource capacity, and the current state of the epidemic.

Per capita PEPFAR funding for people living with HIV/AIDS also varies widely by focus country. For example, in 2006 Guyana, with an estimated 12,000 people living with HIV/AIDS, was receiving roughly $1,800 in PEPFAR funds per person living with HIV/AIDS. In contrast, South Africa, which has an estimated 5.5 million people living with HIV/AIDS, was receiving about $40 in PEPFAR funds per person living with HIV/AIDS. OGAC reported that the Deputy Principals Group decides on the total funding per fiscal year per country, but provided the Committee with no information on the process used in making these decisions. The per person allocations presented above do not take into account important factors, including the country's own capacity to fund its programs, but they suggest a need for more transparent budgeting and planning so the rationale for these allocations can be better understood.

CONCLUSION

PEPFAR has been responsive to the Leadership Act's challenging mandate to coordinate all U.S. international HIV/AIDS activities and has made progress in coordinating among the agencies of the U.S. government involved in the program and with other global HIV/AIDS donors at both the headquarters and country levels. The program has also made progress in harmonizing with the focus countries. The virtual organization created by OGAC, the implementing agencies, and the Country Teams exhibits many of the positive features of a learning organization and has evolved considerably during the initial years of the program. With the improvements in transparency and accountability for marginalized groups of people recommended by the Committee, and with the increased flexibility that would be afforded by removal of the congressional budget allocations, the U.S. Global AIDS Initiative should be able to make even greater progress toward achieving the goals of the Leadership Act.

REFERENCES

Bunnell, R., J. Ekwaru, P. Solberg, and N. Wamai. 2006. Changes in sexual behavior and risk of HIV transmission after antiretroviral therapy and prevention interventions in rural Uganda. *AIDS* 20:85–92.

Dybul, M. 2005 (May 24). *Integrated prevention, treatment and care: Network systems.* Presentation at the PEPFAR Second Annual Field Meeting, Addis Ababa, Ethiopia.

Dybul, M. 2006 (July 13). *The President's Emergency Plan for AIDS Relief: Looking back and looking forward.* Remarks as prepared to the Center for Strategic and International Studies. Washington, DC: U.S. Office of the Global AIDS Coordinator. http://www.pepfar.gov (accessed July 13, 2006).

Furguson, A., M. Pere, C. Morris, E. Ngugi, and S. Moses. 2004. Sexual patterning and condom use among a group of HIV vulnerable men in Thika, Kenya. *Sexually Transmitted Infection* 80:435–439.

GAO (Government Accountability Office). 2006. *Global health: Spending requirement presents challenges for allocating prevention funding under the President's Emergency Plan for AIDS Relief* (GAO-06-395). Washington, DC: GAO.

Garvin, D. 2000. *Learning in action: A guide to putting the learning organization to work.* Boston, MA: Harvard Business School Press.

Martinson, N. 2006. *Outpatient provider costs of treating adults with ARVs in Soweto.* Presentation at the PEPFAR 3rd Annual Meeting. Durban, South Africa: Martinson and University of the Witwatersrand.

McKinsey and Company. 2005. *Global health partnerships: Assessing country consequences.* Seattle, WA: Bill and Melinda Gates Foundation.

Moloney-Kitts, M. 2005 (April 19). *Office of the Global AIDS Coordinator.* Presentation at the Second Meeting of the Institute of Medicine Committee for the Evaluation of PEPFAR Implementation, Washington, DC.

OECD (Organisation for Economic Co-operation and Development). 2003. *Harmonising donor practices for effective aid delivery good practice papers: A DAC reference document.* Paris, France: OECD.

OGAC (Office of the U.S. Global AIDS Coordinator). 2004. *The President's Emergency Plan for AIDS Relief: U.S. five-year global HIV/AIDS strategy.* Washington, DC: OGAC.

OGAC. 2005a. *PEPFAR first annual report to Congress.* Washington, DC: OGAC.

OGAC. 2005b. *The President's Emergency Plan for AIDS Relief: Defining US support for national strategies* (PowerPoint Presentation). Washington, DC: OGAC. http://www.pepfar.gov (accessed July 19, 2005).

OGAC. 2005c. *FY2005 funded targeted evaluation studies: Status update.* Washington, DC: OGAC.

OGAC. 2005d. *FY2005 country operational plans.* Washington, DC: OGAC.

OGAC. 2006a. *PEPFAR second annual report to Congress.* Washington, DC: OGAC.

OGAC. 2006b. *PEPFAR: Technical considerations for the FY2007 country operational plans.* Washington, DC: OGAC.

OGAC. 2006c. *PEPFAR FY2007 COP resource guide.* Washington, DC: OGAC.

OGAC. 2006d. *FY2006 funded targeted evaluation studies: Status update.* Washington, DC: OGAC.

OGAC. 2006e. *Centrally-funded targeted evaluation studies: Status update.* Washington, DC: OGAC.

OGAC. 2006f. *FY2006 country operational plans.* Washington, DC: OGAC.

OGAC. 2006g. *A blueprint for public health evaluations in the President's Emergency Plan for AIDS Relief.* Washington, DC: OGAC.

OGAC. 2007. Office of the Global AIDS Coordinator's Suggested Factual Changes to the PEPFAR Implementation: Progress and Promise Report. Email communication to IOM staff on March 29, 2007.

OGAC, Global Fund to Fight AIDS, Tuberculosis, and Malaria, and World Bank. 2006. *Report: Joint coordination meeting on HIV/AIDS, January 10–11, 2006.* Washington, DC and Geneva, Switzerland: OGAC, Global Fund to Fight AIDS, Tuberculosis and Malaria, and World Bank.

OMB (Office of Management and Budget). 2007a. *Program assessment rating tool (PART).* http://www.whitehouse.gov/omb/part/ (accessed February 19, 2007).

OMB. 2007b. *Program assessment for the President's Emergency Plan for AIDS Relief: Focus countries.* http://www.whitehouse.gov/omb/expectmore/summary/10004619.2005.html (accessed February 19, 2007).

Riedner, G., O. Hoffman, M. Rusizoka, D. Mmbando, L. Maboko, H. Grosskurth, J. Todd, R. Hayes, and M. Hoelscher. 2006. Decline in sexually transmitted infection prevalence and HIV incidence in female bar workers attending prevention and care services in Mbeya region, Tanzania. *AIDS* 20:609–615.

The Rome Declaration on harmonization. 2003. High level forum on harmonization, February 24–25, 2003, Rome, Italy. http://www.aidharmonization.org (accessed November 10, 2006).

Rugg, D., G. Peersman, and M. Carael. 2004. *Global advances in HIV/AIDS monitoring and evaluation.* Minneapolis, MN: Wiley Periodicals, Inc.

Shakow, A. 2006. *Global Fund–World Bank HIV/AIDS programs comparative advantage study.* Washington, DC and Geneva, Switzerland: Global Fund to Fight AIDS, Tuberculosis, and Malaria, and World Bank. http://www.cgdev.org/doc/event%20docs/2.7.06%20HIV/GFWBReportFinalVersion.pdf (accessed November 3, 2006).

Stanton, B., X. Li, J. Kahihuata, A. Fitzgerald, S. Neumbo, G. Kanduuombe, I. B. Ricardo, J. S. Galbraith, N. Terreri, I. Guevara, H. Shipena, J. Strijdom, R. Clemens, and R. F. Zimba. 1998. Increased protected sex and abstinence among Namibian youth following a HIV risk reduction intervention: A randomized, longitudinal study. *AIDS* 12:2473–2480.

UNAIDS (Joint United Nations Programme on HIV/AIDS). 2004a. *"Three ones" key principles.* Conference paper 1, Washington consultation of April 4, 2004. Geneva, Switzerland: UNAIDS. http://www.unaids.org/NetTools/Misc/DocInfo.aspx?LANG=en&href=http://gva-doc-owl/WEBcontent/Documents/pub/UNA-docs/Three-Ones_KeyPrinciples_en.pdf (accessed September 20, 2006).

UNAIDS. 2004b. *Clearing the common ground for the "three ones": Report of a consultation process.* Conference paper 2, Washington consultation of April 25, 2004. Geneva, Switzerland: UNAIDS.

UNAIDS. 2005a. *Global task team on improving AIDS coordination among multilateral institutions and international donors: Final report.* Geneva, Switzerland: UNAIDS.

UNAIDS. 2005b. *The "three ones" in action: Where we are and where we go from here.* Geneva, Switzerland: UNAIDS.

UNAIDS. 2006. *Considerations for countries to set their own targets for AIDS prevention, treatment, and care.* Geneva, Switzerland: UNAIDS.

UNAIDS, African Union, WHO (World Health Organization). 2006. *Brazzaville commitment on scaling up towards universal access to HIV and AIDS prevention, treatment, care and support in Africa by 2010.* Geneva, Switzerland: UNAIDS.

USAID. 2005. *Office of the Inspector General: Audit of USAID's implementation of the President's Emergency Plan for AIDS Relief.* Audit report number 9-000-05-009-P. Washington, DC: USAID.

USAID (U.S. Agency for International Development). 2006a. *Quality assurance and workforce development project: Year four annual report: Performance period: July 1, 2005–June 30, 2006, July 31, 2006.* Washington, DC: USAID.

USAID. 2006b. *Quality assurance project.* Washington, DC: USAID. http://www.qaproject.org (accessed November 3, 2006).

USAID. 2006c. *Office of the Inspector General audit of USAID's progress in implementing the President's Emergency Plan for AIDS Relief.* Audit report number 9-000-07-004-P. Washington, DC: USAID.

USAID, UNAIDS, UNICEF (United Nations Children's Fund). 2004. *Children on the brink: A joint report of new orphan estimates and a framework for action.* Washington, DC: USAID.

4

PEPFAR's Prevention Category

Summary of Key Findings

- PEPFAR's ambitious prevention target—to support the prevention of a total of 7 million infections in the 15 focus countries—differs from the treatment and care targets in several respects: the target represents long-term impact, it is to be estimated at the national level by modeling, and it is to be measured for the year 2010. To achieve this target, PEPFAR is implementing a wide variety of HIV prevention activities, including those related to preventing mother-to-child transmission, preventing sexual transmission and transmission through injecting drug use, and reducing the risk of transmission through blood transfusion and medical injection. While many of these activities have been shown to lead to a decrease in the transmission of HIV, it is difficult to report on short-term progress for most prevention activities because of the long-term nature of their impact and a lack of indicators that can easily be linked to national declines in incidence.
- PEPFAR is making progress in prevention of mother-to-child transmission, one of the few areas of preventive activity for which specific indicators exist that allow relatively direct estimation of infections averted. Thus far, PEPFAR has supported the provision of services aimed at preventing mother-to-child transmission to women during more than 6 million pregnancies. These efforts have included providing prophylactic antiretroviral therapy to more than 530,000 women, estimated to have resulted in more than 100,000 infant infections averted.
- PEPFAR's approach to achieving the prevention target involves planning and implementing prevention programs and activities that are evidence-based, harmonized with country plans and priorities, and appropriate to each country's unique epidemiologic and cultural context. However, the abstinence-until-marriage budget allocation in the Leadership Act hampers these efforts and thus PEPFAR's ability to meet the target. Despite the efforts of the Office of the U.S. Global AIDS Coordinator to administer the allocation judiciously, it has greatly limited the ability of Country Teams to develop and implement comprehensive prevention programs that are well integrated with each other and with counseling and testing, care, and treatment programs and that target those populations at greatest risk.
- PEPFAR has contributed substantially to improvements in HIV surveillance that enables an overview of the epidemiologic context in the focus countries and can be used to measure progress. However, the focus countries are not conducting adequate behavioral surveillance surveys, which are critical for obtaining information on patterns of exposure and at-risk populations. PEPFAR could provide more support for such surveys.
- PEPFAR is supporting targeted evaluation of some prevention programs, but could be doing more program evaluation and operations research, particularly for unproven interventions, to ensure that prevention funds are being used most efficiently to have the greatest impact on the focus countries' HIV/AIDS epidemics.

Recommendation Discussed in This Chapter

Recommendation 4-1: The U.S. Global AIDS Initiative should enhance and intensify HIV prevention through a planning process that links timely national information on the epidemic to the selection of the most appropriate intervention packages and to the optimal targeting of interventions to populations in whom infections are most likely to occur. The U.S. Global AIDS Coordinator should enhance current data on HIV prevalence by supporting quality behavioral surveys to identify patterns of risk. The Coordinator should support country plans to identify where infections are to be averted to achieve prevention targets and should track progress toward achieving prevention goals by measuring risk behaviors, the prevalence and incidence of other sexually transmitted infections, and ultimately the prevalence and incidence of HIV.

4

PEPFAR's Prevention Category

CATEGORY, TARGET, AND RESULTS

The Prevention Category

The prevention category encompasses five funding and reporting subcategories: (1) abstinence/be faithful, (2) condoms and other prevention, (3) prevention of mother-to-child transmission, (4) blood safety, and (5) injection safety. Funding for these subcategories for fiscal years 2004–2006 is shown in Table 4-1. Corresponding to these subcategories are four types of prevention activities funded by the President's Emergency Plan for AIDS Relief (PEPFAR): promotion of behavior change aimed at risk avoidance and risk reduction, provision of comprehensive programs for people who engage in high-risk behavior, prevention of mother-to-child transmission of HIV, and reduction of medical transmission of HIV by ensuring safe blood supplies and safe medical injections and providing training in universal medical precautions (see Table 4-2). Strategies guiding these activities include scaling up existing prevention programs, advancing policy initiatives that support prevention of HIV infection, and collecting strategic information needed to monitor and evaluate progress and ensure compliance with PEPFAR policies and strategies (OGAC, 2006d). PEPFAR's authorizing legislation requires that 33 percent of total prevention funding be spent on abstinence-until-marriage activities; PEPFAR allocates these funds under the abstinence/be faithful subcategory.

Voluntary counseling and testing, typically a key component of HIV

TABLE 4-1 PEPFAR Prevention Funding (in millions of U.S. dollars) and Percent by Subcategory for Fiscal Years 2004–2006

	Fiscal Year 2004		Fiscal Year 2005		Fiscal Year 2006		Total Fiscal Years 2004–2006	
Subcategory	Funding	Percent	Funding	Percent	Funding	Percent	Funding	Percent
Abstinence/Be Faithful	63	31	76	26	104	33	243	30
Condoms and Other Prevention	45	22	66	22	72	23	183	22
Prevention of Mother-to-Child Transmission	44	21	66	23	71	23	181	22
Blood Safety	27	13	53	18	31	10	111	14
Injection Safety	27	13	33	11	34	11	94	12
Total*	$207	100	$294	100	$311	100	$812	100

*Numbers may not add to the totals shown because of rounding.

SOURCE: OGAC, 2005d, 2006c.

prevention programs, is listed as a prevention activity in PEPFAR's authorizing legislation. However, PEPFAR budgets and reports on voluntary counseling and testing under the care category, and those activities are therefore discussed in Chapter 6. Also included under the care category is secondary preventive care for HIV-positive people and their family members/caregivers. Likewise, prevention activities specifically targeting orphans

TABLE 4-2 PEPFAR Activities Corresponding to Funding and Reporting Subcategories

Prevention Activities	Prevention Funding and Reporting Categories
Promotion of behavior change aimed at risk avoidance and risk reduction	Abstinence/be faithful; condoms and other prevention
Provision of comprehensive programs for people who engage in high-risk behavior	Condoms and other prevention
Prevention of mother-to-child transmission of HIV	Prevention of mother-to-child transmission of HIV
Reduction of medical transmission of HIV by ensuring safe blood supplies and safe medical injections and providing training in universal medical precautions	Blood safety; injection safety

SOURCE: OGAC, 2004, 2005a, 2006a.

and other vulnerable children are included in that category and thus are discussed in Chapter 7.

Target

The overall target for PEPAR prevention programs, as described in the legislation, is to prevent approximately 7 million HIV infections in the 15 focus countries by 2010. Each country has a target that represents roughly 50 percent of the expected incidence of HIV. These country targets are to be achieved through both PEPFAR-supported activities and the prevention activities of the host government and other donors.

The Office of the U.S. Global AIDS Coordinator (OGAC) plans to measure achievement of the prevention target by using U.S. Census Bureau statistical models of country-level prevalence trends at intervals until 2010. Mathematical models of 10 transmission dynamics of the virus will play a central role in calculating HIV infections averted. A range of models representing the spread of HIV through populations have been developed and used over the course of the HIV/AIDS pandemic (Anderson and Garnett, 2000). Models for the expected trends in HIV can be compared with observed trends to determine whether reductions in incidence have occurred. To calculate the expected infections averted by interventions, the predicted HIV epidemic without changes in patterns of exposure is compared with that predicted when interventions are in place. Such a modeling exercise requires epidemiologic and behavioral data to capture patterns of risk and measures of the efficacy of interventions in changing behaviors among individuals and populations. PEPFAR's initial targets for HIV prevention were based on mathematical models of this type, which used the best available epidemiologic evidence (Stover et al., 2002).

To evaluate achievements in HIV prevention, models are used to predict the prevalence of HIV in the near future, which is compared with the estimated prevalence. The latter estimates are based on HIV prevalence in antenatal clinics and in general populations-based surveys, such as the Demographic and Health Surveys, as well as in generalized HIV epidemics. In concentrated epidemics, the size of high-risk groups and the prevalence of HIV in these groups is estimated. The models, developed in part by the Joint United Nations Programme on HIV/AIDS (UNAIDS), use a highly simple representation of an epidemic, which is fit to prevalence data. Such a model extrapolates the previous epidemic trend and determines whether the current trend has diverged from this. Such an approach is reasonable for evaluation, but cannot distinguish between the natural dynamics of an HIV epidemic and the impact of interventions (UNAIDS, 1999, 2002; Garnett et al., 2006). A conservative approach would be to use models to predict the lowest prevalence expected from natural dynamics and see whether observed trends fall below this prediction. Such an approach has been used to identify the impact of changes in risk behavior on epidemics in Uganda, Zimbabwe, and urban Kenya (Kilian et al., 1999; Hallett et al., 2006).

PEPFAR has established intermediate targets for the focus countries by setting yearly, country-level targets that are used to estimate numbers of infections prevented in infants. These numbers represent part of the total 7 million infections the program aims to prevent.

Results

As noted above, achievement of the prevention target will be measured in 2010. In the interim, the only result framed in terms of infections prevented is the infections averted through prevention of mother-to-child transmission. The other results are similar to those for treatment and care in that they provide a count of people who have received prevention services, but do not allow determination of the quality of those services or whether they will translate into infections prevented. PEPFAR's prevention results are summarized in Table 4-3.

PEPFAR's indicators for activities related to prevention of sexual transmission, though generally consistent with globally agreed-upon indicators, have changed over time. The program's first annual report included measures in addition to those shown in Table 4-3, such as number of mass media HIV/AIDS prevention programs, but these indicators were subsequently dropped in the evaluation guidance published by OGAC and not reported in subsequent annual reports. In 2005, the Center for Strategic and International Studies studied the indicators being used by PEPFAR, comparing them with those included in the United Nations General Assembly Special Session on HIV/AIDS, Global Fund guidance, and Millennium Challenge Goals. The study found that, with regard to indicators for activities related to prevention of sexual transmission, PEPFAR was the only initiative to collect program data based on the components of the ABC model.[1] While many of the initiatives did collect information on condom distribution and outlets separately, none of the other initiative separated A, B, and C in the tracking of prevention activities (Morrison et al., 2005).

The Committee was unable to evaluate data related to specific at-risk populations because the data collected by PEPFAR are not broken down by these populations. See Chapter 3 for further discussion.

---

[1]The ABC model was developed by the Government of Uganda in 1986 for a national prevention program encouraging Ugandans to abstain from sex until marriage (A), be faithful to one partner (B), and use condoms (C). Uganda's program is referenced in the Leadership Act.

TABLE 4-3 PEPFAR Prevention Results by Fiscal Year, 2004–2006

Subcategory	Fiscal Year 2004	Fiscal Year 2005	Fiscal Year 2006
Abstinence/Be Faithful			
Number of people reached by PEPFAR-supported abstinence-only community outreach programs for HIV/AIDS prevention	11,530,400	Not available	Not available
Number of people reached by PEPFAR-supported abstinence/be faithful community outreach programs for HIV/AIDS prevention	24,041,800	24,861,700	40,247,500
Number of people receiving PEPFAR-supported training or retraining to promote HIV/AIDS prevention through abstinence and/or being faithful	116,600	174,400	299,300
Condoms and Other Prevention			
Number of people reached with community outreach programs that promote HIV/AIDS prevention through condom promotion, related, and other services	11,899,900	17,941,100	21,203,300
Number of people receiving PEPFAR-supported training or retraining to provide condoms and related services	51,200	93,200	129,300
Prevention of Mother-to-Child Transmission			
Number of women receiving prevention of mother-to-child transmission services	1,271,300	1,957,900	2,814,700
Number of women receiving a complete course of antiretroviral prophylaxis for prevention of mother-to-child transmission	125,100	122,600	285,600
Number of infant infections averted	23,800	23,400	54,400
Number of people receiving PEPFAR-supported training or retraining in prevention of mother-to-child transmission	24,600	28,600	32,600
Number of service outlets supported by PEPFAR providing the minimum package of prevention of mother-to-child transmission services according to national or international standards	2,200	2,500	4,863
Blood Safety			
Number of service outlets related to blood safety supported by PEPFAR	249	585	3,848
Number of people receiving PEPFAR-supported training or retraining in blood safety	2,200	8,000	6,600
Injection Safety			
Number of people receiving PEPFAR-supported training or retraining in injection safety	4,300	12,300	52,100

SOURCE: OGAC, 2005b, 2006b, 2007a, 2007b.

REVIEW OF PROGRESS TO DATE

This section reviews the progress of PEPFAR's activities to prevent HIV infection according to the primary routes of transmission of HIV: sexual, through injecting drug use, from mother-to-child, and medical. Also discussed is PEPFAR's progress in the crucial area of removing gender barriers to prevention.

Prevention of Sexual Transmission of HIV

Promotion of Behavior Change

Sexual transmission accounts for more than 80 percent of all HIV infections worldwide (Piot et al., 1988). Behavioral interventions designed to reduce the risk of sexual transmission of HIV are tailored to specific groups and to be effective require a current understanding of HIV epidemiology, in particular those people at highest risk of infection. These interventions include providing counseling and testing; encouraging risk reduction in people who are both HIV-positive and HIV-negative; and reducing HIV risk cofactors, such as the presence of another sexually transmitted infection (JHU AIDS Service, 2006).

The Leadership Act describes activities to be supported by the U.S. Global AIDS Initiative to prevent HIV transmission. These activities focus on "delay of sexual debut, abstinence, fidelity and monogamy, reduction of casual sexual partnering, reducing sexual violence and coercion, including child marriage, widow inheritance, and polygamy, and where appropriate, use of condoms" (P.L. 108-25, p. 729).

As described in the strategy for the program, PEPFAR's primary approach to preventing sexual transmission of HIV is aimed at changing ABC behaviors. Largely in response to the Leadership Act's requirement that 33 percent of funding for prevention of sexual transmission go to support abstinence-until-marriage (A) programs, PEPFAR divides activities related to preventing sexual transmission into two funding and reporting subcategories: abstinence/be faithful and condoms and other prevention (GAO, 2006).

Abstinence/Be Faithful

Operational plans for the 15 focus countries incorporate a variety of activities funded under the abstinence/be faithful subcategory, including school-based, community, and media interventions aimed at delaying sexual activity among youths; promoting fidelity and reduction of the number of partners among sexually active adults; addressing gender norms and HIV-related issues, such as intergenerational and coercive sex; increasing family and community involvement in HIV prevention; and promoting counseling and testing, especially for family members of people living with HIV/AIDS (OGAC, 2006c). Funding under abstinence/be faithful also supports technical assistance and capacity building activities, such as the formulation of culturally appropriate school curriculum focused on developing students' life skills, training of adults (teachers and community counselors) to promote abstinence/be faithful messages in their communities, and strengthening of the capacity of local organizations to enable them to receive U.S. government funding under the abstinence/be faithful subcategory (OGAC, 2006c). Examples of abstinence/be faithful activities in selected focus countries are presented in Box 4-1.

BOX 4-1
Selected Examples of PEPFAR-Supported Abstinence/Be Faithful Activities

In **Ethiopia,** PEPFAR is funding programs that address negative social norms that lead to increased risk of HIV infection for young girls. Behavior change activities are directed at older men who seek sexual relationships with younger girls and the communities that explicitly or implicitly condone such relationships.

In **South Africa,** a number of PEPFAR partners are bringing tailored AB messages into communities with door-to-door counseling on risk assessment and behavior change, as well as the use of traditional healers to deliver prevention messages that reinforce traditional values.

In **Uganda,** PEPFAR has supported the development and tailoring of school-based prevention curriculum. Support for the Presidential Initiative on AIDS Strategy for Communication to Youth, a school-based HIV/AIDS communication initiative for youths, has provided training for a large number of primary school teachers on abstinence and life skills messages, as well as related teaching and reading materials.

In **Namibia,** a PEPFAR partner is focusing on prevention by strengthening AB messages at counseling and testing sites in the community setting, providing counseling and testing for partners and family members of people who are HIV-positive, offering risk reduction counseling, and stressing the importance of being faithful to a partner of known HIV status.

SOURCE: OGAC, 2006c.

Condoms and Other Prevention

Activities aimed at preventing sexual transmission of HIV under the condoms and other prevention subcategory include interventions for a number of priority groups, such as sero-discordant couples, people living with HIV, the military, police, commercial sex workers and their clients, truck drivers, and refugees. These interventions include mass media campaigns, peer-to peer counseling, condom promotion, and communication interventions targeting behavior change in high-risk venues and along transportation corridors. There are a number of examples of comprehensive and appropriate PEPFAR-funded programs addressing the needs of these populations. However, because of a lack of systematic data on these programs and on the needs of populations most at risk in the focus countries, it is not possible to determine the extent to which these programs are addressing the needs.

According to OGAC, the total number of U.S. government–funded male and female condoms shipped to the focus countries increased from 115 million in 2001 to 198 million in 2005 (OGAC, 2006b) with a total of nearly 407 million condoms purchased for the focus countries in the first 3 years of PEPFAR (OGAC, 2007). The number of U.S. government–funded condoms shipped to individual focus countries in 2005 ranged from 0 to nearly 70 million (OGAC, 2006b). It is unclear how much of the increase in condoms provided to the focus countries is due to PEPFAR. The relevant data for 2002 through 2004 were not available to the Committee, and in many of the countries, U.S. government agencies are funding other development programs, such as family planning programs, that include the distribution of condoms. As of June 2006, PEPFAR had supported nearly 86,000 condom outlets (OGAC, 2006a).

OGAC reports that the lack of data with which to determine the number of condoms provided specifically under PEPFAR is linked to rules that apply to the focus countries' access to a commodities fund that is generally used to purchase condoms for U.S. Agency for International Development (USAID) programs. According to discussions with OGAC and Country Teams, USAID programs in countries other than the PEPFAR focus countries typically pool worldwide condom orders and procure the condoms centrally for both family planning and HIV prevention programs. Because the focus countries are reportedly not eligible to receive condoms from the commodities fund because of the interpretation of legislative intent, a number of PEPFAR-supported programs use their PEPFAR funds to purchase condoms. OGAC officials also reported that family planning and HIV prevention programs promote the use of condoms for health generally, including prevention of both disease and pregnancy. Thus all of the condoms shipped to the focus countries are used for both purposes.

In addition to the interventions described above, PEPFAR is supporting the development of a number of new prevention technologies, such as microbicides (female-controlled chemical barriers to prevent transmission of HIV). The U.S. Global AIDS Initiative, through the National Institutes of Health, supports scaling up for clinical trials of three microbicide candidates as well as the HIV Prevention Trials Network, a worldwide collaborative that develops and tests the safety and efficacy of nonvaccine interventions designed to prevent HIV transmission (OGAC, 2005b).

A variety of other prevention activities are funded under the condoms and other prevention subcategory. For example, PEPFAR is supporting studies of risk reduction associated with male circumcision and of alcohol consumption as a risk factor for HIV transmission in a few of the focus countries. PEPFAR is also supporting the training of clinicians and peer counselors in how to communicate comprehensive ABC-based prevention messages. Workplace prevention programs funded by PEPFAR are focused on the development of workplace strategies and training for how to deal with the personal and potential commercial impacts of HIV/AIDS in the workplace.

Comprehensive and integrated approaches drawing on all components of ABC and targeting specific populations have been shown to be effective in increasing healthy behaviors and decreasing transmission of HIV, especially when integrated with other HIV services, such as counseling and testing, treatment of other sexually transmitted infections, and antiretroviral therapy (ART) (Stanton et al., 1998; Furguson et al., 2004; Bunnell et al., 2006; Riedner et al., 2006). There is, however, little evidence to show that ABC when separated out into its components is as effective as the comprehensive approach (Bollinger et al., 2004).

Examples of condoms and other prevention activities in selected focus countries are presented in Box 4-2.

Information Campaigns and Training

Overall, OGAC has reported reaching more than 140 million people in the 15 focus countries with messages intended to prevent the sexual transmission of HIV, a number that represents over one-fourth of the combined population of more than half a billion people in the focus countries. Of this total, roughly two-thirds of people received abstinence-until-marriage/be faithful messages and roughly one-third received condoms and other prevention messages. PEPFAR has supported the training or retraining of more than 864,000 people for prevention programs related to preventing sexual transmission of HIV. Roughly two-thirds of those trained were trained for abstinence-until-marriage/be faithful programs (OGAC, 2005b, 2006a,b, 2007).

BOX 4-2
Selected Examples of PEPFAR-Supported Condoms and Other Prevention Activities

In **Mozambique,** PEPFAR has supported a condom social marketing program through which condoms are sold in bars, hotels, and shops along transportation corridors and other areas of high-risk behavior. The program includes behavior change communication targeting those most at risk of transmission, such as uniformed services and mobile populations.

In **South Africa,** a PEPFAR-funded program is supporting the scale-up of postrape services, including postexposure HIV prophylaxis. This program also includes policy development and training for health and social workers and police.

In **Haiti,** a comprehensive PEPFAR-funded program targets commercial sex workers. The sex workers are provided some services, including counseling and testing and condoms, on site, and are referred to sex worker–friendly sites for the provision of other services, including counseling and testing and clinical treatment of sexually transmitted and opportunistic infections. People who are HIV-positive and their partners are referred through strong networks for care and treatment services, as needed.

In **Botswana,** PEPFAR is supporting two programs aimed at reducing the contribution of alcohol use to the HIV/AIDS epidemic—one targeting health care workers and another targeting drinking establishments and their patrons.

In **Uganda,** PEPFAR is funding a number of prevention programs focused on prevention for sero-discordant couples in which counseling and testing, including a door-to-door counseling and testing program piloted in 2005, is the key entry point for other prevention programming.

In **Namibia,** PEPFAR has partnered with the Namibian Defense Force and the Ministry of Defense to fund "edutainment" events; training of Ministry of Defense personnel in home-based care, peer education, and gender sensitivity; policy discussions with the Ministry's higher echelons; and provision of materials for information, education, and communication.

SOURCE: OGAC, 2006c.

Prevention of HIV Transmission Through Injecting Drug Use

One of the most-at-risk populations for HIV transmission is people who use injection drugs. Current U.S. policy prohibits the U.S. Global AIDS Initiative from funding needle or syringe exchange programs (OGAC, 2006f), and thus from supporting all aspects of the complete recommended comprehensive package of services for people who use injection drugs (UNAIDS, 2005b). However, the PEPFAR strategy acknowledges the need for comprehensive HIV prevention and care programs for people who use injection drugs, especially in countries such as Vietnam where HIV infection is at low levels in the general population, and those who use injection drugs are pivotal in increasing HIV infection rates among the general population (OGAC, 2004). PEPFAR-supported activities targeted to people who use injection drugs include working with ministries of health on relevant national policies and supporting assessments of the contribution of substance use to the HIV epidemic globally; development of culturally appropriate 12-step programs to decrease drug use; education of health professionals and policy makers regarding best practices for HIV prevention strategies for people who abuse substances; peer-to-peer counseling on HIV; confidential, routine HIV counseling and testing in substance abuse programs; community-based outreach that addresses HIV prevention, risk reduction, and substance use with links to appropriate care services; prevention education on the risks of injecting drugs and sharing syringes; education and counseling on how to reduce or stop injecting drugs; HIV treatment or referral to treatment for an HIV-infected person who uses drugs; and substance abuse treatment programs for HIV-infected people, including medication-assisted treatment with methadone, buprenorphine, and naltrexone. For people who are HIV-negative, PEPFAR can only support medication-assisted treatment on a pilot basis, and support for all medication-assisted substance abuse therapy requires prior approval from OGAC (OGAC, 2006f).

Prevention of Mother-to-Child Transmission

In 2005, approximately 700,000 children under age 15 worldwide became infected with HIV, mainly through mother-to-child transmission. Approximately 90 percent of these infections due to mother-to-child transmission occurred in Africa. Studies have shown that transmission can take place during pregnancy, labor, or delivery and through breastfeeding. In the absence of any intervention, rates of mother-to-child transmission of HIV can vary from 15 to 30 percent without breastfeeding and from 30 to 45 percent with prolonged breastfeeding (WHO, 2002a). A comprehensive set of activities—including counseling and testing, prophylactic antiretroviral therapy in late pregnancy and delivery, as well as for the newborn; safe delivery practices; and use of breastmilk substitutes when safe water is available—has been found to be effective in preventing transmission of HIV to infants. The United Nations Children's Fund (UNICEF) has estimated that only 9 percent of pregnant women who were HIV-positive in low- and middle-income countries received antiretroviral prophylaxis for prevention of mother-to-child transmission in 2005 (UNICEF et al., 2007).

Successful prevention of mother-to-child transmission of HIV requires that each mother–infant pair participate in a cascade of events that begins with HIV testing and continues through postdelivery follow-up and testing for the infant at age 18 months (Stringer et al., 2005). Dadian and colleagues (2003) have identified the following steps in the process: attendance at an initial antenatal care visit, pretest counseling related to HIV and mother-to-child transmission, receipt of an HIV test, provision of antiretroviral prophylaxis, counseling on methods for reducing transmission through breastfeeding, follow-up with mother and child postdelivery, and HIV testing or assessment for the infant after age 18 months. Declines in participation have been found at each of these steps as the result of a variety of factors, including denial of HIV infection, opposition from male partners, women's fear of disclosure of HIV status to their partner and fear of being "found out" if they are taking drugs or not breastfeeding, concern about taking drugs in pregnancy, failure to return for checkups in the month before delivery, home delivery, and premature delivery before treatment can be given (GHPWG, 2004). Because failure to complete all steps can result in reduced coverage and diminished program effectiveness, it is crucial to collect information at each step to enable tracking of the points at which mothers are discontinuing services (Stringer et al., 2005).

Country Operational Plans describe PEPFAR support for national efforts to prevent mother-to-child transmission through a number of avenues. At the national level, PEPFAR provides technical assistance to host governments in the development and adoption of guidelines and policies aimed at improving the standardization and quality of such efforts. In addition, by helping to strengthen commodity management systems, PEPFAR partners increase the availability of many commodities essential to these prevention efforts, including antiretroviral medications and test kits (OGAC, 2006c).

At the community level, PEPFAR-funded programs are expanding the numbers of sites providing services related to prevention of mother-to-child transmission and antenatal care in an attempt to expand the utilization of these services. Such services are crucial in settings where relatively few women give birth in health care facilities and would otherwise miss the opportunity to receive prophylactic antiretroviral medications at birth and reduce the risk of transmission to their infants. PEPFAR programs are working with national leaders and local health care workers to find ways of providing the medications and of offering follow-up and postpartum care in nontraditional settings, including giving the medications to pregnant women to take home and training traditional birth attendants in prevention of mother-to-child transmission. PEPFAR programs also give pregnant women information on how to reduce the risk of transmission to their infants through breastfeeding. Finally, in some focus countries, PEPFAR is supporting the improvement and expansion of information management systems and conducting evaluations to assess the effectiveness of specific preventive programs for mothers (OGAC, 2006c). Box 4-3 provides some examples of PEPFAR-supported activities aimed at preventing mother-to-child transmission in selected focus countries.

BOX 4-3
Selected Examples of PEPFAR-Supported Activities Aimed at Preventing Mother-to-Child Transmission

In **Kenya,** PEPFAR-supported programs are adopting a family approach to reduce stigma, increase uptake of services, and improve adherence to ART through couples counseling and testing, male involvement, and community-based promotion of HIV care. In addition, pregnant women with World Health Organization (WHO) stage III and IV disease will be referred to comprehensive care centers for ART as a strategy for preventing mother-to-child transmission; these services will be provided in provincial, district, and high-volume health centers.

In **Rwanda,** PEPFAR is supporting the national program through interpersonal and mass media communications that promote early antenatal clinic attendance, delivery in health care facilities, safe infant feeding practices, early infant diagnosis, and male involvement.

In **Nigeria,** PEPFAR is supporting antenatal services, laboratories, and training of personnel involved in counseling and testing and obstetric and gynecologic services at designated hospitals. PEPFAR funding also covers the procurement of prophylactic antiretroviral medications and breastmilk substitutes, as well as the costs of laboratory tests for diagnosis and monitoring.

In **Botswana,** PEPFAR is supporting the expansion of psychosocial support services for women who are HIV-positive, their partners, and their families that include encouraging partners to be tested. This multicomponent project also supports a peer-counseling program, trains counselors to promote adherence to ART, offers support services to other people living with HIV/AIDS who are receiving ART, and links between ART programs and programs focused on prevention of mother-to-child transmission.

SOURCE: OGAC, 2006c.

According to OGAC, since the start of the program, PEPFAR has supported services to women during 6 million pregnancies to prevent mother-to-child transmission of HIV; and more than 533,000 of these women received antiretroviral prophylaxis. Overall, in the focus countries the proportion of eligible women who are receiving services to prevent mother-to-child transmission has increased from 2004 to 2006. Specifically, the proportion of eligible pregnant women receiving services such as counseling and testing has increased from 7 to 16 percent, and the proportion of HIV-positive pregnant women receiving antiretroviral prophylaxis has increased from 9 to 21 percent (OGAC, 2007).

Prevention of mother-to-child transmission is the only subcategory of prevention activities that has specific targets per country per year. Yet it is unclear how PEPFAR will factor these results into the model being used to measure progress toward the overall prevention target. Given results thus far and the targets through 2007, it appears that the contribution of this subcategory to the overall target may be small. OGAC estimates infant infections averted by assuming, based on the cascade discussed earlier, that only 19 percent of the women who have been provided with antiretroviral prophylaxis will subsequently give birth to an infant who is HIV-negative. Through September 30, 2006, OGAC has estimated that PEPFAR-supported programs have prevented 101,500 infant infections (OGAC, 2007).

Training for prevention of mother-to-child transmission supported by PEPFAR has included in-service training of health care providers in antenatal clinics in counseling and testing and in the administration of antiretroviral medications. In addition, PEPFAR is working to expand the capacity of training facilities to meet personnel needs for these preventive programs by supporting the development of related curriculum. OGAC reports that PEPFAR has funded the training of more than 85,000 people to provide a variety of these preventive services, including HIV counseling and testing for pregnant women, antiretroviral prophylaxis, counseling and support for safe infant feeding practices, and family planning counseling and referral (OGAC, 2005b, 2006b, 2007).

Prevention of Medical Transmission of HIV

Blood Safety

The safety and availability of blood for transfusions has been negatively affected by the emergence and spread of HIV. Unsafe blood disproportionately impacts women (who often need transfusions for pregnancy-related complications) and children (who experience high rates of malnutrition, malaria, and severe life-threatening anemia). An inadequate supply of safe blood products results in many deaths in medical settings in developing countries (WHO, 2006a).

PEPFAR sees improving the availability and safety of blood as crucial to reducing the spread of HIV and to enabling the focus countries to develop basic infrastructure and strengthen their health care systems (Ryan, 2006). PEPFAR's blood safety activities have included supporting the development of associated governance structures, increasing laboratory capacity to screen blood supplies for HIV and other diseases, training health care workers in safe blood transfusion methods, increasing the number of voluntary donors through awareness campaigns, and conducting quality evaluations to ensure the effective implementation of blood safety procedures. OGAC reports that PEPFAR funds have contributed to the establishment of more than 4,600 blood safety service outlets in the focus countries through support for infrastructure, equipment, and supplies; donor recruitment activities; blood collection and distribution logistics; testing, screening, and transfusion; waste management; training; and management to ensure a safe and adequate blood supply. In addition, PEPFAR has supported the training of more than 16,700 people in blood safety procedures and services (OGAC, 2005b, 2006b, 2007). Examples of PEPFAR-supported blood safety activities in selected focus countries are presented in Box 4-4.

Injection Safety

Among sources of HIV infection associated with health care, injections with nonsterile equipment are of particular concern. In addition, protection of health care workers is an essential component of any strategy to prevent workers from discriminating against HIV-infected patients (WHO, 2006b).

PEPFAR has identified medical injection safety as a key component of its prevention strategy. Related activities provide a wide range of support to host countries, including the development of improved policies for safe injection practices and medical waste management, enhanced training of health workers, procurement of safe injection supplies, and support for the development and dissemination of communications addressing safe medical practices for both medical professionals and the public. OGAC reports that PEPFAR has supported the training of more than 68,000 people in injection

BOX 4-4
Selected Examples of PEPFAR-Supported Blood Safety Activities

In **South Africa,** PEPFAR supports the National Blood Service Program, which is coordinating with the National Department of Health and the Department of Education to provide prevention education to potential young donors to assist them in protecting themselves from infection and enable them to be "certified" as safe donors.

In **Namibia,** PEPFAR supported the addition of a blood donation site and a laboratory. PEPFAR funds also supported training in the recruitment of donors, processing of donated units, and purchase of blood safety equipment.

In **Haiti,** PEPFAR has supported a number of blood safety activities, including introducing new legislation to return supervision of the blood transfusion system to the Ministry of Health, increasing participation of voluntary donors through blood collection and public awareness campaigns, renovating blood clinics, increasing blood screening, and training clinicians and nurses in the clinical use of blood.

SOURCE: OGAC, 2006c.

safety procedures and services (OGAC, 2005b, 2006b, 2007). Other accomplishments, such as supporting the establishment of government entities responsible for adopting national guidelines, monitoring injection safety practices, and overseeing the development of nursing school curriculum on medical injection, are described in the Country Operational Plans (OGAC, 2005d, 2006a,c). Examples of PEPFAR-supported injection safety activities are presented in Box 4-5.

Increased Focus on Gender Issues in Prevention

OGAC has provided Country Teams with guidance on ways to address gender issues in prevention programming appropriate to the context of each country. The Gender Technical Working Group identified review criteria for PEPFAR-supported prevention activities for the fiscal year 2007 Country Operational Plans. These include the following (OGAC GTWG, 2006):

- Ensure equitable access to gender-appropriate prevention messages and services by girls and boys, women and men.
- Support comprehensive, integrated efforts to reduce the practices of cross-generational and transactional sex, multiple sexual partners,

BOX 4-5
Selected Examples of PEPFAR-Supported Medical Injection Safety Activities

In **Mozambique,** PEPFAR has supported the Ministry of Health Biosafety Program and provided technical assistance and training to Ministry of Health staff to introduce a standards-based approach to biosafety in central and provincial referral hospitals, as well as technical assistance and training on injection safety at all levels of health facilities.

In **Uganda,** PEPFAR supported the development of a comprehensive medical safety program that included strengthening national leadership and medical safety bodies; implementing related policy and guidelines; constructing 10 incinerators in 10 districts in partnership with WHO; and procuring adequate supplies, such as auto-disabling syringes and needles.

In **Vietnam,** PEPFAR supports collaboration with the National Institute of Occupational and Environmental Health in Hanoi on medical safety that has been ongoing since 1999. Currently, PEPFAR supports staff exchanges aimed at training institute staff in occupational safety and health research techniques.

SOURCE: OGAC, 2006c.

and gender-based violence, including activities to change male norms and behaviors.

- Support interventions aimed at eradicating gender-based violence and the exploitation of women and girls by prostitution, sex trafficking, rape, and sexual abuse; provide postrape prophylaxis.
- Ensure that vulnerable girls and women are reached by services that empower them to prevent HIV infection, including strategies to increase women's access to employment and income generation.
- Provide behavior change education on male norms, violence, and alcohol abuse to military, uniformed services, and mobile populations.
- Address the unique needs of male and female users of injection drugs.

OGAC has identified the need to design prevention programs targeting women and girls, such as programs to prevent mother-to-child transmission of HIV and to provide voluntary counseling and testing. OGAC is also suggesting that PEPFAR programs create opportunities to establish connections with nonpregnant women and adolescent girls by using reproductive health and family planning programs as entry points. Many gender issues are being addressed in some PEPFAR-supported activities. The fiscal year 2006 Country Operational Plans contain many examples of PEPFAR prevention programs that include gender components. Without specific gender indicators or good data on which gender-focused interventions work best, however, OGAC will be unable to report what impact these programs are having on women's risk of contracting HIV (OGAC GTWG, 2006; OGAC, 2006e). Moreover, programmatic barriers remain to reaching women who are at risk of contracting HIV, such as young girls engaging in transactional sex, commercial sex workers, and sero-discordant couples. Examples of gender-related activities supported by PEPFAR in selected focus countries are presented in Box 4-6.

ISSUES AND OPPORTUNITIES FOR IMPROVEMENT

Although it is difficult to report on the short-term progress of national prevention activities supported by PEPFAR, the Committee identified a number of issues and associated adjustments to the program that could enhance the quality, accountability, and flexibility of PEPFAR's prevention efforts. These include collection of surveillance data, integration of prevention with treatment and care, greater flexibility to select country-appropriate prevention activities through removal of the abstinence-until-marriage budget allocation, and targeting of populations at greatest risk. Evaluation of prevention interventions, discussed in Chapter 8, represents another opportunity for improvement.

BOX 4-6
Selected Examples of PEPFAR-Supported Prevention Activities That Include Gender Components

In **Botswana,** a PEPFAR-supported call center used to link people with HIV/AIDS services is being expanded to offer anonymous counseling for mental health problems and gender-based violence.

In **Zambia,** PEPFAR is supporting a weekly interactive national radio show, Club New Teen Generation, which is designed to promote a dialogue among and between youth, parents, teachers, and some high-profile public figures. Key themes of the show include gender issues such as cross-generational sex and means of improving sexual negotiation skills.

In **Ethiopia,** PEPFAR is supporting a program focused on addressing sexual violence against women, the delivery of postexposure prophylaxis, cross-generational and coercive sexual relationship behaviors, and substance abuse and sexual risk-taking behaviors.

SOURCE: OGAC, 2006c.

Collection of Surveillance Data

Data from sentinel and behavioral surveillance surveys are essential if national policy makers are to design responses to HIV/AIDS that appropriately address the risk behaviors fueling their country's epidemic. For PEPFAR, such data are necessary to identify and target programs to those most at risk of contracting HIV. PEPFAR highlights the need to incorporate these data in the planning of prevention programs in each focus country in its guidance to the Country Teams. According to this guidance, the following steps are to be followed in the planning stage (OGAC, 2005e):

- Estimate the proportion of new infections that are associated with specific behaviors, such as prostitution, early onset of sexual activity among youths, and transmission through sexual networks.
- Review prevalence data available from national serosurveys, antenatal clinic surveillance, and/or voluntary counseling and testing clinics to assess infection burdens by age and gender.
- Understand who is engaging in risk-related activities, how to reach these people, and what individual and structural factors can be leveraged to promote change.

PEPFAR and other U.S. government–funded programs before it have supported the collection of surveillance data in many of the focus countries. However, the collection, analysis, and appropriate application of both sentinel and behavioral surveillance data pose a number of challenges. For example, methodological issues arise, such as low utilization of antenatal clinics, which compromises the representativeness of surveillance data, and the difficulty of accurate sampling of at-risk and/or marginalized groups for behavioral surveys of at-risk populations. Host countries' capacity to analyze the data collected and apply the findings may be limited, and there may be political opposition to collecting accurate information on the epidemic.

Since 2000, a majority of the 15 focus country governments have been leading the collection of sentinel surveillance data, primarily in antenatal clinics. In addition, the Demographic and Health Surveys have been conducted in the majority of focus countries in the last 6 years. However, only a few of the countries have conducted behavioral surveys focused specifically on high-risk populations. Without behavioral data on these populations, it is difficult for countries and donors to know what specific factors are driving each epidemic and what particular interventions would be most successful for each country in preventing the further spread of HIV.

PEPFAR funds have directly supported the collection of surveillance data in all of the focus countries through technical assistance; updating of infrastructure to manage the data collected; and procurement of supplies, such as test kits, to be used in conducting the surveys. In addition, grantees are working to strengthen the capacity of ministries of health and the national AIDS agencies to develop and conduct surveys both on a national scale and for targeted populations. In a number of countries, PEPFAR has supported the placement of experts in the ministry of health or other relevant agencies to assist with specific projects, as well as to train staff in how to improve their data collection activities. PEPFAR has also supported the focus countries in appropriate use of the data being collected and to develop strategies for dissemination (OGAC, 2005c). In addition, slots have been created for PEPFAR Country Team staff with expertise in surveillance to coordinate all PEPFAR-funded surveillance activities and help direct the gathering of data at the country level (OGAC, 2005c).

In accordance with its own guidance, PEPFAR will need to use all available information on key risk behaviors and vulnerable populations in planning and implementing tailored prevention programs that address the needs of each focus country. PEPFAR's continued support for the collection of sentinel surveillance and Demographic and Health Survey data in the focus countries, as well as for Country Operational Plans to conduct more frequent behavioral surveillance surveys, is required to ensure the availability of this information.

Recommendation 4-1: The U.S. Global AIDS Initiative should enhance and intensify HIV prevention through a planning process that links timely national information on the epidemic to the selection of the most appropriate intervention packages and to the optimal targeting of interventions to populations in whom infections are most likely to occur. The U.S. Global AIDS Coordinator should enhance current data on HIV prevalence by supporting quality behavioral surveys to identify patterns of risk. The Coordinator should support country plans to identify where infections are to be averted to achieve prevention targets and should track progress toward achieving prevention goals by measuring risk behaviors, the prevalence and incidence of other sexually transmitted infections, and ultimately the prevalence and incidence of HIV.

Integration of Prevention with Treatment and Care

PEPFAR has increasingly emphasized the importance of integrating its prevention, treatment, and care interventions. However, the separation of counseling and testing from prevention in both budgeting and reporting creates a challenge to implementing the optimal package of integrated prevention activities. Even so, PEPFAR programs are working to improve the integration of services. It is, however, difficult to assess the success of these efforts as information on the extent of such programmatic linkages is not being collected.

Integration of HIV/AIDS prevention, treatment, and care programs has become more important with the scale-up of treatment and care programs, which has created opportunities to capitalize on prevention interventions (GHPWG, 2004). If countries do not succeed in stemming the tide of new infections, the need for treatment will continue to increase and outpace their ability to develop the capacity to meet it (Mathers and Loncar, 2006). Key integration points include ART, counseling and testing, prevention of mother-to-child transmission, and diagnosis and treatment of sexually transmitted infections. The Global HIV Prevention Working Group (2004) made the following recommendations for integrating HIV prevention and treatment programs:

- Integrate HIV prevention and treatment. Health care settings, including HIV treatment sites, should deliver HIV prevention services that will train health care workers in the delivery of HIV prevention interventions. There should be significant expansion and aggressive promotion of voluntary HIV testing and counseling, which should be universally offered in all health care settings. Conversely, prevention programs should promote HIV testing, educate communities about HIV treatments, and facilitate linkages to ART and other care.

- Develop prevention strategies for people who are HIV-positive. Programs tailored to the needs of people living with HIV/AIDS should be developed and implemented. These programs should involve people living with HIV/AIDS and combat stigma with enforceable laws.
- Adapt prevention for people who are HIV-negative. New strategies must emphasize the continued importance of risk reduction and stress that ART is not a cure.
- Monitor impact. Surveillance systems should closely monitor the behavioral impact of ART.

Integrated HIV/AIDS programs have been shown to improve the effectiveness of national programs in decreasing rates of HIV infection and death from AIDS. A UNAIDS (2005a) study projects numbers of new HIV infections and AIDS deaths through 2019 based on models for treatment-centered, prevention-centered, and joint prevention/treatment global responses. The latter model results in the largest number of infections averted and the lowest number of AIDS deaths over a 15-year projection. Similarly, an optimistic model developed by Mathers and Loncar (2006), which assumes increased prevention activity, projects a decline in HIV/AIDS deaths as of 2030 from an estimated baseline of 6.5 million to 3.7 million. Likewise, a conference of Christian Aid HIV partners underscored the need to shift the focus of HIV interventions from a prevention-specific ABC approach to a comprehensive approach developed by the African Network of Religious Leaders Living with or Personally Affected by HIV/AIDS called SAVE (*S*afer practices, *A*vailable medications, *V*oluntary counseling and testing, and *E*mpowerment).

In most of the focus countries, HIV infection is hyperendemic, with transmission occurring from those unaware of their infection status to others unaware of the risk (often spouses of either gender). Counseling and testing are therefore essential to achieving a long-term, sustainable impact on reducing HIV transmission, as well as meeting treatment and care goals. Given its placement in the care category, it appears that PEPFAR views counseling and testing primarily as a means of identifying HIV/AIDS cases eligible for treatment and care. In addition to case finding, however, counseling and testing represents an opportunity to provide HIV education, including prevention messages to people testing both positive and negative for HIV.

PEPFAR continues to struggle with how to integrate prevention, treatment, and care activities and how to measure the level of integration both among PEPFAR-funded services and between those services and the broader health care system in each focus country. For example, OGAC has endeavored to afford Country Teams greater flexibility in planning and budgeting their fiscal year 2007 ABC programs. Country Teams will be able to use combined abstinence/be faithful and condoms and other prevention funds from the same partner to implement integrated interventions. PEPFAR's continued attention to the barriers involved is required to improve the integration of prevention with treatment and care services, especially with regard to counseling and testing.

Greater Flexibility to Select Country-Appropriate Prevention Activities

In addition to epidemiologic data and evidence on specific interventions typically used in the development of prevention programs, PEPFAR's prevention planning is controlled in part by budgetary allocations outlined in its authorizing legislation. The variability of the epidemics in the focus countries underscores the need for specific and timely information in designing prevention programs that address the most important needs and can result in the most infections averted. Even when sufficient data are available, however, Country Teams are not completely free to target funding and interventions to those at greatest risk of acquiring HIV and to prevent transmission from people living with HIV and within sero-discordant couples through improved integration with counseling and testing, care, and treatment.

Since the beginning of the program, concern has been raised about the ability to implement appropriate, integrated, and comprehensive prevention programs given the restriction created by the 33 percent abstinence-until-marriage budgetary allocation. In 2005, OGAC provided guidance to Country Teams for implementing this allocation. This guidance included the implementation definitions of abstaining from sex until marriage (A), being faithful to one partner (B), and using condoms (C), as well as details on how to fund tailored, country-specific prevention activities through the appropriate mix of those components. Nonetheless, confusion and frustration in the field caused by the abstinence-until-marriage allocation have persisted, as reflected in the Committee's discussions with PEPFAR Country Teams during its country visits in which staff indicated that the allocation did not allow them sufficient flexibility to create the appropriate prevention portfolio based on the available data. The Government Accountability Office (GAO, 2006) reached a similar conclusion. OGAC has attempted to provide the Country Teams with greater flexibility through a variety of management policies, but the problem remains. See Chapter 3 for further discussion of and the Committee's recommendation related to the budget allocations.

Targeting Prevention Interventions

The proportions of total PEPFAR prevention funding allocated to each subcategory—abstinence/be faithful (30 percent), condoms and other prevention (22 percent), prevention of mother-to-child transmission (22 percent), blood safety (14 percent), and medical injection safety (12 percent)—are not well-aligned with the estimated proportions of new infections from the major routes of transmission. For example, it is estimated that in sub-Saharan Africa, transmission through sexual contact, from mother-to-child, and via health care procedures (including blood transfusions and medical injections) account for 80–90 percent, 5–35 percent, and 5–10 percent of new infections, respectively, with regional variation (NAS, 1994; Quinn et al., 1994; Quinn, 1996, 2001; WHO, 2002b; Askew and Berer, 2003; Bertozzi et al., 2006).

Together, the two subcategories related to sexual transmission—abstinence/be faithful and condoms and other prevention (which also includes funds for activities related to people who use injecting drugs), account for approximately 52 percent of PEPFAR's prevention funding, well below the estimated contribution of sexual transmission to new infections. In contrast, the blood safety and safe injection subcategories make up 25 percent of PEPFAR prevention funding but are responsible for a much smaller proportion of new infections.

CONCLUSION

In its effort to achieve the target of preventing 7 million infections in the 15 focus countries by 2010, PEPFAR supports the implementation of various prevention interventions, including voluntary counseling and testing, prevention of mother-to-child transmission, and many ABC-related programs, that have been shown to lead to a decrease in the transmission of HIV when targeted to the appropriate populations. It is difficult to know whether these activities will lead to the necessary national declines in incidence, however, because of a lack of information on both the short-term progress of the interventions and the extent to which PEPFAR has been able to target these interventions to those populations most at risk. To support the implementation of comprehensive and evidence-based prevention interventions appropriate to each country's unique epidemiologic and cultural context in order to achieve the prevention target, PEPFAR will need to make a number of adjustments to enhance its surveillance efforts, integrate prevention with treatment and care, and allow greater flexibility in its prevention programs.

REFERENCES

Anderson, R. M., and G. P. Garnett. 2000. Mathematical models of the transmission and control of sexually transmitted diseases. *Sexually Transmitted Diseases* 27:636–643.

Askew, I., and M. Berer. 2003. The contribution of sexual and reproductive health services to the fight against HIV/AIDS: A review. *Reproductive Health Matters* 11(22):51–73.

Bertozzi, S., P. Padian, J. Wegbreit, L. M. DeMaria, B. Feldman, H. Gayle, J. Gold, R. Grant, and M. T. Isbell. 2006. HIV/AIDS prevention and treatment. In *Disease control priorities in developing countries*. 2nd ed., edited by D. T. Jamison, J. G. Breman, A. R. Measham, G. Alleyne, M. Claeson, D. B. Evans, P. Jha, A. Mills, and P. Musgrove. New York and Washington, DC: Oxford University Press and World Bank.

Bollinger, L., K. Cooper-Arnold, and J. Stover. 2004. Where are the gaps? The effect of HIV-prevention interventions on behavior change. *Studies in Family Planning* 35(1):27–38.

Bunnell, R., J. Ekwaru, P. Solberg, and N. Wamai. 2006. Changes in sexual behavior and risk of HIV transmission after antiretroviral therapy and prevention interventions in rural Uganda. *AIDS* 20:85–92.

Dadian, M., M. Siwale, C. Kankasa, R. Nduati, D. Mbori Ngacha, J. Oyieke, N. Rutenberg, S. Geibel, and S. Kalibala. 2003. *Prevention of mother-to-child transmission assessing feasibility, acceptability, and cost of services in Kenya and Zambia*. Horizons Report December 2003. Washington, DC: The Population Council, Inc.

Furguson, A., M. Pere, C. Morris, E. Ngugi, and S. Moses. 2004. Sexual patterning and condom use among a group of HIV vulnerable men in Thika, Kenya. *Sexually Transmitted Infection* 80:435–439.

GAO (Government Accountability Office). 2006. *Global health: Spending requirement presents challenges for allocating prevention funding under the President's Emergency Plan for AIDS Relief* (GAO-06-395). Washington, DC: GAO.

Garnett, G. P., S. Gregson, and K. A. Stanecki. 2006. Criteria for detecting and understanding changes in the risk of HIV infection at a national level in generalised epidemics. *Sexually Transmitted Infections* 82(Suppl. 1):i48–i51.

GHPWG (Global HIV Prevention Working Group). 2004. *HIV prevention in the era of expanded treatment access*. http://www.gatesfoundation.org/nr/downloads/globalhealth/aids/PWG2004Report.pdf (accessed January 31, 2007).

Hallett, T. B., J. Aberle-Grasse, G. Bello, L.-M. Boulos, M. P. A. Cayemittes, B. Cheluget, J. Chipeta, R. Dorrington, S. Dube, A. K. Ekra, J. M. Garcia-Calleja, G. P. Garnett, S. Greby, S. Gregson, J. T. Grove, S. Hader, J. Hanson, W. Hladik, S. Ismail, W. Kassim, W. Kirungi, L. Kouassi, A. Mahomva, L. Marum, C. Maurice, M. Nolan, T. Rehle, J. Stover, and N. Walker. 2006. Declines in HIV prevalence can be associated with changing sexual behaviour in Uganda, urban Kenya, Zimbabwe and urban Haiti. *Sexually Transmitted Infections* 82(Suppl. 1):i1–i8.

JHU AIDS Service (Johns Hopkins University AIDS Service). 2006. *Elements of successful HIV prevention programs*. http://www.hopkins-aids.edu/prevention/prevention7.html#1a (accessed January 31, 2007).

Kilian, A. H. D., S. Gregson, B. Ndyanabangi, K. Walusaga, W. Kipp, G. Sahlmuller, G. P. Garnett, G. Asiimwe-Okiror, G. Kabagambe, P. Weis, and F. von Sonnenberg. 1999. Reductions in risk behaviour provide the most consistent explanation of declining HIV-1 prevalence in Uganda. *AIDS* 13:391–398.

Mathers, C., and D. Loncar. 2006. Projections of global mortality and burden of disease from 2002 to 2030. *PLoS Medicine* 3(11):e442.

Morrison, S., J. Kates, and P. Nieburg. 2005. *Prevention indicators for the President's Emergency Plan for AIDS Relief: A report of the CSIS task force on HIV/AIDS working committee on prevention*. Washington, DC: Center for Strategic and International Studies.

NAS (National Academy of Sciences). 1994. Population migration and the spread of types 1 and 2 human immunodeficiency viruses. *Proceedings of the National Academy of Sciences (USA)* 91(7):2407–2414.

OGAC (Office of the U.S. Global AIDS Coordinator). 2004. *The President's Emergency Plan for AIDS Relief: U.S. five-year global HIV/AIDS strategy.* Washington, DC: OGAC.

OGAC. 2005a. *The President's Emergency Plan for AIDS Relief: Compassionate action provides hope through treatment success.* Washington, DC: OGAC.

OGAC. 2005b. *PEPFAR first annual report to Congress.* Washington, DC: OGAC.

OGAC. 2005c. *PEPFAR: Quarterly, facility-based HIV care/ART reporting form* (updated July 11). Washington, DC: OGAC.

OGAC. 2005d. *FY2005 Country Operational Plans.* Washington, DC: OGAC.

OGAC. 2005e. *ABC guidance #1 for United States government in-country staff and implementing partners applying the ABC approach to preventing sexually-transmitted HIV infections within the President's Emergency Plan for AIDS Relief.* http://www.state.gov/s/gac/partners/guide/ (accessed January 31, 2007).

OGAC. 2006a. *PEPFAR semi-annual report, FY2006.* Washington, DC: OGAC.

OGAC. 2006b. *PEPFAR second annual report to Congress.* Washington, DC: OGAC.

OGAC. 2006c. *FY2006 Country Operational Plans.* Washington, DC: OGAC.

OGAC. 2006d. *OGAC website emergency plan basics—Prevention.* http://www.state.gov/s/gac/plan/prevention/ (accessed January 31, 3007).

OGAC. 2006e (June 1). *PEPFAR gender consultation meeting.* Washington, DC: OGAC.

OGAC. 2006f. *The President's Emergency Plan for AIDS Relief HIV prevention among drug users guidance #1: Injection heroin use.* Washington, DC: OGAC.

OGAC GTWG (OGAC Gender Technical Working Group). 2006. *2006 work plan April 3, 2006 gender annex B FY07 country operational plan review criteria.* Washington, DC: OGAC.

OGAC. 2007a. *PEPFAR third annual report to Congress.* Washington, DC: OGAC.

OGAC. 2007b. Office of the Global AIDS Coordinator's Suggested Factual Changes to the PEPFAR Implementation: Progress and Promise Report. Email communication to IOM staff on March 29, 2007.

Piot, P., F. A. Plummer, F. S. Mhalu, J. L. Lamburay, J. Chin, and J. M. Mann. 1988. AIDS: An international perspective. *Science* 239(4840):573–579.

Quinn, T. C. 1996. Global burden of the HIV pandemic. *The Lancet* 348:99–106.

Quinn, T. C. 2001. AIDS in Africa: A retrospective. *Bulletin of the World Health Organization* 79(12):1156–1167. Geneva, Switzerland: World Health Organization.

Quinn, T. C., A. Ruff, and N. Halsey. 1994. Special considerations for developing nations. In *Pediatric AIDS: The challenge of HIV infection in infants, children, and adolescents.* Edited by P. A. Pizzo and C. M. Wilfert. Baltimore, MD: Williams & Wilkins. Pp. 31–49.

Riedner, G., O. Hoffman, M. Rusizoka, D. Mmbando, L. Maboko, H. Grosskurth, J. Todd, R. Hayes, and M. Hoelscher. 2006. Decline in sexually transmitted infection prevalence and HIV incidence in female bar workers attending prevention and care services in Mbeya region, Tanzania. *AIDS* 20:609–615.

Ryan, C. 2006. *Written testimony to the Committee on International Relations, June 27, 2006.* http://wwwc.house.gov/international_relations/109/rya062706.pdf#search=%22Blood%20Safety%20PEPFAr%22 (accessed January 31, 2007).

Stanton, B., X. Li, J. Kahihuata, A. Fitzgerald, S. Neumbo, G. Kanduuombe, I. B. Ricardo, J. S. Galbraith, N. Terreri, I. Guevara, H. Shipena, J. Strijdom, R. Clemens, and R. F. Zimba. 1998. Increased protected sex and abstinence among Namibian youth following a HIV risk reduction intervention: A randomized, longitudinal study. *AIDS* 12:2473–2480.

Stover, J., N. Walker, G. P. Garnett, J. A. Salomon, K. A. Stanecki, P. Ghys, N. C. Grassly, R. M. Anderson, and B. Schwartlander. 2002. Can we reverse the HIV/AIDS pandemic with an expanded response? *Lancet* 360:73–77.

Stringer, J., M. Sinkala, C. C. Maclean, J. Levy, C. Kankasa, A. Degroot, E. M. Stringer, E. P. Acosta, R. L. Goldenberg, and S. H. Vermund. 2005. Effectiveness of a city-wide program to prevent mother-to-child HIV transmission in Lusaka, Zambia. *AIDS* 19(12):1309–1315.

UNAIDS (Joint United Nations Programme on HIV/AIDS). 1999. *Trends in HIV incidence and prevalence: Natural course of the epidemic or results of behaviour change?* UNAIDS Best Practice Collection. Geneva, Switzerland: UNAIDS.

UNAIDS. 2002. The UNAIDS reference group on estimates, modelling and projections. Improved methods and assumptions for estimation of the HIV/AIDS epidemic and its impact: Recommendations of the UNAIDS reference group on estimates, modelling and projections. *AIDS* 16:W1–W16.

UNAIDS. 2005a. *Policy position paper: Intensifying HIV prevention.* Geneva, Switzerland: UNAIDS.

UNAIDS. 2005b. *Guidelines for measuring national HIV prevalence in population-based surveys 2005.* Geneva, Switzerland: UNAIDS.

UNICEF (The United Nations Children's Fund), UNAIDS, and WHO (World Health Organization). 2007. *Children and AIDS: A stocktaking report.* New York: UNICEF.

WHO (World Health Organization). 2002a. *Prevention of HIV in infants and children review of evidence and WHO activities (WHO/HIV/2002.08).* Geneva, Switzerland: WHO.

WHO. 2002b. *Blood safety: Aide-memoire for national blood programmes.* Geneva, Switzerland: WHO.

WHO. 2006a. *Blood transfusion safety.* http://www.who.int/bloodsafety/en/ (accessed January 31, 2007).

WHO. 2006b. *HIV/AIDS.* http://www.who.int/hiv/topics/precautions/universal/en/ (accessed January 31, 2007).

5

PEPFAR's Treatment Category

Summary of Key Findings

- PEPFAR narrowly defines treatment as antiretroviral therapy (ART) and includes in this category only activities that directly support the provision of ART. PEPFAR has supported rapid expansion of the availability of ART to people living with HIV infection. By September 2006, PEPFAR was supporting ART for 822,000 women, men, and children in the focus countries.
- PEPFAR is supporting ART within national treatment plans that are consistent with the World Health Organization's guidelines for ART in resource-constrained settings. However, PEPFAR has not always been able to support national plans for purchases of antiretroviral medications.
- PEPFAR is supporting ART programs in addressing the critical issue of adherence to therapy, and limited observational studies show that adherence in the focus countries compares favorably with that observed earlier in Western Europe and North America. PEPFAR is also supporting sentinel surveillance to monitor for resistance.
- Among people receiving ART supported by PEPFAR, 61 percent are women and 9 percent children. PEPFAR's Pediatric Treatment Initiative is attempting to address real and perceived barriers to pediatric treatment.
- The observed rapid clinical response to ART has, in a number of the programs the Committee visited, reportedly resulted in increased interest by people in obtaining HIV testing, followed by ART when indicated.
- PEPFAR is supporting programs in addressing the rapid resurgence of tuberculosis in both child and adult populations throughout sub-Saharan Africa. This resurgence has been fueled by HIV-associated immunodeficiency. In some communities, as many as 80 percent of people newly diagnosed with active tuberculosis have concomitant HIV infection.
- While the success of PEPFAR-supported roll-out of ART has been gratifying, many obstacles remain and will require continued concerted attention at all levels. These obstacles include shortages of trained medical and paramedical personnel, insufficient quantities of antiretroviral medications, difficulties in delivering ART in many rural districts, weak supply chains for antiretroviral medications and other commodities, and inadequate laboratory capacity.

Recommendations Discussed in This Chapter

Recommendation 5-1: The U.S. Global AIDS Coordinator should ensure that adequate medications are available to place 2 million people on sustained antiretroviral therapy to achieve PEPFAR's stated 5-year treatment target. To achieve this target, the Coordinator should also ensure that adequate linkages are established among prevention, treatment, and care programs and rapidly expand the availability of antiretroviral therapy to both children and adults.

Recommendation 5-2: To support countries' ownership of their responses to their HIV/AIDS epidemics, the U.S. Global AIDS Initiative should maintain its commitment to harmonization and participate fully in the development of harmonized procedures. To this end, the U.S. Global AIDS Coordinator should work to support World Health Organization (WHO) prequalification as the accepted global standard for assuring the quality of generic medications. Specifically, the Coordinator should provide an analysis of WHO prequalification that determines whether it can adequately assure the quality of generic antiretroviral medications for purchase under PEPFAR. If the analysis shows that WHO prequalification needs strengthening to provide a sufficient guarantee of quality for PEPFAR, the U.S. Global AIDS Initiative should work with other donors to support strengthening of the process, and work to transition from U.S. Food and Drug Administration approval to WHO prequalification as rapidly as feasible.

5

PEPFAR's Treatment Category

CATEGORY, TARGET, AND RESULTS

The Treatment Category

The President's Emergency Plan for AIDS Relief (PEPFAR) defines treatment narrowly as antiretroviral therapy (ART), and for purposes of budgeting and performance targets, ART is categorized separately from all other related care services. PEPFAR's treatment category includes only activities that directly or indirectly support the provision of ART, including procurement of antiretroviral medications (ARVs), essential laboratory monitoring, equipment and training of personnel for the provision of ART and laboratory monitoring, development of adequate laboratory infrastructure, and support for supply chain management systems for ARVs and related commodities. For purposes of budgeting, complying with budget allocations, and counting progress toward targets, PEPFAR categorizes other services in the care continuum under its other categories. For example, PEPFAR includes most treatment for the prevention of mother-to-child transmission in its prevention category[1] (see Chapter 4), and therapy for coinfections such as tuberculosis and malaria, as well as nonclinical care, in its care category (see Chapter 6). The consequences of this definition and categorization are discussed further in this chapter and in Chapter 8 in the section

[1]Only services in which the mother is receiving ART (termed prevention of mother-to-child transmission plus) are included under the treatment category. Provision of ARVs solely to prevent transmission of HIV from mother to infant is included under the prevention category.

on integration. Funding for PEPFAR-supported treatment activities includes ART and laboratory infrastructure and has roughly tripled from 2004 to 2006 (see Chapter 3).

Target

PEPFAR's 5-year treatment target, as described in the program's authorizing legislation, is to support the focus countries in providing ART to 2 million people. This target represents a count of the number of people receiving ART that is supported directly or indirectly by PEPFAR, and is a globally accepted and widely used early indicator of program implementation. This count provides limited information and does not indicate how well people receiving ART are doing or how the availability of ART affects a country and its HIV/AIDS epidemic. Challenges to obtaining this count are discussed in this chapter; measures of treatment success are addressed in the discussion of impact evaluation in Chapter 8.

Similar to other donor programs, PEPFAR has had to balance its need to be accountable to the U.S. Congress with its accountability to the people of the focus countries within the framework of harmonization. The program has faced the dilemma of needing information that is not readily or routinely available from clinics or ministries of health, and has imposed unprecedented reporting requirements on both urban and rural treatment centers that often have severe shortages of personnel at all levels.

At the global level, PEPFAR requirements for monitoring the number of people receiving ART are reasonably well harmonized with the recommended indicators of the World Health Organization (WHO) and their definitions. PEPFAR generally supports the WHO-recommended tools, including patient records and ART registers, for monitoring and evaluating ART.

Information systems in the focus countries are generally in need of substantial development and strengthening, and PEPFAR is supporting improved HIV-related information systems from the level of rural clinics to that of ministries of health. Although PEPFAR is supporting some innovative information system projects, paper-based records and limited computer access are still the prevailing norm in the focus countries. Provision of even basic monitoring data therefore remains a challenge in most of the countries.

PEPFAR has had to work closely with host countries and other donors to determine which people on ART it can fairly count as having received its support. Host countries are understandably sensitive to donors appearing to take credit for the country's accomplishments, and it is important at both the country and global levels to avoid double-counting if an accurate accounting of the proportion of eligible patients who are receiving ART is to be obtained. Initially, PEPFAR did create ill will in a few focus countries by appearing to take credit for the country's accomplishments. The program has since endeavored to be clear in its reporting that it is claiming credit for having provided some measure of support for a person's ART rather than exclusively and directly providing the treatment. PEPFAR has also been working closely with the Global Fund, as well as with each focus country, to avoid overlaps in attribution. The Committee encourages PEPFAR to continue in this vein, participating in joint attribution and enhancing coordination among all donors and with the host countries.

PEPFAR's strategy for achieving its treatment target includes

- Rapidly scaling up treatment availability using a network model.
- Building capacity for long-term sustainability of quality HIV/AIDS treatment programs.
- Collecting strategic information with which to monitor and evaluate progress and ensure compliance with PEPFAR and national policies and strategies (OGAC, 2004).

To achieve the treatment target, PEPFAR's approach to implementation is to assist countries in the "development of appropriate treatment protocols and policies to ensure safe and effective treatment services, drug supply, and equitable distribution of health resources," and to work with existing clinical programs and develop additional infrastructure, staff, and technical capacity, as needed, to provide "long-term, widespread, high-quality, safe, and essential services to the maximum number of people in need" (OGAC, 2004, p. 11).

Results

According to the Office of the U.S. Global AIDS Coordinator (OGAC), 822,000 people were receiving PEPFAR-supported ART in the focus countries by the end of September 2006, as compared with 155,000 in fiscal year 2004. Approximately 61 percent of this total were women and 9 percent children (OGAC, 2007). These proportions for women and children compare favorably with global averages (WHO and UNAIDS, 2006; UNAIDS, 2006), but may need to increase to reflect actual needs. Recent data indicate that women are disproportionately represented among people living with HIV/AIDS and among the newly infected, particularly in resource-constrained countries, and that children accounted for more than 13 percent of AIDS deaths in 2005 (GAA, 2006; UNAIDS, 2006; WHO and UNAIDS, 2006).

PEPFAR has also supported training in the provision of ART for more than 100,000 health workers and training for more than 17,000 laboratory personnel, as well as significant expansion in the number of ART delivery

TABLE 5-1 PEPFAR Treatment Results by Fiscal Year, 2004–2006

Subcategory	Fiscal Year 2004	Fiscal Year 2005	Fiscal Year 2006
ART			
Number of people receiving ART supported by PEPFAR	155,000	401,000	822,000
Number of ART sites supported by PEPFAR*	300	800	1,912
Number of health workers trained with PEPFAR support in the provision of treatment according to national and/or international standards	12,200	36,500	52,000
Laboratory Infrastructure			
Number of laboratories supported by PEPFAR with the capacity to perform (1) HIV tests and (2) CD4 tests and/or lymphocyte tests	Not available	900	958
Number of people trained with PEPFAR support in the provision of laboratory-related services	3,100	5,700	8,300

*Includes both ART and prevention of mother-to-child transmission plus sites.

SOURCE: OGAC, 2005a, 2006a, 2007.

sites and laboratories that can provide the needed support (see Table 5-1). In addition, PEPFAR has provided funding and technical assistance to strengthen laboratory infrastructure and national procurement and supply chain systems.

REVIEW OF PROGRESS TO DATE

Support for National Programs to Follow the World Health Organization's Guidelines

Nearly all of the focus countries have developed treatment targets and published plans for scaling up ART to meet those targets. While each focus country has a program tailored to its particular circumstances, all the programs are based on WHO's recommendations for delivery of ART in resource-limited settings. PEPFAR has both supported the development of national treatment plans and endeavored to program its activities within the parameters of these national plans and the WHO guidelines. Although concerns have been expressed by several focus countries about the lack of consultation with local authorities during the initial development of PEPFAR treatment programs, and there has been widespread frustration with PEPFAR limits on the procurement of ARVs, PEPFAR's support for ART appears to be generally consistent with national plans in the focus countries.

The 2003 revision of the WHO guidelines is intended to support and facilitate the proper management and scale-up of ART by promoting a public health approach that includes the following elements:

- Scaling up ART, with the objective of universal access.
- Standardizing and simplifying antiretroviral regimens to support efficient implementation of treatment programs in resource-limited settings.
- Ensuring a scientific evidence base for ART programs so as to avoid the use of subpar treatment protocols that could compromise the treatment outcomes of individual patients and create the potential for the emergence of widespread drug resistance.

The WHO guidelines emphasize consideration of the challenges to ART programs posed by working in resource-limited settings, including human resources, health system infrastructure, and socioeconomic conditions. The guidelines include recommendations for when to start ART and with which antiretroviral regimens, reasons for changing the treatment, and what regimens to use if such change is necessary. They also address how treatment should be monitored, with specific reference to the side effects of ART, and make recommendations for particular patient subgroups (WHO, 2006a).

PEPFAR recommends that ART include the following elements (OGAC, 2005a):

- Uninterrupted supply of appropriate ARVs
- General clinical support for patients, including other medications and diagnostics
- Training and support for health care providers
- Infrastructure (clinics, counseling rooms, laboratories, distribution and logistics systems)
- Monitoring and reporting systems
- Appropriate referrals

At the same time, PEPFAR officials have recognized that each nation's needs are unique, and that each nation is therefore in the best position to tailor its plans to fit its particular circumstances. Thus the approach to ART varies considerably among the focus countries. One important factor in this variation is differences in the prevalence of HIV infection; the national HIV prevalence varies more than 20-fold among the 15 focus countries (see Chapter 2). A second salient factor is wide variation in the health care systems already in place. Several countries have well-established medical, nursing, and paramedical education programs, while a few have neither medical nor nursing schools. Access to basic medical services is also highly variable, although most of the focus countries have developed plans for improving access to medical care as an essential element of national policy. In those nations with strong publicly financed health systems, government-supported hospitals were generally able to assume major responsibilities for the initial roll-out of ART, while in others, the process was more dependent on nongovernmental organizations, often faith-based organizations, which provide the majority of health care services in many of the focus countries (GHC, 2005). Integration of those organizations into the national system also varies considerably from country to country.

Diagnosis and Evaluation

As seen among the ART programs the Committee visited, patients diagnosed as HIV-positive are usually scheduled to receive clinical and laboratory evaluation by a health care worker to determine whether they require initiation of ART. Clinical evaluation is uniformly based on the WHO clinical criteria; availability of appropriate laboratory evaluation is variable, however.

Eligibility for ART

Eligibility for ART is determined by country treatment guidelines, which are generally based on the WHO 2006 *Recommendations for Antiretroviral Therapy in Adults and Adolescents in Resource-Limited Settings.* As recommended by WHO, focus country guidelines utilize WHO clinical staging and, when available, CD4 cell count to determine eligibility for ART. Patients with severe HIV-associated clinical disease (WHO clinical stage 4) and those with WHO clinical stage 3 disease with associated tuberculosis or severe bacterial infections are eligible for ART, as are all patients with CD4 counts below 200 cells/mm^3, regardless of WHO clinical stage. In all focus countries visited, the great majority of patients receiving ART have WHO clinical stage 4 disease or clinical stage 3 complicated by major opportunistic infections (usually tuberculosis or severe bacterial disease) or unexplained severe malnutrition. Eligibility criteria for infants and young children are different and are discussed in the section below on treatment of HIV/AIDS in children.

Preparation for ART

Most of the focus countries have developed readiness programs to enhance adherence of eligible patients to ART. Although these programs vary, many are based on the "buddy" concept, by which each patient is required to bring a friend (a family member if possible) to one or more meetings with an adherence counselor prior to the initiation of ART. An essential part of such programs is discussing with the patient and buddy what side effects may be experienced with ART, which of those side effects may be self-limited, and which dictate prompt discontinuation of ART (Nachega et al., 2006). Overall, this approach appears to be working well, but is difficult to accomplish in instances in which access to ART is limited to centers at considerable distances from where patients live.

ART Initiation

Following diagnosis, evaluation, and readiness training, the patient begins ART, usually involving one of the three-drug, first-line regimens recommended by WHO (Gilks et al., 2006). None of the WHO-recommended first-line regimens for adults require refrigeration, and all are now produced in generic form by one or more pharmaceutical companies (FDA, 2006). Although the ART guidelines in all the focus countries are based on the ARV regimens recommended by WHO, other three-drug regimens may be used at the discretion of the supervising physician in some tertiary treatment sites.

Follow-up of Patients Receiving ART

Follow-up is arranged at intervals recommended by WHO and is often reinforced by providing ARVs sufficient to last until the next essential follow-up visit. Most programs visited by the Committee use additional techniques to support adherence during the first few weeks of ART. In some sites, weekly visits to patients' dwellings by an outreach worker are arranged for 4 to 6 weeks after initiation of treatment. In other cases, assigned "buddies," who have received adherence training along with the patients, provide similar support. Although not universal, such techniques for enhancing adherence are employed in the majority of treatment sites. At follow-up visits, the patient is asked about side effects and difficulties with adherence. Continued close adherence to the prescribed regimen is emphasized by the health care worker. If stated adherence is good but improved strength and well-being have not been achieved, potential underlying problems (for example, inadequate caloric intake or concomitant tuberculosis infection, both discussed below) are investigated, and appropriate adjuvant therapy, insofar as possible, is arranged.

Adherence to Therapy

Based on limited observational studies, short-term adherence to ARV regimens in the focus countries appears to be as good as or better than that observed earlier in Western Europe and North America (Farmer et al., 2001; Mills et al., 2006; Nachega et al., 2006; Stringer et al., 2006). As PEPFAR progresses with rapid scale-up and outreach to previously neglected communities, a continued strong emphasis on adherence to therapy is essential. Substantial lack of adherence would not only result in treatment failure, but also would contribute to widespread resistance of the virus to therapy. Failure to adhere would thus not only be harmful to individual patients, but would also necessitate even greater investments of human and financial resources to overcome the resulting resistance problems (IOM, 2005).

PEPFAR does not routinely report on adherence as part of its ongoing program monitoring. However, some relevant data have been obtained from independent observational cohort studies in the focus countries, several of which have reported encouraging levels of adherence (Spacek et al., 2005; Calmy et al., 2006; Stringer et al., 2006; Wools-Kaloustian et al., 2006). Continued support for such evaluations will be critical for determining program effectiveness. Relatively short breaks in adherence (2 to 4 weeks) or repeated breaks for shorter intervals can result in viral resistance to two of the three components of recommended first-line ARV regimens. And a single resistance mutation (K103N) to the non-nucleoside component (either nevirapine or efavirenz) renders the virus resistant to the entire class of non-nucleoside reverse transcriptase inhibitor drugs. The consequence of such resistance patterns is that patients require drugs of a different class—protease inhibitors (Hirsch et al., 2003). The protease inhibitors not only cause more frequent undesirable side effects, but are several-fold more expensive than the WHO-recommended first-line drugs. Few protease inhibitors are now available as generics, and the complexity of their production may cause them to remain relatively expensive for the indefinite future.

Stigma Reduction

Clinicians visited by the Committee reported that the excellent clinical response to ART has in many areas led people in the surrounding communities to be more receptive to obtaining HIV testing and, when appropriate, therapy. This same phenomenon has been reported in other settings as well, including South Africa and Haiti (Castro and Farmer, 2005; Nachega et al., 2006). It appears that a benefit of the response to therapy may be a reduction in stigma associated with HIV testing. Recognition that people receiving effective ART rapidly gain weight and strength and do not suffer from recurrent opportunistic infections reportedly has greatly enhanced the perceived value of the PEPFAR program in the focus countries.

Resistance Monitoring

A previous Institute of Medicine report concluded that general screening for resistance to ARVs was not recommended because the prevalence of resistance in HIV-infected individuals not previously exposed to ART was expected to be very low. However, the report did recommend that coordinated, systematic testing for resistance to ARVs should be conducted among a subset of patients failing treatment (IOM, 2005). The results of testing such patients would aid in determining whether and when routine population-based resistance testing might prove effective. PEPFAR provides support for resistance monitoring; selected examples of such activities in are presented in Box 5-1.

Women as a Proportion of Those Receiving PEPFAR-Supported ART

To ensure that women benefit from equitable access to ARVs and other HIV-related treatments, PEPFAR is working to support treatment programs in addressing the many barriers faced disproportionately by women and girls in accessing health care. Approaches to this end include efforts to shorten waiting times, to provide appropriate appointment schedules and increased numbers of female health workers, and to ensure privacy and confidentiality. These efforts appear to be yielding positive results, and OGAC reported that 61 percent of those receiving PEPFAR-supported ART are women and girls.

BOX 5-1
Selected Examples of PEPFAR-Supported Resistance Monitoring Activities

In **Mozambique,** PEPFAR is supporting a combined tuberculosis/HIV prevalence and drug resistance study.

In **Namibia,** PEPFAR is providing technical assistance and funding for resistance testing for surveillance purposes, and is planning to gradually build local capacity to perform resistance testing in the country over the next 3 to 4 years.

In **Rwanda,** PEPFAR is providing technical assistance and training to laboratory professionals in molecular virology techniques, as well as the development of a quality assurance/quality control program for the HIV drug resistance surveillance program.

In **South Africa,** PEPFAR is supporting surveillance to detect resistant virus in pregnant women.

In **Vietnam,** PEPFAR supported the establishment of a surveillance system for ARV resistance focused on strengthening national collaboration and partnerships for ARV resistance monitoring and assisting in the development of national guidelines for such efforts.

SOURCE: OGAC, 2005b.

Treatment of HIV/AIDS in Children

The Country Operational Plans for fiscal years 2005 and 2006 describe a wide range of PEPFAR-supported pediatric treatment activities. Selected examples of these activities are presented in Box 5-2.

According to the Global AIDS Alliance (GAA, 2006), although PEPFAR has increased funding available for pediatric HIV services, country-level stakeholders still are not mobilizing sufficiently to take advantage of opportunities offered by the Global Fund and PEPFAR to scale up pediatric treatment. Even though the number of countries offering infant testing programs increased in 2005, the laboratory infrastructure for widespread infant testing has not been established (GAA, 2006). PEPFAR's 2007 guidance for Country Operational Plans requests that when setting 2007 targets, Country Teams take into account that pediatric formulations may be limited and that the cost of such formulations may be up to three times that of adult formulations. The guidance suggests that 15 percent of people receiving PEPFAR-supported ART should be children, but recognizes that while some countries may be able to meet this target for 2007, others may be just initiating their pediatric programs and may feasibly be able to target

BOX 5-2
Selected Examples of PEPFAR-Supported Pediatric Treatment Activities

PEPFAR is providing technical assistance to support a number of countries in adapting and implementing international pediatric treatment guidelines.

In **Côte D'Ivoire,** PEPFAR supports a National Pediatric ART Reference Center.

In **Namibia,** PEPFAR is supporting efforts to help make nonpediatricians more comfortable with pediatric HIV/AIDS. These efforts include adapting training materials to the country context as the basis for a new training program in pediatric HIV/AIDS. This training is targeted to medical officers and nurses assigned to pediatric outpatient departments, pediatric wards, and communicable disease clinics.

In **Tanzania,** PEPFAR supports a collaborative aimed at improving quality of care for children with severe illness and HIV/AIDS in three district hospitals. The effort includes strengthening the pediatric components of the national HIV/AIDS care and treatment guidelines and facilitating the training of physicians, nurses, and other caregivers so they can provide higher-quality pediatric services in the context of the collaborative approach to quality improvement.

SOURCE: OGAC, 2005b, 2006d.

the 5–10 percent range, with the goal of increasing to 15 percent (OGAC, 2006e).

To help address the universal challenges involved in pediatric treatment (discussed below in the section on issues and opportunities for improvement), in early 2006 PEPFAR announced a public–private partnership that would be devoted to scientific and technical discussions of solutions for pediatric HIV treatment, formulations, and access. This partnership includes innovator and generic pharmaceutical companies, multilateral organizations such as the Joint United Nations Programme on HIV/AIDS (UNAIDS) and the United Nations Children's Fund (UNICEF), and agencies across the U.S. government. The partners are expected to contribute their diverse expertise to accelerate children's access to treatment. The partnership met twice in 2006. Its initial plans include the following: (1) identify scientific obstacles to pediatric treatment that the partnership could address; (2) take practical steps and share best practices on the scientific issues surrounding dosing of ARVs for pediatric patients; and (3) develop systems for clinical and technical support to facilitate rapid regulatory review, approval, manufacture, and availability of pediatric ARV formulations (OGAC, 2006c).

ISSUES AND OPPORTUNITIES FOR IMPROVEMENT

Limited Availability of ART

Virtually every treatment program that the committee visited in the focus countries was crowded to the point of overflowing, and many programs reported long waiting lists. Many people lamented the lack of availability of ART for large numbers of those identified as eligible and expressed the hope that scale-up of treatment could proceed even more rapidly.

In all focus countries, ART roll-out to rural areas has been slow and challenging. In these areas, transportation is often poor, and trained health care workers and laboratory facilities are either minimal or nonexistent. The inability to reach some health care facilities during the rainy season in several countries is a major challenge. A challenge to PEPFAR is the need to collaborate with host governments to develop means of overcoming these obstacles and to demonstrate to all countries how rural treatment can best be achieved.

> **Recommendation 5-1: The U.S. Global AIDS Coordinator should ensure that adequate medications are available to place 2 million people on sustained antiretroviral therapy to achieve PEPFAR's stated 5-year treatment target. To achieve this target, the Coordinator should also ensure that adequate linkages are established among prevention, treatment, and care programs and rapidly expand the availability of antiretroviral therapy to both children and adults.**

Areas for Improvement in ART Programs

Eligibility for ART

The WHO guidelines state emphatically that "treatment of patients with WHO clinical stage 4 disease should not depend on a CD4 cell count determination; all such patients should initiate ART" (WHO, 2006c, p. 14). In several of the sites visited by the Committee, symptomatic stage 4 patients were required to await a CD4 cell count before initiation of treatment, a sometimes lethal delay. Since CD4 cell count determinations are not available in the majority of treatment sites, PEPFAR can effectively address this issue by supporting countries in ensuring that medical and paramedical personnel at ART sites understand that no CD4 cell count is needed prior to initiation of ART in people with WHO clinical stage 4 and symptomatic clinical stage 3 disease.

Preparation for ART

A practice observed in a few treatment sites was a rigid requirement for a fixed number of readiness or adherence training sessions. Such practices are problematic in areas in which patients must travel long distances and/or have no means of transportation to treatment sites, and thus can pose an insurmountable burden, especially for people with advanced AIDS. PEPFAR can address this problem by supporting treatment sites in building reasonable flexibility into such preparatory programs.

Resistance Monitoring

Although results from the current limited surveillance will be helpful in determining the loci for more extensive resistance testing, the Coordinator has determined that it is now time to establish a more effective, systematic means of resistance monitoring in carefully selected sentinel populations more broadly representative of the focus countries. Both the high cost and the requirement for relatively sophisticated laboratory equipment make it impractical to establish widespread resistance testing at all treatment sites. The Committee supports PEPFAR's plans to address the problem by establishing sentinel systems that monitor specific representative populations on a continuing basis to determine what resistance mutations are emerging and how rapidly, and by supporting the development of simple, inexpensive techniques for resistance monitoring with the potential for utilization at secondary and tertiary treatment sites.

Integration of Treatment with Prevention and Care Programs

Although PEPFAR promotes integration of ART with other needed prevention, treatment, and care services, primarily through referral, PEPFAR's programmatic division into discrete prevention, treatment, and care categories does not facilitate integrated services. The Committee observed and was told about many needed improvements in the integration of ART, for example, with counseling and testing; with treatment programs for other sexually transmitted infections, tuberculosis, and malaria; with reproductive health clinics; with home-based care programs; and with community-based programs. A particular problem resulting from the lack of integration is a disconnect between HIV testing and ART availability. The Committee visited a number of sites where large numbers of people who had been identified as HIV-positive and in need of treatment could not access it. This lack of access was due in part to the rapid scale-up of testing programs not linked to treatment sites and ARV availability. Some of the clinicians with whom the Committee met reported that knowledge of HIV infection in large numbers of people for whom no treatment was available was profoundly demoralizing to they themselves, as well as to those eligible but untreated and those already in treatment in the same areas. The need for evaluations aimed at understanding the appropriate balance between testing and treatment specifically and how to achieve better integration of programs generally is discussed in Chapter 8.

Need for Data on the Effectiveness of ART

Overall, 12- to 18-month follow-up results for ART appear to have exceeded expectations in focus countries for which adequate follow-up data are available (Stringer et al., 2006; Wools-Kaloustian et al., 2006). This, however, is an area to which more attention will need to be directed, with specific information being gathered on such critical issues as ability to return to the workforce and presence or absence of long-term side effects of ART. The effectiveness and sustainability of the PEPFAR program will be dependent on the improved quality of life and return to normal daily activities of a large proportion of patients receiving ART. Data on the effectiveness of ART exist for some cohorts of patients in the focus countries, but are not yet uniformly available. PEPFAR will need to support the focus country ART programs in making such data routinely available.

Challenges for Treatment of Children

Globally, the roll-out of ART to pediatric populations has lagged considerably behind that to adults (GAA, 2006; UNAIDS, 2006). The reasons for this are multiple, and most are currently being addressed by PEPFAR (OGAC, 2005b, 2006d). All elements of treatment have been more difficult in young children than adults. Diagnosis of HIV/AIDS in children has been limited in part because most counseling and testing programs in the focus countries have targeted primarily young adults. The general lack of linkage of prevention of mother-to-child transmission to testing of infants and small children has lessened the likelihood of identifying those who are HIV-positive at that level. Many children who are found to be HIV-positive are orphans or living with orphan heads of households, further complicating adherence to treatment regimens and follow-up clinical visits (GAA, 2006). Treatment has frequently been compromised by initial extreme shortages or absence of U.S. Food and Drug Administration (FDA)-approved generic pediatric formulations of ARVs, especially oral suspensions, which are most helpful for infants and small children, and by the fact that one of the initially utilized pediatric formulations required refrigeration (WHO, 2006a). There still are no available FDA-approved combination preparations in dosages appropriate for small children and infants. This problem is exacerbated by the fact that several focus countries have few if any pediatricians, and general practitioners are often reluctant to assume responsibility for treatment of small children with HIV/AIDS. Even experienced clinicians with whom the Committee visited reported some hesitation in initiating treatment of children because of the complexity of dosing and the need to vary doses over time as the child grows.

A further complicating factor is the very high rate of HIV/tuberculosis coinfection in small children. Such coinfection has been even more common in small children than in adults in the few regions for which relevant data are available (GAA, 2006; UNAIDS, 2006). This has added to the complexity of already difficult dosing schedules. (Tuberculosis/HIV coinfection is discussed further below.)

Despite the many ongoing obstacles to treatment for children, PEPFAR has supported the initiation of pediatric ART programs in all focus countries (OGAC, 2006a,c,d,f,g).

Need for Continued Attention to Marginalized Populations

There is little data available with which to determine how successful PEPFAR-supported ART programs have been in providing access to treatment by especially vulnerable populations in whom HIV prevalence usually exceeds that of the general population. These populations include, but are not limited to, incarcerated people, people who engage in commercial sex work, men who have sex with men, and people who use injection drugs. PEPFAR reported that it is supporting a variety of ART programs that focus on these populations. However, there is a need to further develop and document such programs (see Chapter 3 for discussion of the Committee's recommendation).

Need to Address Tuberculosis/HIV Coinfection

Another large group of people who are benefiting greatly from PEPFAR programs are those coinfected with tuberculosis and HIV. The immunodeficiency associated with HIV/AIDS has fueled a rapid resurgence of tuberculosis in both children and adults throughout sub-Saharan Africa. In several focus countries, the most frequent cause of death in people with HIV/AIDS is rapidly progressive tuberculosis (Elliott et al., 1993; Harries et al., 2001). In some communities, up to 75 percent of people newly diagnosed with active tuberculosis have concomitant HIV/AIDS infection (Lawn et al., 2006), and an effective response to therapy for tuberculosis depends on concomitant treatment of HIV/AIDS. This poses a challenge, since rifampicin, one of the most effective anti-tuberculosis medications, decreases the plasma levels of several first- and second-line ARVs (Aaron et al., 2004). The Committee learned that effective dosing schedules to overcome this problem are now being introduced at PEPFAR-supported treatment sites.

PEPFAR categorizes tuberculosis/HIV coinfection and other opportunistic infections under its care category. Therefore, these issues are discussed more fully in Chapter 6.

Limited Direct Support for Nutrition

Inadequate caloric intake is a major problem in some regions of all the focus countries and has been clearly identified as a principal reason for failure of clinical response to ART in several regions (Wools-Kaloustian et al., 2006). PEPFAR has recognized this problem and supported many programs in undertaking initiatives to address it. Many patients identified as having HIV infection in the focus countries have lost considerable amounts of weight, and are severely malnourished by the time the diagnosis has been established and ART initiated. Several focus country programs are using PEPFAR funds to develop and implement innovative nutritional support programs for patients receiving ARVs, and additional sites have requested that PEPFAR provide funds to increase nutritional support.

OGAC reported that when possible, PEPFAR has been coordinating with other U.S. government partners such as the U.S. Department of Agriculture and with United Nations agencies, private volunteer organizations, and other international and local partners to ensure that nutritional support is being provided to people living with HIV/AIDS. Additionally, in cases where no other food support resources are available, PEPFAR directly funds the provision of nutritional support both to patients receiving ART and to pregnant and lactating women living with HIV/AIDS (OGAC, 2006b). Both the 2005 and 2006 Country Operational Plans describe ongoing and planned nutritional support activities, including collaborations with other, non-PEPFAR U.S. government food funding sources (see Box 5-3).

Need to Harmonize PEPFAR's ARV Purchase Requirements with National Plans

PEPFAR has a stated goal of supporting rapid scale-up of ART and is "committed to funding the purchase of the lowest-cost ARVs from any source, regardless of origin, whether copies, generic, or branded, as long as those drugs are proven safe, effective, and of high quality, and their purchase is consistent with international law" (OGAC, 2006a, p. 47). However, PEPFAR's quality assurance requirement has prevented the program from being fully harmonized with the ART programs of the focus countries and thus has limited PEPFAR's ability to support the purchase of the focus countries' first-choice ARVs.

When PEPFAR was initiated, the U.S. Global AIDS Coordinator determined that FDA approval would be the standard for assuring the quality of PEPFAR-provided ARVs. This standard differs from that of other donors—the Global Fund, the World Bank, and the agencies of the United Nations—as well as that of national HIV/AIDS programs, including those

BOX 5-3
Selected Examples of PEPFAR-Supported Nutritional Support Activities

In **Kenya,** PEPFAR is supporting a demonstration/training farm that fills food prescriptions for eligible patients. The initiative is a public–private partnership between U.S. and Kenyan organizations that involves several comprehensive HIV care clinics in urban and rural centers in western Kenya with close to 4,000 patients on ART.

In **Ethiopia,** PEPFAR coordinates with the U.S. Department of Agriculture food aid program. Funding is managed by USAID and is used to complement care programs for orphans and vulnerable children and people living with HIV/AIDS.

In **Haiti,** PEPFAR coordinates with other U.S. food assistance programs for the nutritional support of orphans.

In **Mozambique,** PEPFAR is supporting HIV-specific nutritional training for improved immune system response in people who are HIV-positive, as well as training on home garden food production specifically for resource-poor households to improve food security for those on ART.

in the focus countries, all of which rely on the WHO Prequalification of Medicines Project to assure the quality of ARVs for purchase under their programs (see Box 5-4).

The majority of the focus countries have chosen to use generic versions of ARVs in their national programs, and a number of generic ARVs have been prequalified by WHO. When PEPFAR started, however, no generic ARVs had FDA approval, and thus the focus countries were unable to use PEPFAR funds to support their purchase—particularly first-line ARVs and medications that combine two or three ARVs into one pill, known as fixed-dose combinations. Consequently, focus countries whose plans called for generic ARVs made arrangements, whenever possible, to use other sources of funding to purchase the desired generics, and used PEPFAR funds for the purchase of ARVs for which no generic version was available—primarily second-line and pediatric formulations.

Subsequently, the Coordinator supported an expedited FDA review process for generic ARVs (DHHS, 2004; DHHS et al., 2006), and since December 2004 when the first such drug was approved, more than 30 generic versions of first-line ARVs have been FDA-approved for purchase by PEPFAR, including several of the two- and three-drug fixed-dosed combinations suitable for adults as well as several pediatric formulations (FDA, 2006; OGAC, 2007). However, some of the fixed-dose combination ARVs most desired by the focus countries were approved by the FDA only within the past year (FDA, 2006). Moreover, because some focus countries rely on WHO prequalification, they require it in addition to FDA approval. To partly address this problem, the FDA has agreed to share its drug files

BOX 5-4
The WHO Prequalification of Medicines Project

The WHO Prequalification of Medicines Project started in 2001 with the mission of facilitating access to medicines that meet unified standards of quality, safety, and efficacy for HIV/AIDS, malaria, and tuberculosis. The United Nations and the World Bank support WHO prequalification as a key contribution to the United Nations' priority goal of addressing widespread diseases in countries with limited access to quality medicines. Prequalification evaluates products submitted by companies around the world according to WHO standards of quality, safety, and efficacy. When products are found to meet those standards, they are added to a list accessible to United Nations organizations, countries, and procurement agencies.

SOURCE: WHO, 2006b.

with WHO to expedite the drugs' addition to WHO's list of prequalified medicines. Nonetheless, PEPFAR's requirement for FDA approval rather than the globally accepted WHO prequalification was the most often-cited impediment to coordination and harmonization during the Committee's visits to the focus countries, and continues to limit harmonization and rapid availability of PEPFAR-supported first-line ARVs. OGAC reported that only 10 percent of all PEPFAR-supported ARV purchases were for FDA-approved generics in fiscal year 2005, increasing to 27 percent in 2006 (OGAC, 2006f, 2007). Across the focus countries in 2006, the proportion of PEPFAR-supported ARV purchases for FDA-approved generics ranged from 0 to 87 percent (OGAC, 2007).

A previous IOM Committee strongly endorsed "a rigorous, standardized international mechanism to support national quality assurance programs for antiretroviral drugs" (IOM, 2005, p. 8). The Coordinator has not yet determined whether WHO prequalification provides such a mechanism and can adequately assure the quality of generic ARVs for purchase under PEPFAR. U.S. participation in such a mechanism would improve both coordination at the global level and harmonization at the country level, and facilitate more rapid availability of ARVs.

Recommendation 5-2: To support countries' ownership of their responses to their HIV/AIDS epidemics, the U.S. Global AIDS Initiative should maintain its commitment to harmonization and participate fully in the development of harmonized procedures. To this end, the U.S. Global AIDS Coordinator should work to support World Health Organization (WHO) prequalification as the accepted global standard for assuring the quality of generic medications. Specifically, the Coordinator should provide an analysis of WHO prequalification that determines whether it can adequately assure the quality of generic antiretroviral medications for purchase under PEPFAR. If the analysis shows that WHO prequalification needs strengthening to provide a sufficient guarantee of quality for PEPFAR, the U.S. Global AIDS Initiative should work with other donors to support strengthening of the process, and work to transition from U.S. Food and Drug Administration approval to WHO prequalification as rapidly as feasible.

Human Resource Limitations

Although PEPFAR has supported the training of large numbers of health and laboratory workers, the human resource limitations facing treatment facilities are increasingly felt as treatment expands. A full discussion of human resource issues and the Committee's related recommendation can be found in Chapter 8.

Limited Laboratory Services

The focus countries have generally accepted the WHO guidelines on minimal basic laboratory requirements for initiating and monitoring ART (Gilks et al., 2006; WHO, 2006d). All focus countries have at least one functioning laboratory that can provide these essential services in a tertiary site. However, these services are not uniformly available in secondary treatment sites (provincial medical centers), are seldom available in primary sites (district medical centers), and are generally lacking in outlying rural areas in every focus country. This situation further limits the achievement of PEPFAR's treatment goals.

PEPFAR's stated goal for laboratory activities and infrastructure is to establish and support national quality-assured networks of tiered laboratory services that provide clear lines of authority and organization for the development of national laboratory policies, quality assurance programs, and standardized training and testing. PEPFAR's approach is to promote the early establishment and regular reinforcement of local referral networks both within and among implementing partners. According to 2007 PEPFAR planning direction (OGAC, 2006e), the laboratory components of Country Operational Plans should emphasize implementing partner efforts to

- Standardize laboratory best practices and provide related training.
- Provide for uniform quality assurance measures among laboratories.
- Provide for common equipment and supportive maintenance testing.
- Support a unified approach to procurement and distribution of laboratory commodities.

A previous Institute of Medicine committee recommended that donors and program managers plan and budget for laboratory activities that can foster more accurate and effective HIV diagnosis and management, using WHO's 2003 guidelines as the initial template (IOM, 2005). PEPFAR's Adult Treatment Technical Working Group advised that the focus of PEPFAR-funded laboratory services should be to support ART, and that funding and activities for laboratory services should therefore be related primarily to supporting patients at sites where they are treated. In addition, the working group advised that laboratory services should demonstrate the adequacy of physical infrastructure, trained staff, equipment, supplies, reagents, and quality assurance for diagnosing and treating HIV and opportunistic infections and evaluating drug toxicities. The working group recommended that PEPFAR promote and support a tiered, public health–focused laboratory network as part of the national laboratory strategy (OGAC, 2006h).

Strengthening the Supply Chain

Both the Leadership Act and the PEPFAR strategy recognized the life-threatening consequences of any interruption to the supply of ARVs, as well as the need to avoid waste and to address such issues as diversion and counterfeiting. During the Committee's visits, the many challenges to securing a reliable supply of ARVs and other HIV/AIDS commodities were evident across all of the focus countries, as were considerable efforts to overcome those challenges, many supported by PEPFAR. Officials in most of the countries visited reported that their ability to predict and maintain supplies had improved, often with assistance from PEPFAR. Some reported past examples of dangerous stock-outs, and all cited the difficulty of obtaining certain drugs or formulations and ongoing concern about maintaining adequate supplies.

PEPFAR has supported the strengthening of supply chain systems and initially planned to support a central supply chain management system (OGAC, 2004, 2005b, 2006b). In late 2005, PEPFAR established the Partnership for Supply Chain Management, a consortium of 17 companies (including those that had previously been providing procurement and logistical support in the focus countries) that is managed under a contract with the U.S. Agency for International Development (USAID) (see Box 5-5). The stated goal of the partnership is to support the provision of an uninterrupted supply of HIV/AIDS commodities flowing through an accountable system.

OGAC funds the central operations of the Partnership for Supply Chain Management from its budget ($15 million for the first year, which includes funds to provide technical assistance to the focus countries in planning for their supply chain needs). The rest of the partnership's funding comes from country budgets and depends on which services the Country Teams opt to purchase. OGAC reported that at the end of 2006, funding from focus country prevention, treatment, and care budgets totaled $94 million (OGAC, 2007). The contract for the Partnership for Supply Chain Management began in October 2005—too late for the 2006 planning cycle; thus its activities would, at the earliest, be part of the 2007 Country Operational Plans. However, Partnership for Supply Chain Management officials told the Committee that all 15 focus countries had opted to work with the partnership to some degree, ranging from procurement of a limited range of ARVs or laboratory supplies to procurement of almost all PEPFAR-funded commodities. Further, officials of the partnership have made initial visits to all focus countries and opened 10 country offices (OGAC, 2007). Also, as part of its effort to collaborate with other global procurement and distribution systems, the Partnership for Supply Chain Management is serving as the technical secretariat of a World Bank, Global Fund, and PEPFAR working group for joint procurement planning.

BOX 5-5
Institutions Comprising the Partnership for Supply Chain Management

- Affordable Medicines for Africa (AMFA)—Johannesburg, South Africa
- AMFA Foundation—St. Charles, Illinois, USA
- Booz Allen Hamilton—McLean, Virginia, USA
- Crown Agents Consultancy, Inc.—Washington, DC, USA
- Fuel Logistics Group (Pty) Ltd.—Sandton, South Africa
- International Dispensary Association—Amsterdam, Netherlands
- JSI Research & Training Institute, Inc.—Boston, Massachusetts, USA
- Management Sciences for Health, Inc.—Boston, Massachusetts, USA
- The Manoff Group, Inc.—Washington, DC, USA
- MAP International—Brunswick, Georgia, USA
- Net1 UEPS Technologies, Inc.—Rosebank, South Africa
- The North-West University—Potchefstroom, South Africa
- Northrop Grumman Information Technology—McLean, Virginia, USA
- Program for Appropriate Technology in Health (PATH)—Seattle, Washington, USA
- UPS Supply Chain Solutions^{SM}—Atlanta, Georgia, USA
- Voxiva, Inc.—Washington, DC, USA
- 3i Infotech, Inc.—Edison, New Jersey, USA

SOURCE: OGAC, 2007.

The Partnership for Supply Chain Management was established too recently for the Committee to be able to judge its performance fairly. However, the Committee shares a number of concerns that have been raised by various stakeholders and urges OGAC to monitor the partnership's implementation carefully to ensure that any problems that develop are addressed immediately. One concern relates to PEPFAR's requirement for FDA approval of medications purchased under the program, discussed elsewhere in this chapter. The Partnership for Supply Chain Management is subject to this requirement, which will likely limit its usefulness to many of the focus countries, its efficiency, and its ability to offer medications at the lowest possible cost.

The Committee also shares the concern expressed by stakeholders such as the advocacy group Health GAP and the Ecumenical Pharmaceutical Network—a broadly based international organization that includes many of the faith-based organizations supported by PEPFAR—that the Partnership for Supply Chain Management could undermine country capacity by creating a parallel system, and thus destabilizing rather than strengthening existing systems; having a brain drain effect by taking personnel from existing systems to work for the partnership; lacking adequate transparency in sharing plans for an exit strategy; and lacking long-term plans for sustainability (Health GAP, 2005; EPN, 2004, 2006). The Partnership for Supply Chain Management has articulated plans to address each of these concerns (Partnership for Supply Chain Management, 2006; OGAC, 2007), but it is too soon to determine how effectively it is carrying out these plans.

The Committee believes it is critical that the Partnership for Supply Chain Management not create a parallel, U.S.-controlled system, but rather strengthen existing local, national, and regional systems, as well as facilitate technology transfer and regional harmonization to ensure sustainability well beyond the life of PEPFAR. To this end, the partnership requires the ability to respond genuinely to local priorities and needs rather than imposing a uniform solution. Evaluating the effectiveness of the partnership in these terms would encourage it to operate in this manner (see Chapter 8).

CONCLUSION

PEPFAR has supported a rapid and substantial expansion of the availability of ART to men, women, and children in the focus countries and has provided support to strengthen the associated workforce, laboratory, procurement, and supply chain systems. The primary early accomplishment of the U.S. Global AIDS Initiative has been to demonstrate that HIV/AIDS services, particularly treatment, can be rapidly scaled up in resource-constrained and otherwise severely challenged environments such as those existing in the focus countries—something many had doubted could be done (UNAIDS, 2001; WHO, 2003a,b; IOM, 2005). But the impact of the expanded availability of ART on the countries' epidemics remains to be demonstrated, and further expansion of treatment and strengthening of related systems are needed. Meeting these needs will continue to be challenging, and continued support from the U.S. Global AIDS Initiative, with the improvements suggested by the Committee, will be necessary to assist the focus countries in sustaining and expanding the gains made against their HIV/AIDS epidemics.

REFERENCES

Aaron, L., D. Saadoun, I. Calatroni, O. Launay, N. Memain, V. Vincent, G. Marchal, B. Dupont, O. Bouchaud, D. Valeyre, and O. Lortholary. 2004. Tuberculosis in HIV-infected patients: A comprehensive review. *Clinical Microbiology and Infection* 10:388–398.

Calmy, A., L. Pinoges, E. Szumilin, R. Zachariah, and N. L. Ford. 2006. Generic fixed-dose combination antiretroviral treatment in resource-poor settings: Multicentric observational cohort. *AIDS* 20(8):1163–1169.

Castro, A., and P. Farmer. 2005. Understanding and addressing AIDS-related stigma: From anthropological theory to clinical practice in Haiti. *American Journal of Public Health* 95:53–59.

DHHS (Department of Health and Human Services), FDA (U.S. Food and Drug Administration), and CDER (Center for Drug Evaluation and Research). 2004. *Guidance for industry: Fixed dose combination and co-packaged drug products for treatment of HIV.* Washington, DC: DHHS.

DHHS, FDA, and CDER. 2006. *Guidance for industry: Fixed dose combinations, co-packaged drug products, and single-entity versions of previously approved antiretrovirals for the treatment of HIV.* Washington, DC: DHHS.

EPN (Ecumenical Pharmaceutical Network). 2004. *A statement of the Ecumenical Pharmaceutical Network (EPN) on the President's Emergency Plan for AIDS Relief (PEPFAR).* http://www.healthgap.org/press_releases/04/100704_EPN_PEPFAR_statement.html (accessed October 2, 2006).

EPN. 2006. *Annual report, 2005.* Kenya: EPN Publications.

Elliott, A. M., B. Halwiindr, R. J. Hayes, N. Luo, G. Tembo, L. Machiels, C. Bem, G. Steenbergen, J. O. Pobee, and P. P. Nunn. 1993. The impact of human immunodeficiency virus on presentation and diagnosis of tuberculosis in a cohort study in Zambia. *The Journal of Tropical Medicine and Hygiene* 96:1–11.

Farmer, P., F. Leandre, J. Mukherjee, R. Gupta, L. Tarter, and J. Y. Kim. 2001. Community-based treatment of advanced HIV disease: Introducing DOT-HAART (directly observed therapy with highly active antiretroviral therapy). *Bulletin of the World Health Organization* 79:1145–1151. Geneva, Switzerland: World Health Organization.

FDA (Food and Drug Administration). 2006. *President's Emergency Plan for AIDS Relief approved and tentatively approved antiretrovirals in association with the President's Emergency Plan.* http://www.fda.gov/oia/pepfar.htm (accessed October 26, 2006).

GAA (Global AIDS Alliance). 2006. *Children left out: Global community failing to scale up the prevention and treatment of pediatric HIV/AIDS.* Washington, DC: GAA.

GHC (Global Health Council). 2005. *Faith in action: Examining the role of faith-based organizations in addressing HIV/AIDS: A multi-country, key informant survey.* Washington, DC: GHC.

Gilks, C. F., S. Crowley, R. Ekpini, S. Gove, J. Perriens, Y. Souteyrand, D. Sutherland, M. Vitoria, T. Guerma, and K. De Cock. 2006. The WHO public-health approach to antiretroviral treatment against HIV in resource-limited settings. *Lancet* 368(9534):505–510.

Harries, A. D., N. J. Hargreaves, J. Kemp, A. Jindani, D. A. Enarson, D. Maher, and F. M. Salaniponi. 2001. Deaths from tuberculosis in sub-Saharan African countries with a high prevalence of HIV-1. *Lancet* 357:1519–1523.

Health GAP (Global Access Project). 2005. *Analysis of the U.S. Global AIDS Program and the PEPFAR Supply Chain Management System (SCMS).* http://www.pepfarwatch.org (accessed February 18, 2007).

Hirsch, M., F. Brun-Vezinet, B. Clotet, B. Conway, D. R. Kuritzkes, R. T. D'Aquila, L. M. Demeter, S. M. Hammer, V. A. Johnson, C. Loveday, J. W. Mellors, D. M. Jacobsen, and D. D. Richman. 2003. Antiviral drug resistance testing in adults infected with human immunodeficiency virus, type 1: Recommendations of an International AIDS Society-USA Panel. *Clinical Infectious Diseases: An Official Publication of the Infectious Diseases Society of America* 37:113–128.

IOM (Institute of Medicine). 2005. *Scaling up treatment for the global AIDS pandemic: Challenges and opportunities.* Washington, DC: The National Academies Press.

Lawn, S. D., L. Myer, L. G. Bekker, and R. Wood. 2006. Burden of tuberculosis in an antiretroviral treatment programme in sub-Saharan Africa: Impact on treatment outcomes and implications for tuberculosis control. *AIDS* 20:1605–1612.

Mills, E. J., J. B. Nachega, I. Buchan, J. Orbinski, A. Attaran, S. Singh, B. Rachlis, P. Wu, C. Cooper, L. Thabane, K. Wilson, G. H. Guyatt, and D. R. Bangsberg. 2006. Adherence to antiretroviral therapy in sub-Saharan Africa and North America: A meta-analysis. *JAMA: The Journal of the American Medical Association* 296:679–690.

Nachega, J. B., A. R. Knowlton, A. Deluca, J. H. Schoeman, L. Watkinson, A. Efron, R. E. Chaisson, and G. Maartens. 2006. Treatment supporter to improve adherence to antiretroviral therapy in HIV-infected South African Adults. *Journal of Acquired Immune Deficiency Syndromes* 206(43):S127–S133.

OGAC (Office of the U.S. Global AIDS Coordinator). 2004. *The President's Emergency Plan for AIDS Relief: U.S. five-year global HIV/AIDS strategy.* Washington, DC: OGAC.

OGAC. 2005a. *PEPFAR first annual report to Congress.* Washington, DC: OGAC.

OGAC. 2005b. *FY2005 Country Operational Plans.* Washington, DC: OGAC.

OGAC. 2006a. *PEPFAR second annual report to Congress.* Washington, DC: OGAC.

OGAC. 2006b. *PEPFAR report on food and nutrition for people living with HIV/AIDS.* Washington, DC: OGAC.

OGAC. 2006c. *Building a new public-private partnership for pediatric AIDS treatment.* http://www.state.gov/s/gac/rl/fs/2006/62974.htm (accessed August, 3, 2006).

OGAC. 2006d. *FY2006 Country Operational Plans.* Washington, DC: OGAC.

OGAC. 2006e *PEPFAR FY2007 COP resource guide.* Washington, DC: OGAC.

OGAC. 2006f. *Bringing hope: Supplying antiretroviral drugs for HIV/AIDS treatment: The President's Emergency Plan for AIDS Relief Report on antiretroviral drugs for HIV/AIDS treatment.* Washington, DC: OGAC.

OGAC. 2006g (June 12–15). *Building on successes: Ensuring long-term solutions.* Annotated version of rapporteur presentations at the President's Emergency Plan for AIDS Relief HIV/AIDS Implementers' Meeting, Durban, South Africa.

OGAC. 2006h. *Proposed plan for the Adult Treatment Technical Working Group in 2006.* Washington, DC: OGAC.

OGAC. 2007. *PEPFAR third annual report to Congress.* Washington, DC: OGAC.

Partnership for Supply Chain Management. 2006. *The supply chain management system.* http://scms.pfscm.org (accessed January 11, 2007).

Spacek, L. A., M. S. Hasan, M. R. Kamya, D. Mwesigire, A. Ronald, H. Mayanja, R. D. Moore, M. Bates, and T. C. Quinn. 2005. Response to antiretroviral therapy in HIV-infected patients attending a public, urban clinic in Kampala, Uganda. *Clinical Infectious Diseases: An Official Publication of the Infectious Diseases Society of America* 42:252–259.

Stringer J., I. Zulu, J. Levy, E. M. Stringer, A. Mwango, B. H. Chi, V. Mtonga, S. Reid, R. A. Cantrell, M. Bulterys, M. S. Saag, R. G. Marlink, A. Mwinga, T. V. Ellerbrock, and M. Sinkala. 2006. Rapid scale-up of antiretroviral therapy at primary care sites in Zambia: Feasibility and early outcomes. *JAMA: The Journal of the American Medical Association* 296:782–793.

UNAIDS (United Nations Programme on HIV/AIDS). 2001. *The global strategy framework on HIV/AIDS.* Geneva, Switzerland: UNAIDS.

UNAIDS. 2006. *2006 report on the global AIDS epidemic.* Geneva, Switzerland: UNAIDS.

WHO (World Health Organization). 2003a. *A public health approach for scaling up antiretroviral (ARV) treatment.* http://www.who.int/hiv/toolkit/arv/en/index.jsp (accessed September 7, 2006).

WHO. 2003b. *Treating 3 million by 2005, making it happen: The WHO strategy.* http://www.who.int/hiv/toolkit/arv/en/index.jsp (accessed September 7, 2006).

WHO. 2006a. *Antiretroviral therapy of HIV infection in infants and children in resource-limited settings, towards universal access: Recommendations for a public health approach.* Geneva, Switzerland: WHO.

WHO. 2006b. *Prequalification project: Ensuring the quality, safety and efficacy of HIV/AIDS medicines and diagnostics.* http://mednet3.who.int/prequal/ (accessed September 1, 2006).

WHO. 2006c. *Antiretroviral therapy for HIV infection in adults and adolescents: Recommendations for a public health approach, 2006 revision.* Geneva, Switzerland: WHO.
WHO. 2006d. *Patient monitoring guidelines for HIV and antiretroviral therapy (ART).* Geneva, Switzerland: WHO.
WHO and UNAIDS (2006). *Progress in scaling up access to HIV treatment in low- and middle-income countries, June 2006. Fact Sheet.* Geneva, Switzerland: WHO and UNAIDS
Wools-Kaloustian, K., S. Kimaiyo, and L. Diero. 2006. Viability and effectiveness of large-scale HIV treatment initiatives in sub-Saharan Africa: Experience from western Kenya. *AIDS* 20:41–48.

6

PEPFAR's Care Category

Summary of Key Findings

- As of September 30, 2006, PEPFAR was supporting care services to nearly 2.5 million people, not including orphans and other vulnerable children. Its 5-year target is care for 10 million people (including orphans and other vulnerable children, see Chapter 7). PEPFAR's care domains and the services within them are largely consistent with those recommended by the World Health Organization for comprehensive care, with several exceptions—the most notable being antiretroviral therapy, which PEPFAR places in the separate category of treatment.
- Care services include clinical, social, and spiritual care; prevention for people who are HIV-positive; psychological support; and voluntary counseling and testing—all of which are offered in a variety of settings. Counseling and testing services, however, are not counted toward PEPFAR's 5-year care target. Given its importance as the point of entry for care, prevention, and treatment, counseling and testing is being scaled up in all of the focus countries.
- The majority of care is offered in the home, but PEPFAR's model for the home-care workforce has three elements that both have advantages and present challenges: heavy reliance on World Health Organization–recommended community health workers; the focus of its training resources on existing health professionals; and heavy reliance on unpaid volunteers, who are usually familial caregivers—most often women, young girls, and elderly grandmothers. The variability in the quality and length of the training of community health workers raises concern about their ability to provide needed levels of care, particularly for patient assessments for advanced care or administration of medications. PEPFAR's training focus does not increase the pool of new health workers, contributing to heavy patient loads of paid skilled nurses. And heavy reliance on unpaid volunteers poses problems for sustainability.
- The quality of care services and the integration of care with prevention and treatment services are difficult to judge because of the great variability in the skills of service providers and the services offered. Efforts to develop and provide comprehensive services are hampered by nascent infrastructures and a lack of necessary resources and commodities, but continued efforts to improve and provide integrated, community-based, family-centered care services are needed. An issue of particular note is the comprehensiveness of PEPFAR's efforts to address the nutritional and food security needs of people living with and affected by HIV/AIDS.
- PEPFAR has encouraged Country Teams to standardize preventive care services for those living with and affected by HIV/AIDS. Preventive care services can play a vital role in keeping people healthier longer, particularly when they are not eligible for antiretroviral therapy.

Recommendation Discussed in This Chapter

Recommendation 6-1: The U.S. Global AIDS Coordinator should continue to promote and support a community-based, family-centered model of care in order to enhance and coordinate supportive care services for people living with HIV/AIDS, with special emphasis on orphans, other vulnerable children, and people requiring end-of-life care. This model should include integration as appropriate with prevention and treatment programs and linkages with other public-sector and nongovernmental organization services within and outside of the health sector, such as primary health care, nutrition support, education, social work, and the work of agencies facilitating income generation.

6

PEPFAR's Care Category

CATEGORY, TARGET, AND RESULTS

The Care Category

The President's Emergency Plan for AIDS Relief (PEPFAR) defines care as "palliative care" (see Box 6-1); care for children orphaned or made vulnerable due to HIV/AIDS (discussed in Chapter 7) is explicitly included in the definition (OGAC, 2004). The Office of the U.S. Global AIDS Coordinator (OGAC) provided further clarification of operational definitions and strategies for care in *Final Draft HIV/AIDS Palliative Care Guidance #1: An Overview of Comprehensive HIV/AIDS Care Services in the President's Emergency Plan for AIDS Relief* (OGAC, 2005c), issued in final form in February 2006.

In the United States, the term "palliative care" denotes end-of-life or hospice care provided by trained health professionals and volunteers in the last 6 months of a person's life. The definition adopted by PEPFAR is broader and based on that of the World Health Organization (WHO). According to WHO, palliative care is "an holistic approach to improve the quality of life of patients with incurable disease and their families through the prevention and relief of suffering by means of early identification and careful assessment and treatment of pain and other problems, physical, psychosocial and spiritual" (WHO, 2004c, p. 7). PEPFAR defines palliative care as encompassing five domains: clinical, psychological, spiritual, social, and preventive care for HIV-infected people. The PEPFAR definition

BOX 6-1
PEPFAR's Definition of Palliative Care

PEPFAR defines palliative care as:

> . . . patient and family-centered care [which] optimizes the quality of life of adults and children living with HIV though the active anticipation, prevention, and treatment of pain, symptoms and suffering from the onset of HIV diagnosis through death. It also provides the routine monitoring that is essential to determine the optimal time to initiate ART, but continues during and after the initiation of treatment. [It] includes and goes beyond medical management of infections, neurological, or oncological complications of HIV/AIDS to comprehensively address symptoms and suffering throughout the continuum of HIV disease. Routine, confidential counseling and testing is an essential component of palliative care to identify those who need or will need palliative care, family members who could also be infected and in need of care, and family members and partners not infected and in need of prevention.

SOURCE: OGAC, 2006d, p. 3.

is consistent with the WHO standard with several exceptions, the most significant of which are in the domain of clinical care. WHO includes both antiretroviral therapy (ART) and services to prevent mother-to-child transmission of HIV in the clinical care domain. By contrast, OGAC includes in that domain only routine follow-up to determine the best timing for initiation of ART, placing ART itself in PEPFAR's treatment category, and includes services to prevent mother-to-child transmission in the prevention category. In addition, pain management and prevention/management of opportunistic infections are funded under PEPFAR's care category, but are placed operationally under the treatment category. The Committee was unable to determine whether this creates challenges to ensuring that these services are a consistent part of home-based care and programs. OGAC also supports voluntary counseling and testing activities with funds from the care category, but the Leadership Act places these activities in the prevention category (OGAC, 2004). One last difference is what WHO describes as the domains of "socioeconomic care" and "human rights and legal support." It appears that PEPFAR combines these activities into one domain that it calls "social care." Table 6-1 shows a comparison of the WHO and PEPFAR definitions of comprehensive care; the types of providers for the services listed are shown in parentheses if they are identified.

PEPFAR divides care services into three budgeting and reporting subcategories: (1) routine care for HIV/AIDS and care for tuberculosis (TB),

(2) voluntary counseling and testing, and (3) care-related training. These services can be provided in a variety of settings, including individual homes and community facilities, such as day care centers, outpatient clinics, health centers, workplace facilities, hospice centers, and university/hospital-based centers. The Leadership Act mandates that 15 percent of all funds allocated to the focus countries be designated for palliative care services (OGAC, 2004). Funding for the care category (including funds for services to orphans and other vulnerable children) as a percentage of all resources allocated for prevention, treatment, care, and other program support activities has remained steady (see Chapter 3).

Target

Unlike the prevention and treatment categories, the care category was not assigned a specific target in the Leadership Act. The 5-year target of care for 10 million people, including orphans and other vulnerable children, was identified in the PEPFAR strategy (OGAC, 2004). Note that although millions of people have received counseling and testing services, which are seen as the point of entry for care and treatment services, OGAC is counting these people toward neither the target of 10 million people receiving care nor any other PEPFAR target.

Like the treatment target, the care target is a count of people receiving services and does not provide information about the quality or impact of those services. With the data currently available, it is not possible to determine whether the care services PEPFAR is supporting are of sufficient and equal quality, duration, and type; offered by knowledgeable and skilled providers who receive adequate and appropriate supervision at all levels (a question that applies especially to in-home volunteers and community health workers); or meet the needs of those being served. It is also difficult to determine how people served have been counted toward the care target as the definition of a person served has changed over the life of PEPFAR to become more rigorous and to be more consistent with global norms.

Results

As shown in Table 6-2, the number of people OGAC reported as having received routine care services has steadily increased each year. By fiscal year 2005, the number of people receiving routine care more than doubled. In fiscal year 2006, however, there was a decline in the number of people who received TB treatment as part of their care services, compared to the previous fiscal year. Through September 30, 2006, PEPFAR had cumulatively supported voluntary counseling and testing for nearly 19 million men, women, and children (OGAC, 2007a). Of equal significance for the

TABLE 6-1 Comparison of WHO and PEPFAR Definitions of Comprehensive Care for Adults and Children Affected by HIV/AIDS

Domain	WHO	PEPFAR
Clinical Care (accessible to everyone regardless of age and gender)	(Medical and nursing staff) • Voluntary counseling and testing • Prevention of mother-to-child transmission • Preventive therapy (opportunistic infections [OIs] and tuberculosis [TB]) • Management of sexually transmitted infections and OIs • Palliative or end-of-life care • Support systems (laboratories, drug management) • Nutritional support • Antiretroviral therapy • Health education measures • Adequate universal precautions in facilities • Postexposure prophylaxis	(Physicians, clinical officers, nurses, midwives, traditional healers, community health workers, volunteers) • Voluntary counseling and testing • Preventive therapy (OIs, TB) • Management of OIs and pain • Time-limited nutritional support for clinically malnourished people living with HIV/AIDS • Follow-up for initiation of antiretroviral therapy and support for adherence • Behavior change communication • End-of-life and bereavement care
Psychological Support (patient and family support to assist in disclosure)	• Initial and follow-up counseling services for emotional and spiritual needs • Support groups, post-test clubs • Other peer, volunteer, or outreach approaches within communities	• Mental health counseling • Family care and support groups • Support for HIV status disclosure • Bereavement care • Treatment for mood and anxiety disorders • Development and implementation of culturally and age-appropriate psychological initiatives
Socioeconomic Support (material support, economic security, food security to meet daily living needs)	• Micro-credit schemes • Housing • Food support • Helping hands in the household • Health insurance schemes • Schemes that include HIV/AIDS care and treatment • Planning and support for orphans and other vulnerable children in households and communities	Equivalent activities are in the "social care" domain (WHO's "human rights and legal support" domain—see below)

TABLE 6-1 Continued

Domain	WHO	PEPFAR
Human Rights and Legal Support (available in health facilities, communities, and in the workplace to promote equal access to care)	• Stigma and discrimination reduction • Succession planning and property protection • Participation of people living with HIV/AIDS	(PEPFAR calls this domain "social care") • Community-based support groups • Efforts to reduce stigma and discrimination • Community development and mobilization of people living with HIV/AIDS • Legal services (succession planning, legal documents, inheritance rights) • Assistance to secure government grants, housing, or health care • Linkages to food support and income generation programs • Efforts to increase community awareness of prevention, treatment, and care services • Other activities designed to strengthen affected households and communities, including income generation activities
Spiritual Care (culturally appropriate and sensitive to individual and community religious beliefs and practices)	Equivalent activities are in the "psychological support" domain	• Life reviews and assessments • Counseling related to fear, hope, forgiveness, meaning of life • Life-completion tasks
Prevention for HIV-infected Individuals	Not a separate category, but addressed by services and activities in several domains	• Counseling and testing for sero-discordant couples • Case management services • Reinforcement messages from providers for encouragement of disclosure, correct and consistent use of condoms, and attendance at support groups

SOURCE: OGAC, 2006f; WHO, 2004c.

TABLE 6-2 PEPFAR Care Results by Fiscal Year, 2004–2006

Category	Fiscal Year 2004	Fiscal Year 2005	Fiscal Year 2006
Total people receiving VCT services[a]	**1,791,900**	**4,653,200**	**6,426,500**
Routine care for HIV/AIDS (2004–2005)[b]	455,800	1,397,200	Not applicable
Routine care for HIV/AIDS (2006)[b]	Not applicable	Not applicable	2,464,000
TB treatment and care	241,100	369,000	301,600
Total people receiving care	**696,900**	**1,766,200**	**2,765,600**
Training—routine/TB care	36,700	86,000	93,900
Training—VCT	14,100	22,200	33,500
Total people receiving care-related training	**50,800**	**108,200**	**127,400**
Service outlets—VCT	2,100	4,200	6,466
Service outlets—routine/TB care	5,400	6,800	8,019

NOTE: Figures shown do not include services to orphans and vulnerable children. VCT = voluntary counseling and testing in settings not providing services to prevent mother-to-child transmission of HIV.

[a]The total number of people receiving VCT services are neither counted towards the number of people receiving care nor included in the total number of people receiving care services in this table, but people who were counseled and tested and found positive would presumably be referred to and receive care services.

[b]In 2004 and 2005, prophylaxis and treatment were excluded from routine care. In 2006, tuberculosis (TB) prophylaxis was included in the routine care indicator, and treatment of TB and HIV remained separate.

SOURCE: OGAC, 2005a, 2006b, 2007a, 2007b.

inclusion of voluntary counseling and testing in the care domain is that the Leadership Act places these services in the prevention category, although OGAC supports them with funds allocated for care (OGAC, 2004). The number of people receiving care-related training has also increased each year, with a cumulative total of more than 286, 000 people being trained. The service outlets for voluntary counseling and testing more than tripled from 2004 to 2006 and the outlets for routine and TB care have increased by more than 1,000 from year to year.

BACKGROUND: MODELS OF CARE

PEPFAR's Network Model

PEPFAR's network model (OGAC, 2004) comprises central medical facilities, district-level hospitals, and local health clinics, supplemented by private, often faith-based facilities to rapidly scale up existing palliative care services for adults, orphans, and other vulnerable children (see Chapter 2). In accordance with national health and HIV/AIDS strategies, PEPFAR intends to build long-term sustainability and capacity by strengthening network-wide linkages among central facilities, international and private donors, community-based services, and home-based programs. The aim is to deliver quality services to intended recipients while following uniform protocols for HIV/AIDS treatment and care and for referrals among the programs. The ultimate goal of the network model is to ensure that technical support and products flow from the center to care facilities at the periphery to expand coverage, especially to rural and underserved areas. In the model's description, well-functioning, adequately staffed facilities with sufficient physical infrastructure and research capabilities at the core are linked with a referral network of smaller regional hospitals and district facilities down to the community level, which features satellite clinics, mobile units, and community-based services. Facilities and staff within the network identify and refer patients needing more complex care to the more advanced central facilities. Information systems would have regular feedback loops linking facilities at all levels of the network, providing solid data to health providers and policy makers for use in decision making.

This model is mainly a medical one, with much of the emphasis being placed on free-standing clinical facilities that offer medical or health services, but not necessarily social or psychological services. The lack of attention to the latter services, whether formal or informal (such as support groups), is of concern to the Committee. OGAC has stated that implementation of the model will strengthen and utilize linkages among the levels of support, but has not articulated how this will occur. Not all facilities in a community provide the same levels and types of care (OGAC, 2004, 2005b, 2006b). Moreover, supervision of care providers is essential in all settings, particularly in home-based care, which over time has required an escalating level of skill (Foster et al., 2005). As early as the PEPFAR strategy document, PEPFAR began to articulate the approach of training and using community health workers to deliver essential supplies, including medications, to people in need in their communities (OGAC, 2004). Their training, along with that of nurses, was to include routine care, symptom management, and monitoring for treatment adherence. According to the strategy, home-based care programs have provided support to large numbers of people and because of their cost-effectiveness were to play a significant role in service delivery as part of the program's community-based approach. Yet the strategy also acknowledges that the capacity of these programs is currently limited beyond provision of the minimum standards of palliative care.

PEPFAR's intent to begin rapid scale-up of care services was founded on the use of existing services and providers. However, the strategy acknowledges that many of the health and social service systems in the focus countries need strengthening and in some cases are practically nonexistent. In addition, weak health systems could exacerbate the effects of stigma and discrimination for people accessing care (OGAC, 2004).

PEPFAR has worked with many faith-based and community-based organizations that have historically been "first responders" not only to HIV/AIDS, but also to other health and social conditions (GHC, 2005). The chronicity of HIV/AIDS taxes fragile systems of care more than any other condition. However, PEPFAR is partnering with these organizations, other donors, and the government sector to build on and strengthen national strategies, organizations, and programs to provide care and essential supplies to those in need. To this end, PEPFAR has provided technical assistance to governmental and nongovernmental organizations and training to personnel, while also expecting the Country Teams to support programs in their Country Operational Plans that are aligned with the national plans and strategies of the host governments. At the same time, PEPFAR has faced challenges in finding and funding local and central service contractors that can provide comprehensive care services. This challenge is compounded by contractors that specialize in particular services and pursue niche funding for their activities. This situation could lead to the funding of multiple contractors to roll out the essential services, and present challenges to the integration of services within the care category and between care and prevention and treatment services. PEPFAR has also attempted to build or strengthen care capacity by providing technical assistance to organizations and training to personnel for not only the provision of services, but also for advocacy for reform of human resources policy and development and expansion of access to and use of pain-relieving medications (OGAC, 2005a, 2006b).

Community-Based, Family-Centered Care

According to OGAC's palliative care guidance, community-based care is "provided in a variety of community settings, including free-standing outpatient clinics, day care centers, school- or university-based clinics, community health centers, workplace clinics, or stand-alone hospices. These delivery sites provide a wide range of interventions, including primary care, management of acute and chronic medical conditions, and supportive care" (OGAC, 2006d, p. 6). OGAC has also stated its expectation that community-based programs supported by PEPFAR establish linkages with inpatient facilities to facilitate referrals, as described in the network model. OGAC provides the example of a linkage model for community-based care consisting of "links with an orphan and other vulnerable children program, a palliative care provider, a food assistance program, a voluntary family planning program, and ART programs within the home and or community" to demonstrate how a patient can be referred to various programs to access comprehensive care at the community level (OGAC, 2006d, p. 7).

Comprehensive care does not simply denote the scope of services a program attempts to provide to intended recipients, although a wide range of support services is essential for care to be comprehensive. It is also necessary to identify specific types of services a person will need over the course of the illness, the linkages and referrals necessary to meet complex service needs, whether services are readily accessible in communities, and quality services provided by all professional and volunteer providers. Timeliness, affordability, availability, access, and cultural appropriateness are critical elements of comprehensive services (Ro et al., 2003; WHO, 2004a).

Family-centered care focuses on priorities defined by the family through its active participation and identification of problems that compromise its functioning and well-being. Family-centered care is based on a core set of values, beliefs, and principles that include compassion, timeliness of services, flexibility (one size does not fit all, especially in the context of providing core services), cultural competence, and individualization. Other characteristics of family-centered care are team planning, development, and support; a focus on outcomes; planning driven by needs; and a community-based setting (FSPC, 2004). OGAC's guidance documents and the Committee's observations during its country visits provide evidence that PEPFAR is incorporating the core principles of family-based care into its community-based approach. For example, the program is increasingly focusing on secondary preventive care services; income generation and economic stability for households; services aimed at helping people be as healthy as possible for as long as possible, with the added goal of keeping families intact; and increased flexibility in individual and community service planning, driven by the needs of the diverse communities within and across the focus countries.

As described in Chapter 2, interventions at the community level involving the active engagement and participation of the community have the greatest likelihood of success. A community-based, family-centered model of HIV/AIDS care extends from HIV diagnosis to care for orphans and other survivors. It recognizes the importance of the community context and family resources in the care of people living with HIV/AIDS. Community-based, family-centered care conceptualizes the continuum of care needs and creates and supports services to meet these needs at appropriate times. The goal is to support those living with and affected by HIV/AIDS in living as well as possible for as long as possible, which includes delaying the need for treatment through the use of preventive care services, initiating appropriate services when indicated, and maximizing the quality of life for all affected by the disease. Services may also be required at some point to support end-of-life care that focuses on appropriate pain management, dignity, grief counseling, and security for those left behind (OGAC, 2006d).

Care Planning

Care planning is initiated upon receipt of an HIV-positive test result or diagnosis of an AIDS-defining opportunistic infection, as well as identification of the stage or severity of illness to determine the immediate level of services needed. Stage of illness is often assessed by CD4 count or symptoms.

Figure 6-1 provides examples of the types of services that may be needed at the various stages of illness (based here on CD4 count). Such a continuum could also be envisioned from a different perspective with different eligibility criteria, and additional social, economic, and psychological needs for children, a family unit, a family member who is HIV-negative, a woman, or an elderly grandmother who is a caregiver. The continuum could similarly be envisioned according to the impact of each stage of disease on an entire family's needs as well as the individual's. The emphasis of services might be different, might have different starting and end points, and might be based on varying durations of need. For example, for a person who is HIV-negative and belongs to the same family as one who is HIV-positive, the continuum would emphasize primary and secondary prevention and other services needed to remain HIV-negative, including access to health care, food, housing, and potable water, with the eventual need for bereavement care. Moreover, individuals who are HIV-negative could be directly affected by the services offered to a family member who is HIV-positive. For example, a child who is HIV-negative could be the focus of succession planning, guardianship decisions, and memory book making. If an elderly grandmother is HIV-negative, she could be the one who assumes responsibility for the care of orphans and other vulnerable children.

There are challenges involved in planning, implementing, and evaluating family-centered care. Perhaps the first of these is to develop and support a culturally sensitive concept of community-based, family-centered care in which community groups are actively involved in the process of formulating and selecting services and service providers. The community is best able to profile its strengths and its contributions so as to identify the support needed to strengthen its response to the epidemic. WHO's studies on palliative care in Africa found that the most successful community initiatives for palliative care and support have been developed and implemented by communities themselves. For this reason, WHO strongly urges that "health sector actions should be community-centered, engaging communities and people living with HIV/AIDS as full and equal partners in the provision of palliative care and other responses to the epidemic. Communities, families,

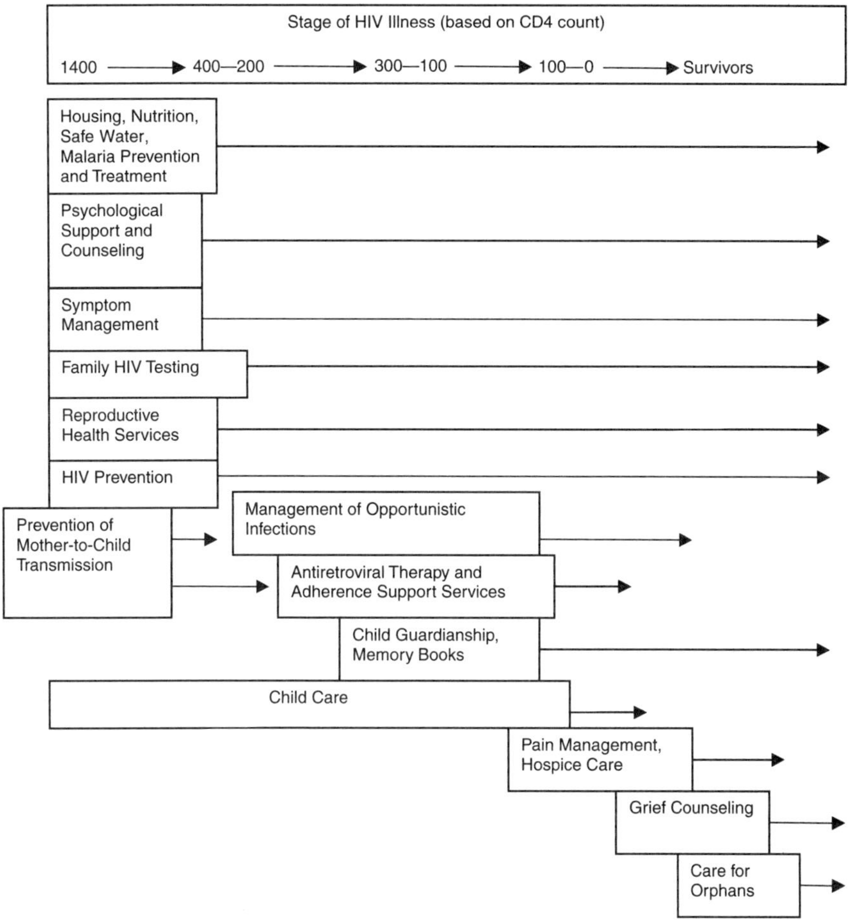

FIGURE 6-1 Stages of illness and appropriate HIV/AIDS care services.

and caregivers should be strengthened and supported in order to increase their capacity to participate in that partnership" (WHO, 2004c, p. 11). At the same time, however, long-term sustainability may be enhanced if resources support this model of care.

REVIEW OF PROGRESS TO DATE

This section reviews progress to date in the subcategories of routine care for HIV and tuberculosis, voluntary counseling and testing, and care-related training, as well as in the transition to sustainability.

Routine Care for HIV and Tuberculosis

Home-Based Care for HIV/AIDS

Home-based care can be provided by a variety of providers with varying levels of clinical and nursing care skills. Much of home-based care, by necessity, focuses on the family affected by HIV/AIDS—not only because the entire household has needs resulting from a family member having the illness, but also because the family is the primary source of support and care for sick and dying family members (WHO, 2004c; Donahue, 2005). Given the increasing demands for care as the epidemic continues to grow, PEPFAR is relying on home-based programs—which are relatively available and affordable—to provide the majority of palliative care to those in need (OGAC, 2004). Global human workforce shortages, particularly acute in Africa, exacerbate the limited availability of skilled clinicians to provide home-based care; thus the majority of this burden falls to family members, particularly women and girls. (These issues are discussed later in the chapter.)

Preventive Care for People Living with HIV/AIDS

Critical elements of a family-based preventive care package include family counseling and testing, cotrimoxazole, a safe water vessel, bed nets, TB prophylaxis, multivitamins, and home-based ART and TB care (Mermin, 2005; Yengi, 2005). As discussed below, PEPFAR supports these critical elements in its secondary preventive care service package.

In April 2006, OGAC released two sets of guidance for secondary preventive care services for both adults and children aged 0–14 born to mothers who are HIV-positive. This guidance was produced under the leadership of several of OGAC's technical working groups—the Palliative Care Technical Working Group, the Food and Nutrition Technical Working Group, and the Orphans and Vulnerable Children Technical Working Group. PEPFAR's second annual report to Congress acknowledged the difficulty of determining or assessing the quality of care services. These guidance documents represent an attempt to address this problem by encouraging the implementation of standardized preventive care services in palliative care programs (OGAC, 2006b).

Preventive care services have reduced mortality and morbidity not only for those living with HIV/AIDS, but also for their family members and children. Parental death associated with HIV/AIDS has been found to triple the risk of death of HIV-negative children in the home, while cotrimoxazole prophylaxis has been shown to decrease mortality for children younger than age 10 if their parent/caregiver is HIV-positive. Moreover, no association has been found between prophylaxis and increased antimicrobial resistance among diarrheal pathogens infecting family members. For US$4 per year, clean water and storage in the home can reduce diarrheal days and episodes. Moreover, bed nets that cost about US$5 can prevent malaria and its complications and reduce malarial prevalence among children who are HIV-negative (nets have seldom been tested for beneficial use with adults who are HIV-positive) (Mermin, 2005; Yengi, 2005). Malaria is an opportunistic infection of particular concern in developing countries. Abu-Raddad and colleagues (2006), for example, found that transient and repeated increases in viral load resulting from recurrent coinfection with malaria may play an important contributory role in the spread of HIV in sub-Saharan Africa.

OGAC has acknowledged the unlikelihood that packages of care services can be standardized for all situations and countries, given variations in setting and in the capacity of partners who are implementing programs (OGAC, 2006f). In accordance with the principle of one national action framework, as well as alignment with international standards, OGAC has specifically acknowledged that "prioritization and selection of components of a preventive care package must be performed locally, and should be consistent with national guidelines and those sponsored by the World Organization operative within the country" (OGAC, 2006f, p. 3). OGAC's guidance documents clarify specific preventive care services PEPFAR will fund directly, as well as their expectations for linking preventive care interventions to other key health care services, such as routine medical care and voluntary family planning (see the discussion of integration of services later in the chapter). Directly funded services for both adults and children (unless otherwise specified) include the following (OGAC, 2006f):

- Technical assistance for developing guidelines and training for the use and provision of cotrimoxazole for prophylaxis of Pneumocystis pneumonia and diarrhea.
- Effective TB interventions for people living with HIV/AIDS including skin tests, treatment of latent TB infection for adults who are HIV-positive and exposed/infected children, screening for active TB, and referral and linkage to TB diagnostic and treatment centers.
- Services related to safe drinking water and personal hygiene, including provision of supplies to treat and store water, soap, and instructions for hand washing.
- Provision of insecticide-treated nets (via linkages with the President's Malaria Initiative and the Global Fund for the Treatment of AIDS, Tuberculosis and Malaria).
- Nutrition services and micronutrient supplementation, including daily supplements for people living with HIV/AIDS—especially pregnant

women, lactating women, and children, as indicated by dietary assessments—as well as nutrition counseling linked to clinic- and home-based care.

- Services and counseling to prevent transmission of HIV to others, including technical assistance for developing national policies and training for the implementation of prevention programs; ongoing counseling for people living with HIV/AIDS related to behavior change; and provision of condoms and referrals to other preventive services, such as family planning and clinics for the diagnosis and treatment of sexually transmitted infections.
- HIV counseling and testing of family members and other contacts, including sero-discordant couples, sex partners of people who are HIV-positive, and referrals to care and prevention services for those who are identified as HIV-positive.

Management of Opportunistic Infections

HIV/AIDS weakens a person's immune system and its ability to fight disease. As a result, many people who are HIV-positive develop bacterial, mycobacterial, fungal, protozoan, and viral infections, as well as neurological conditions, malignancies, and other conditions and complications (e.g., mood and anxiety disorders, wasting syndrome) as they progress through the continuum of the disease (AVERT, 2006). Many of these conditions are called "opportunistic infections" because they take advantage of the opportunity offered by a weakened immune system (the example of malaria was noted above). People with healthy immune systems may contract the same diseases, but people living with HIV/AIDS have a more difficult time recovering from them. One of the goals of clinical HIV care is to quickly assess and manage opportunistic infections to keep patients as healthy as possible for as long as possible. Highly active antiretroviral therapy (HAART) can reduce the amount of HIV in the body and restore immune functioning. In resourced-constrained settings where access to HAART may be limited, however, and in some cases even where HAART is available, diagnosis and treatment of opportunistic infections remains essential to improve health. Prevention of opportunistic infections is, of course, optimum, and in some cases may be achieved by avoiding pathogens that may be found in water sources, uncooked food, domestic animals, and human excrement. While PEPFAR usually addresses medical management and prophylaxis of opportunistic infections in its treatment category, it also addresses prophylaxis through activities under its secondary preventive care package related to safe drinking water, personal hygiene, and training in and use of cotrimoxazole.

Tuberculosis Treatment and Prophylaxis

The global incidence of TB continues to rise, and rates of the disease are growing exponentially in Africa because of the HIV/AIDS epidemic. Given that 50–80 percent of TB patients in sub-Saharan Africa are HIV-positive (OGAC, 2006e), TB clinics are seen as important entry points for identifying candidates for both TB treatment and initiation of ART. In some countries, nurses and lower-level workers are able to provide voluntary counseling and testing for HIV/AIDS for TB patients, but in others they are prohibited from doing so by legislative or policy restrictions. While the uptake of these services is high in some focus countries, fewer than 10 percent of TB patients know their HIV status (OGAC, 2006e). Additional challenges are in adequate diagnostic capability in resource-poor settings; prohibitive patient fees associated with some diagnostics; the difficulty of diagnosing children; the complexity of managing coinfected patients on ART (especially pregnant women); limited or no access to care and treatment because of weak referral systems; costs to patients of services from multiple sites; the dissonance between centrally provided HIV/AIDS services and TB services delivered at the primary care level; nonstandardized TB screening; and limited use of or nonexistent standard surveillance and reporting systems for comorbidities and exposure (OGAC, 2006e). Innovative approaches for addressing these challenges include co-locating services in the same facility, especially in TB clinics and during directly observed therapy in HIV clinics; using mobile units in rural areas; and using community and home-based services to jointly supervise ART and TB treatment. Limited data are available about the consistent provision of routine testing for people exposed to and being treated for TB; as well as about the frequency and success of co-located testing and TB services in PEPFAR-supported programs. The United States and WHO have worked together to formulate strategies for joint TB/HIV activities at the international, national, and subnational levels, but WHO's new algorithms for accelerating diagnosis of sputum smear–negative TB are presenting their own challenges (OGAC, 2006e).

Voluntary Counseling and Testing

Definition

WHO defines voluntary counseling and testing as a confidential dialogue between a client and a care provider aimed at enabling the client to cope with stress and to make personal decisions related to HIV/AIDS (Rehle et al., 2000). According to international standards, dedicated programs for counseling and testing for diagnostic purposes are a critical component of a comprehensive approach to HIV/AIDS care and support (WHO, 2004c).

Voluntary counseling and testing can be offered in a variety of settings—static settings such as clinics and hospitals, or alternative settings such as the home and mobile vans that travel throughout communities. Sessions at PEPFAR's third annual meeting in Durban, South Africa, revealed that the uptake of mobile voluntary counseling and testing is high—much higher compared with static sites. Other data presented at the meeting showed that the availability of routine and diagnostic voluntary counseling and testing in clinical settings leads to high uptake—as high as 97 percent in some hospitals—with 55 percent of patients tested being HIV-positive (OGAC, 2006d). Moreover, many programs are offering couples counseling and testing (OGAC, 2006d), although limited data exist on the uptake of these services. Voluntary counseling and testing has several components, including group or individual pretest education, individual pretest counseling, and individual post-test counseling. In pretest education, a health educator can provide basic information about HIV/AIDS and safer sex and reinforcement messages about behavior change, as well as answer questions and recognize the need for individual counseling and referral. Pretest counseling can be used to clarify information from pretest educational sessions and provide all the information a person needs to give informed consent for the actual testing. Post-test counseling focuses on providing positive, negative, or inconclusive test results to the individual. Counselors are trained to expect a range of emotional responses regardless of the test result; to be prepared to make referrals for prevention, treatment, and care services; to provide risk reduction information and disease education; to provide information on and support for serostatus disclosure; and to be prepared to provide several counseling sessions to the individual if needed (WHO, 2004b). During the Committee's country visits, interest was expressed at the country level in moving toward conducting more group pretest education in hopes of making pretest counseling sessions more efficient, which in turn could help increase the number of people who can be tested. Such group pretest education would not replace individual pretest counseling.

Although funded under the care category, voluntary counseling and testing also plays an important role in prevention and treatment. It can be used for case finding for care, prevention, and treatment services. In prevention, for example, estimating HIV prevalence and targeting prevention messages to people who are both HIV-negative and HIV-positive based on serologic and behavioral surveys are critical activities. In treatment, voluntary counseling and testing is helpful for identifying those eligible for ART. In care, voluntary counseling and testing can be used to identify those in need of palliative care, particularly those not eligible for ART or for whom ART is not available. There may be additional objectives for voluntary counseling and testing, such as supporting surveillance, promoting behavior change, enabling public education, and functioning as a gateway to facilitate referrals to treatment and care services (Rehle et al., 2000). To date, the number of people tested exceeds the numbers who have received care services (OGAC, 2005a, 2006b).

Testing of Infants

PEPFAR is using various methods to identify HIV-exposed or infected children who are in need of services, including pediatric treatment. To advance testing and diagnosis of infants (6 weeks and older) who are HIV-exposed and HIV-positive, PEPFAR is collaborating with some of its implementing partners to pilot and develop the use of dried blood spot testing with polymerase chain reaction testing in several focus countries (OGAC, 2006b; Kaiser Family Foundation, 2006). Previously and with a different testing method, infants were tested at 18 months when they could already be at an advanced stage of the disease. In 2006, one PEPFAR focus country that successfully conducted pilot dried blood spot testing programs in 11 clinics and 1 referral hospital received $54 million from PEPFAR to support the continuation of the testing program (Kaiser Family Foundation, 2006). Results of the country's PEPFAR-supported pilot studies presented at the 16th International AIDS Conference indicate that dried blood spot testing is not only diagnostically specific and sensitive, but also cost-effective because of the simplicity of the supplies and skills needed to perform the procedure: a finger prick (versus phlebotomy) provides enough of a blood sample, the samples (which do not need refrigeration) are dried on a paper card, and they are sent by courier envelope to the nearest testing facility. Given this simplicity, the investigators estimated that a technician could perform 13,000 such tests annually (Gass et al., 2006). The success of this testing method thus has important implications for the scaling up of infant testing and treatment. PEPFAR has supported the adoption of national policies to incorporate dried blood spot testing to improve diagnosis of HIV in infants in 10 of the focus countries (OGAC, 2007a).

Ethical issues are associated with HIV testing for infants, as well as older children and adolescents. Of concern is disclosing positive test results of infants and younger children, which indicate the positive serostatus of their biological mothers, who may not yet have been tested or consented to testing. The major issue of access to children and adolescents to be tested is compounded by other issues, including how to determine at what age obtaining informed consent is appropriate, how to know when a child or adolescent can understand the information provided and discussed in the counseling session well enough to give informed consent, what potential consequences disclosing test results can have, and whether it is appropriate to disclose results to the child or adolescent (HIV Insite, 2006).

Capacity Issues for Counseling and Testing

OGAC has reported that a growing number of best practices for sustainability and scaling up of quality counseling and testing have been identified to assist Country Teams and implementing partners (OGAC, 2006b). PEPFAR is increasing its support to countries in their efforts to integrate counseling and testing into routine care as a means of scaling up testing efforts, especially in programs for pregnant women, clinics that treat TB and sexually transmitted infections, hospitals, and other clinical settings (OGAC, 2006b). PEPFAR is also supporting what it describes as local initiatives to scale up counseling and testing—among them, home-based testing that can test all family members, testing programs for partners or couples, mobile testing, and hotlines linking callers to test sites. PEPFAR has increased its support for the use of rapid tests by encouraging country teams to include such testing in their national plans.

Care-Related Training

The majority of care-related training has been in-service training or retraining for existing health workers, including community health workers (OGAC, 2006b). It is difficult to determine the ratio of in-service to preservice training supported by PEPFAR, as well as whether the training being provided is exponentially increasing the number of skilled or lay workers and paid or unpaid health workers, because information is generally unavailable on the categories of workers involved (nurses, clinical officers, physicians, community health workers, home health workers, and familial caregivers), the type of remuneration, whether the workers are being newly trained or retrained, and whether the same workers are being retrained. There is also little information available about the content of the training curriculum; whether people are completely, partially, or serially trained in knowledge and skill development to provide comprehensive care in home-based settings; and whether those trained receive backup and ongoing supervision from trained health workers, such as nurses.

Preservice support includes curriculum development by incorporating HIV/AIDS care into nursing school curricula, and in some cases a limited number of scholarships and postgraduate fellowships (OGAC, 2006c). Preservice support for highly skilled health workers is expensive and takes several years to produce a newly trained professional. The demand for care in both community and home-based programs necessitates an examination of the contributions made by all donors to human capacity development.

While PEPFAR acknowledges that the ultimate solution to workforce issues rests with the host country, and while PEPFAR may be contributing its fair share to support preservice training, the ratio of in-service to preservice support may need to be re-examined as the program continues.

PEPFAR is relying on the community health worker model of care for a variety of reasons, but primarily because its use can rapidly scale up the immediate pool of people available to provide services. As the term implies, the workers are community members who work in community settings and serve as a liaison between those who need health services and those who provide the services. Community workers often provide basic health services while promoting the key principles of primary health care—equity, multisectoral collaboration, and the use of appropriate technology (JLI, 2004). The goal of the community health worker model is to promote health among those populations and groups who have traditionally lacked access to adequate health and social services, usually due to lack of both financial and human resources. These communities are usually unable to maintain a health program of their own (Ro et al., 2003; UNICEF and WHO, 2006). In the majority of these programs, the communities are not responsible for the initiation and implementation of the program. Their role is mainly participating in some aspects of development (if they are involved in early program planning), implementation, and maintenance of programs (UNICEF and WHO, 2006). Though there are concerns about the reliance on volunteers to scale up care services, as well as some hard-learned consequences when utilizing this model, this model has successfully demonstrated the effectiveness of community health workers in helping underserved individuals access health services in appropriate ways (Ro et al., 2003). In Ethiopia alone, PEPFAR has supported the national strategy of training more than 30,000 community health workers to be placed throughout 15 regions, serving 5,000 people per area (Dybul, 2006; OGAC, 2006c).

Policy reforms supported by PEPFAR—including task shifting and altering the scope of practice for some highly skilled health workers to prioritize and increase the time they can spend providing more complex clinical care—reinforce the use of the community health worker model. Other salient policy reform activities include advocacy for eliminating mandatory retirement for skilled health workers, especially nurses, who are being re-employed to provide clinical services (OGAC, 2006c). Task shifting permits less specialized but trained health workers to assume some of the tasks of those who are more specialized. Examples of task shifting specifically related to care activities include using community health workers to offer counseling and testing services so that nurses can provide other, more complex clinical services. In some focus countries, laws have been changed to allow specially trained nurses or clinical medical officers to prescribe ARVs and medications for management of opportunistic infections, and some community health workers to administer pain-relieving medications, cotrimoxazole prophylaxis, and other treatments for opportunistic infections to enable widespread distribution of services in community and home-based programs. Other community health workers are trained to provide nursing care; deliver refills of medications for ART and treatment of TB and opportunistic infections to patients' homes; monitor adherence to these medications; provide condom education; engage in health promotion; provide compassionate end-of-life care; and offer peer support to meet the psychosocial needs of people living with HIV/AIDS, orphans, and other vulnerable children (OGAC, 2006c). PEPFAR also uses formal partnerships among ministries of health, organizations for people living with HIV/AIDS, and community-based organizations to enable people living with HIV/AIDS to be trained as community health workers who can provide adherence support and prevention services.

Transition from Emergency Aid to Sustainability

During its initial roll-out, PEPFAR utilized established providers that were either already providing similar services or had historically been involved in medical or social health services and held the trust of many people in the communities in which they operated. This translated into a heavy reliance on international nongovernmental organizations, including community- and faith-based organizations (OGAC, 2005a, 2006b). Over its years of operation, PEPFAR has engaged in many activities aimed at building the capacity of communities to plan, implement, and monitor care services. These activities have included providing small grants for local organizations to provide services; strengthening referral systems for social service needs; and supporting the development and operation of networks for people living with HIV/AIDS to be involved in not only the provision of care, but also the development of long-term sustainable programs (OGAC, 2005a, 2006b).

ISSUES AND OPPORTUNITIES FOR IMPROVEMENT

The Committee identified issues and opportunities for improvement in PEPFAR's care category in the following areas: home-based care programs, addressing the psychosocial and spiritual needs of people affected by HIV/AIDS, reliance of volunteers, pain management, addressing the needs of women and girls, voluntary counseling and testing, and integration of services. However, limited data are available about the consistent provision of voluntary counseling and testing as part of home-based services in PEPFAR-supported programs.

Home-Based Care Programs

In addition to coping with the physical and emotional demands of caregiving, according to OGAC, all home-based caregivers also need to learn skills necessary to recognize symptoms of advancing disease or opportunistic infections; to determine whether patients need more advanced care and know how to access the needed services from wherever they may be available; to administer medications; to employ universal precautions to minimize risk exposure for the entire household; to be able to arrange or provide transportation and child care to the extent available; to communicate with the patient and other caregivers, both formal and informal; and to provide emotional support for those who are ill. OGAC recognizes that many home-based care services and programs lack a number of these critical aspects of care (OGAC, 2006d). Therefore, OGAC's palliative care guidance specifically acknowledges that the introduction of comprehensive care into home-based programs requires training and education of medical providers (nurses, clinical officers and physicians, including pediatric nurses and physicians), and community care providers (see Box 6-2).

BOX 6-2
Training Specifications for Introducing Comprehensive Care into PEPFAR Home-Based Programs

- **Clinical diagnosis and care:** assessment and management of pain, symptoms, and opportunistic infections.
- **Medication delivery:** delivery of pain medication and other clinical interventions within the community and home.
- **Basic nursing care:** patient and household hygiene and promotion of disease prevention in the home.
- **Patient protocols:** use of established patient management protocols and standards.
- **Referral procedures:** use of such procedures for diagnostics, care, and treatment.
- **Communication skills:** patient education in local languages on HIV/AIDS and HIV prevention; counseling on disclosure of HIV status; and grief, anxiety, and bereavement care.
- **Interdisciplinary teams:** established to address physical, psychosocial, and spiritual needs of clients.
- **Quality care:** use of other standards and procedures to provide quality care.

SOURCE: OGAC, 2006d.

The Country Operational Plans and PEPFAR's strategic documents, guidance, and annual reports do not provide adequately detailed information on the extent to which PEPFAR is conducting this training and building this capacity at the home and community levels. Concern has been raised in particular, however, about the training received by community health workers. Although there are no international or national certifications for community health workers (OGAC, 2006c), the Committee is concerned about the variability of their training in both quality and length, as well as about the levels of ongoing supervision these workers receive, especially if they are providing the services PEPFAR has identified as critical to the provision of comprehensive care in community- and home-based settings. During country visits, the Committee heard from program implementers about a lack of timely and comprehensive programmatic guidance for family-based care services, which has resulted in delays in program planning, implementation, and evaluation, as well as great variability in the type, quantity, and quality of care services throughout the focus countries. On the African continent in particular, the Joint Learning Initiative has reported that community health workers have taken on more specialized roles in the areas of malaria control, reproductive health, and nutrition and have increased their coverage of a range of services over the last three decades; they have also assumed broader roles as change agents and community advocates. The Joint Learning Initiative has also suggested that historical constraints on the effectiveness of the community health worker model have included lack of attention to primary care and a lack of government support (JLI, 2004). PEPFAR could address some of these issues by building on the recommendations of WHO and the Joint Learning Initiative, which include improving the design, management, monitoring, and evaluation of community health worker programs, with greater emphasis on support, supervision, and community participation and ownership (JLI, 2004).

Addressing the Psychosocial and Spiritual Needs of People Affected by HIV/AIDS

Despite treatment for HIV/AIDS, the burden of pain persists, and people with HIV/AIDS continue to have psychological and spiritual needs. PEPFAR has identified resources necessary to meet these needs in providing care (OGAC, 2004). During the Committee's country visits, however, these services appeared to be the least visible and in need of greater emphasis.

Complications of advanced disease can include neurological sequelae that can result in cognitive, affective, and motor dysfunctions that occur in up to 90 percent of people who are HIV-positive (Kalichman, 1995). Makoae and colleagues (2005) have documented the number and complexity of symptoms experienced by people in sub-Saharan Africa who are

HIV-positive, from initial diagnosis through late-stage illness. According to Holzemer (2002), the available evidence indicates that the term "asymptomatic" as used by the medical community is an unsatisfactory description of the experience of living with symptoms early in the course of HIV infection.

Emotional and spiritual needs include those arising from environmental, physical, and social stressors, as well as grief and bereavement; culturally appropriate treatment of existing or new mood and anxiety disorders; treatment of other mental disorders, including substance abuse and addiction; and the need to deal with issues related to meaning of life, control, and self-esteem. Several studies have documented the challenges faced by people living with HIV infection as they attempt to manage common symptoms, including peripheral neuropathy (Nicholas et al., 2007), fatigue (Corless et al., 2002), depression (Eller et al., 2005), and anxiety (Kemppainen et al., 2006).

Social sequelae can include having to deal with fears of contagion, sickness, and death, as well as with stigma and discrimination, and the need to develop coping strategies (Kalichman, 1995). Harding and colleagues (2005) report that despite treatment, there is the recognition that the burden of pain continues and people with HIV continue to have psychological and spiritual needs, though community burden in providing home care and psychological needs are under explored (Harding et al., 2005). Coleman et al. (2006) describes how prayer is often used as a symptom management strategy for people living with HIV in an ethnically diverse sample.

Reliance on Volunteers

An important issue related to care is the heavy reliance on volunteers to provide home-based care. Many of these are women, young girls, and elderly grandmothers who are "default volunteers" by virtue of their cultural roles and status as familial caregivers. In Africa, women are typically responsible for health care; produce 70 percent of the food consumed; and are more likely to use their incomes to meet children's needs, including schooling. Children are likely, in the short term, to replace the labor of a women who dies (Donahue, 2005), and are often as vulnerable and in as much need of assistance as the people for whom they are caring. The phenomenon of these women and girls, and countless thousands more, who are helping those in greater need has been described as "the poor helping the destitute" (Donahue, 2005, p. 38). Anecdotal evidence suggests that they may be unable to continue in these roles for long for a variety of reasons, including burnout, lack of resources for support, increasing needs for care, failing health, and aging.

Because of their critical importance to community- and home-based care, the sustained use of volunteers for the provision of care is a worthy subject for targeted evaluation. Harding and colleagues (2005) found that the reliance of African palliative care services on volunteers to provide community and home-based care has been largely successful for palliative care, but that community capacity and the resources and clinical supervision necessary to sustain quality care are lacking. They note that it is not yet clear how much trained professional input is needed for supervision of lay workers and patients, what the community's maximum capacity for care is, and what level of skills can be expected from lay workers providing palliative care. Further exploration of these issues is critical to the sustainability of community and home-based services.

Some PEPFAR-supported partners who were operating prior to the program's initiation described to the Committee retention and assistance strategies for volunteers, which to some degree mirror PEPFAR's retention strategies for highly skilled health workers. These strategies include providing transportation to places where care services are offered, reimbursing volunteers' health expenses, providing ART for those in need, and offering psychosocial support. These strategies are not widespread, however, and not all organizations have the resources to adopt them. Some suggest that all volunteers be paid with some form of remuneration, but the effects this might have on the management and sustainability of community and country programs are unknown. Regardless of what strategies are adopted, it would be sensitive of PEPFAR to strike an appropriate balance with the cultural beliefs and customs of familial caregiving for ill and dying family members.

Pain Management

Issues related to pain management include government policies related to the availability of opioids in many types of care settings, professional practice standards that specify who is legally allowed to administer pain medications, and concerns about the illegal redirection of medications made available for pain management (OGAC, 2006d) As previously mentioned, management of pain symptoms is included in PEPFAR's care category, but is operationalized in the treatment category (OGAC, 2004).

Seminal research conducted by WHO (2004c) and Harding and Higginson (2005) examined palliative care and pain management in sub-Saharan Africa in the hopes of illuminating issues and practices that could reduce "the historical inadequacy of pain and symptom control in HIV/AIDS home based-care, which has been called 'home-based neglect'" (Harding and Higginson, 2005, p. 1973). Harding reports that there continues to be misperceptions that ART obviates the need for palliative care; whereas better integration of palliative care in HAART programs is needed (Harding and Higginson, 2004, 2005). Additional research by Harding and colleagues (2005) found significant limitations in and a pressing need for the expansion of current HIV/AIDS palliative and end-of-life care. According to the authors, among the five key strategies needed, "pain control remains a primary challenge [that must be addressed] and requires development of pain medication regulation, procurement and distribution polices, and education of health professionals, community workers, and affected people in their purpose and use" (Harding et al., 2005, p. 5). Since traditional healers are often the first point at which help is sought by both cancer and HIV patients, it is suggested that alliances be forged between traditional healers and palliative care providers; the authors note that educational programs for traditional healers have been associated with improved support for patients with HIV (Harding and Higginson, 2004, 2005). PEPFAR is supporting initiatives to build alliances between traditional healers and other health professionals, but the extent of these partnerships throughout the focus countries is unknown.

OGAC has provided specific guidance on pain management for children. According to this guidance, pain management for children should follow the principles of the WHO analgesic ladder, but special attention should be paid to nonverbal symptoms associated with pain and its intensity, since children often are not able to describe pain adequately to permit appropriate treatment (OGAC, 2006g).

During PEPFAR's third annual meeting in Durban, it was noted that many patients and providers report that pain is undertreated in the majority of patients surveyed, and the African Palliative Care Association, a major south-to-south twinning partner, has reported that opioids are unavailable to the majority of providers—in some cases, even mild analgesics are unavailable for adequate pain management (OGAC, 2006e). The Palliative Care Technical Working Group's fiscal year 2006 plan identified intentions to "gather and disseminate information on simplified tools to ascertain severity of symptoms and pain related to HIV disease in resource poor settings and encourage support for the development of template curricula for pain/symptom management" (OGAC, 2006g, p. 19). The plan also indicated intentions to participate in a number of national and international symposia to learn more about the latest innovations in palliative care, including the 7th Clinical Team and Conference and Scientific Symposium of the National Hospice and Palliative Care Organization in April 2006 (OGAC, 2006g).

Harding and Higginson (2005, p. 1975) note that "palliative care worldwide has been evolving to address integrated management of patients through the course of the disease." They suggest that funders may wish to consider opportunities to improve patient management.

Addressing the Needs of Women and Girls

PEPFAR has expressed a commitment to increasing gender equity in all of its interventions in partnership with both national governments and the civil sector (OGAC, 2005a, 2006b). Women and girls have a number of needs to be met in any concerted and effective response to HIV/AIDS. Many advocates emphasize the urgency of focusing on inheritance and property rights for women and girls since increased financial independence would not only reduce their vulnerability to HIV exposure, but also improve their ability to serve successfully as head-of-households after the death of their male spouses/partners, fathers, and adult children (ICRW, 2005; UNAIDS and UNICEF, 2004; UNICEF, 2006).

Of particular importance given the emphasis of family-centered care is that many women, young girls, and elderly grandmothers may need services while simultaneously serving as primary caregivers for other ill and dying family members. Interventions are necessary to reduce their vulnerability to HIV infection, as well as to enhance their ability to shoulder the long-lasting, caregiving burden. It may be unreasonable to expect women and girls to manage the physical and emotional demands of end-of-life care without skilled assistance. Moreover, women and girls, as well as other caregivers, frequently rely on their community network for assistance, which makes strong, effective, and comprehensive community-based care a necessity.

Restoration of fertility for women on ART is a growing phenomenon with some programs reporting that up to 90 percent of the pregnancies among HIV-positive women are unplanned pregnancies and 81 percent of those unplanned pregnancies are among the women receiving ART. It is essential to address linkages among HIV/AIDS treatment and care, reproductive health, and family planning services (OGAC, 2006e). Strategies are needed to support women in voluntary family planning and reproductive health, which requires integration with prevention of mother-to-child transmission of HIV, voluntary counseling and testing in family planning settings, access to ART and other necessary medications, and care in community- and home-based settings. As part of its commitment to addressing the needs of women and girls, PEPFAR has articulated opportunities for developing such linkages. While PEPFAR funds for contraception are restricted to the purchase of condoms, linkages to existing family planning and reproductive health programs are encouraged (OGAC, 2006h). Reproductive health covers a broad range of women's health issues, including the detection and treatment of sexually transmitted infections and support for the desire of a woman or couple who are HIV-positive or a sero-discordant couple to have children safely (Fleischman, 2006). In addition, integration with treatment programs and training of ART providers to meet the reproductive health needs of their clients may be critical in addressing family planning needs since 61 percent of those receiving ART are women (OGAC, 2005a,

2006h). Conversely, if programs are not implemented with sensitivity to these issues, both women and men may drop out of care and treatment.

PEPFAR's 5-year strategy includes a clear commitment to addressing gender issues and reducing the vulnerability of women and girls to HIV/AIDS (OGAC, 2004). However, program results for voluntary counseling and testing is the only category that is currently required to be disaggregated by gender. Much of the gender focus in counseling and testing for diagnostic purposes is in initiatives to prevent mother-to-child transmission. By the end of fiscal year 2006, OGAC reports that cumulatively 70 percent of those receiving counseling and testing services supported by the U.S. government in prevention of mother-to-child and all other settings were women (OGAC, 2007a).

Voluntary Counseling and Testing

The past 2 years has seen increasing interest in moving toward a model of counseling and testing that makes the HIV test a routine part of medical care. In 2004, both the United Nations Programme on HIV/AIDS (UNAIDS) and WHO recommended that "health care providers routinely offer HIV testing to all patients seen in clinical and community-based health service settings where HIV is prevalent and antiretroviral therapy is available (WHO, 2006, p. 11). Such provider-initiated testing also gives the patient the opportunity to refuse the test or "opt out." While OGAC has stated that PEPFAR will promote and support routine or opt-out testing in appropriate settings, particularly for prevention of mother-to-child transmission (OGAC, 2006b), human rights advocates have raised concern as to whether people are truly able to provide informed consent and not be coerced to undergo testing. This concern appears to stem from questions about whether patients are ready for disclosure of their status and whether stigma, discrimination, and even violence against women may result from undergoing the test and receiving the results (HIV Insite, 2006). Questions also arise about how and whether expanded programs can provide the right amount of information during counseling sessions when human resources are stretched and whether marginalized populations would become more vulnerable to human rights abuses if testing became routine. Other ethical issues, raised above with respect to children and adolescents, include discerning when people are the appropriate age to give consent, when they can understand the information provided and discussed in the counseling session well enough to give informed consent, and given the potential consequences, whether it is appropriate to disclose results to the person being tested.

OGAC has reported several key barriers to counseling and testing, including a lack of routine availability of the services in health care settings, stigma and discrimination, shortages of laboratory personnel, long distances of patients from testing sites, inadequate access to providers, and lack of availability of rapid tests (OGAC, 2006b). At PEPFAR's third annual meeting, several challenges related to scaling up counseling and testing services were identified, including shortages of test kits; lengthy pretest counseling sessions; referrals for care, support, and treatment for difficult-to-reach populations; logistical complications associated with the increased demand for mobile services; and lack of consensus on age of consent for HIV testing and how to communicate HIV test results to children (OGAC, 2006d). OGAC reported that 30–40 million counseling and testing sessions are needed to meet their treatment target of 2 million people. PEFAR efforts to scale-up and integrate counseling and testing services include linking counseling and testing to other HIV services, improving access to these services for the general population, and home-based testing and door-to-door counseling to reach families and sero-discordant couples (OGAC, 2007a).

During its country visits, the Committee heard reports of problems similar to those raised at the annual meeting. Receipt of test results, for example, is critical to effecting behavior change and initiating care. Yet long waits for test results were often cited as the reason people did not return for their results; the use of rapid tests reduced the numbers of people who were tested but remained ignorant of their status. Limited availability of test kits makes it difficult to respond to the demand for testing, while many test kits are past their expiration date. In its second annual report to Congress, OGAC described its intent to provide an uninterrupted supply of high-quality rapid test kits through the supply chain management system.

OGAC has reported that it is contributing to improved quality of counseling and testing services by supporting improved training and greater numbers of counselors, with an emphasis on including information on prevention during counseling sessions (OGAC, 2006b). The quality and impact of those trained to provide counseling and testing and the functioning of testing sites are difficult to determine, however, since OGAC has provided little information in this regard other than numbers. According to OGAC's guidance, counseling and testing are to be provided according to national and international standards. However, there are few descriptions of the training providers receive, about their ongoing supervision, or about follow-up for those who have received a positive test result and have been referred to care and treatment programs.

Integration of Services

Through its disease-specific focus, PEPFAR allows for a concentrated response to all aspects of HIV/AIDS and to an individual's needs throughout the continuum of the illness. At the same time, the program makes choices about eligibility for services because of its limited resources and the magnitude of the needs of those affected by the disease. These unavoidable limitations make it essential that PEPFAR's activities be integrated with and maximize opportunities for referrals to other programs and agencies, including the focus countries' larger health systems. PEPFAR refers to such linkages as "wrap-arounds" and believes its funds can be used to leverage other resources to meet the needs of those affected by HIV/AIDS.

Wrap-around services benefit not only people living with HIV/AIDS, but also family and household members and others in the community. Some of these programs are funded by the U.S. government and some by other donors. Examples are the President's Malaria Initiative; the Global Fund to Fight AIDS, Tuberculosis and Malaria; the United Nations Children's Fund (UNICEF); other bilateral and multilateral family planning programs; and food security programs such as the United Nations World Food Program and Food for Peace (OGAC, 2006d). Wrap-around initiatives address such needs as promotion of gender equity; prevention of opportunistic and parasitic infections (e.g., malaria); strengthening of households' capacity to generate income; strengthening of non-HIV-specific health programs, such as those focused on family planning, child health and immunization, food security and nutrition; substance abuse treatment; and provision of clean water and improved sanitation in communities (OGAC, 2006d). Wrap-arounds were added as an area of emphasis for fiscal year 2006 in OGAC guidance documents.

Beyond providing an opportunity for comprehensive services, integration allows for joint problem solving, reduced workload for staff, savings and better targeting of resources, continued improvement of skills for service providers, improved coordination, and the ability to coordinate in the development of annual plans (Peng, 2006). Integration can also facilitate enhanced monitoring and evaluation to improve program planning and make it possible to gauge the quality of services provided.

PEPFAR provides a wide range of services in its prevention, treatment, and care categories, but many of these services have been fragmented by budgetary allocations. This fragmentation, coupled with poor linkages and inconsistent/incomplete referrals internally and to external providers for services not supported by PEPFAR, creates missed opportunities for integration along the continuum of care and raises concern about whether patients who are receiving such fragmented services are being well served. PEPFAR guidance emphasizes comprehensive and integrated services at the community level, but much of the program's planning is being done by partners at the national rather than the local level. For example, PEPFAR has provided technical assistance at the national level for building sustainable palliative care systems. Through this work, a common set of home-based care services is being identified. However, program planning, implementation, and evaluation have been delayed by a lack of comprehensive programmatic guidance for family-based care services. PEPFAR, working with its partners, needs to plan strategically to implement comprehensive services and build capacity at the community level.

In the care category, PEPFAR's program guidance is inconsistent in terms of integration of services, as evidenced by the exclusion of the services of traditional healers from what are identified as key areas of training for the provision of comprehensive care through home-based programs. At the same time, PEPFAR does have training programs targeting the development of partnerships with traditional healers to address issues related to adherence to ART and discussion of the effectiveness of ART with patients (OGAC, 2005d, 2006a). In addition, the Committee believes further work is needed to incorporate in PEPFAR's training curricula and programmatic guidance cross-cutting issues and services such as nutrition and adherence to ART and other medications. Moreover, integration of palliative and preventive care guidance would have positive benefits in supporting overall wellness before and during ART. Other benefits could include impeding the synergism recently reported between malaria and high rates of transmission of HIV. Given the known concomitant effects of malaria and HIV, intensification of scaling-up efforts of PEPFAR's secondary preventive care services and improving their linkages to services for comorbid infections is necessary. Doing so could contribute to efforts to keep people healthier longer, regardless of whether they are eligible for ART. Such linkages may be imperiled, however, if funding for these other key health care services lags far behind the enormous increases in funding for HIV/AIDS services from multiple sources.

Recommendation 6-1: The U.S. Global AIDS Coordinator should continue to promote and support a community-based, family-centered model of care in order to enhance and coordinate supportive care services for people living with HIV/AIDS, with special emphasis on orphans, vulnerable children, and people requiring end-of-life care. This model should include integration as appropriate with prevention and treatment programs and linkages with other public-sector and nongovernmental organization services within and outside of the health sector, such as primary health care, nutrition support, education, social work, and the work of agencies facilitating income generation.

CONCLUSION

As discussed at PEPFAR's third annual meeting in Durban, South Africa (OGAC, 2006e), challenges to PEPFAR's care services include the limited attention care has received as a result of confusion about what PEPFAR means by palliative care, as well as budgetary constraints; implementation issues related to preventive care, such as the cost and replenishment of consumables; the integration of palliative care with other services; concern about the ability of programs to meet the increased demand for services resulting from voluntary counseling and testing; questions about how to measure the quality of services and define who can be counted as receiving care; expansion of care services to primary health centers; and the difficulty of ensuring adequate and appropriate commodities, such as medications for pain and management of opportunistic infections, especially TB (OGAC, 2006e).

OGAC's continued inclusion of global care-related guidance in PEPFAR-supported programs underscores its commitment to harmonization and collaboration with other global stakeholders. As the evidence base grows and communities learn more about how best to deal with the epidemic, these practices need to be scaled up and tailored to the needs of other communities. If international standards indicate that insecticide-treated bed nets are effective and should be provided to members of all households to decrease exposure to opportunistic infections such as malaria, for example, PEPFAR-supported preventive care services need to be linked with wrap-around programs that will support such interventions. If specific pharmaceuticals are recommended to treat opportunistic infections such as TB and malaria, establishing linkages with regional and national program managers with responsibility for supply chain management to ensure their timely availability will be necessary. More widespread and consistent inclusion of international guidance may contribute to improved integration of services within service categories, as well as across the continuum of services.

PEPFAR-supported care programs need to support and promote community-based, family-centered care. Although this is part of the program's approach to care delivery, all program implementers could benefit from improved articulation of these expectations. Consensus guidance that is well articulated will facilitate the development of clear standards for the provision and quality of community-based services for families that will contribute to a sustainable response to the epidemic. The Committee is cognizant that its recommendation to this end could have the unintended consequence of increasing the caregiving burden of women and girls; therefore, careful attention to the need for concomitant interventions to ameliorate this effect is essential.

PEPFAR's success in achieving its 5-year target of providing care to 10 million people, as well as in providing care services thereafter, is contingent upon how it defines what it means to have received care services. A simple numerical count is inadequate because an evaluator or program manager cannot know just what services a person has received beyond "care" or whether the count provides an accurate number of people receiving specific types of services or the number of times a person has been served.

In addition, the Committee believes OGAC recognizes that PEPFAR faces challenges in measuring the quality of services rendered by providers of varying levels of skills. Issuance of PEPFAR's preventive care package was a step toward defining quality care by standardizing basic preventive care services, and efforts to train service providers according to national and international standards where they exist contribute to standardization of care, but challenges remain in the way quality of care services is measured.

Finally, the Committee believes it is critical for OGAC to improve integration of services both within service categories and across the continuum of illness regardless of budget constraints. Successful integration can facilitate the provision of comprehensive services from the facility to the household and community levels, and ensure that everyone living with and affected by HIV/AIDS will be able to access services that are culturally appropriate, affordable, and timely.

REFERENCES

Abu-Raddad, L. J., P. Patnaik, and J. Kublin. 2006. Dual infection with HIV and malaria fuels the spread of both diseases in sub-Saharan Africa. *Science* 314:1603–1606.

AVERT. 2006. *HIV-related opportunistic infections: Prevention and treatment.* http://www.avert.org/aidscare.htm (accessed October 31, 2006).

Coleman, C. L., L. S. Eller, K. M. Nokes, E. Bunch, N. Reynolds, I. Corless, P. Dole, J. K. Kemppainen, D. Wantland, K. Kirksey, L. Seficik, P. Nicholas, J. J. Hamilton, Y.-F. Tsai, and W. L. Holzemer. 2006. Prayers as a complimentary health strategy for managing HIV related symptoms among an ethnically diverse sample. *Holistic Nursing Practice* 20(2):65–72.

Corless, I. G., E. H. Bunch, J. K. Kemppainen, W. L. Holzemer, K. M. Nokes, L. S. Eller, C. J. Portillo, E. Butensky, P. K. Nicholas, C. A. Bain, S. Davis, K. M. Kirksey, and F.-Y. Chou. 2002. Self-care for fatigue in HIV disease. *Oncology Nursing Forum* 29(5):E60–E69).

Donahue, J. 2005. Strengthening households and communities: The key to reducing the economic impacts of HIV/AIDS on children and families. In *A generation at risk: The global impact of HIV/AIDS on orphans and vulnerable children.* Edited by G. Foster, C. Levine, and J. Williamson. New York: Cambridge University Press. Pp. 37–65.

Dybul, M. 2006 (July 13). *The President's Emergency Plan for AIDS Relief: Looking back and looking forward.* Remarks as prepared to Center for Strategic and International Studies. http://www.pepfar.gov (accessed January 3, 2007).

Eller, L. S., I. B. Corless, E. H. Bunch, J. K. Kemppainen, W. L. Holzemer, K. Nokes, C. J. Portillo, and P. Nicholas. 2005. Self-care strategies for depression in persons with HIV disease. *Journal of Advanced Nursing* 51(12):119–130.

Fleischman, J. 2006. *Integrating reproductive health and HIV/AIDS programs: Strategic opportunities for PEPFAR.* Washington, DC: Center for International and Strategic Studies.

Foster, G., C. Levine, and J. Williamson. 2005. *A generation at risk: The global impact of HIV/AIDS on orphans and vulnerable children.* New York: Cambridge University Press.

FSPC (Family Strengthening Policy Center). 2004. *Policy brief: Introduction to family strengthening.* Washington, DC: National Human Services Assembly.

Gass, R. N, C. Luo, N. Ngongo, S. Crowley, G. Tene, G. Sherman, and A. Harries. 2006. *Scaling up pediatric HIV care and treatment in resource-constrained settings.* Presentation at the XVI International AIDS Conference, Toronto, Canada.

GHC (Global Health Council). 2005. *Faith in action: Examining the role of faith-based organizations in addressing HIV/AIDS.* Washington, DC: GHC.

Harding, R., and I. Higginson. 2004. *Palliative care in sub-Saharan Africa: An appraisal.* London: King's College London, University of London.

Harding, R., and I. Higginson. 2005. Palliative care in sub-Saharan Africa. *Lancet* 365:1971–1977.

Harding, R., D. Karus, P. Easterbrook, V. H. Raveis, I. J. Higginson, and K. Marconi. 2005. Does palliative care improve outcomes for patients with HIV/AIDS? A systematic review of the evidence. *Sexually Transmitted Infections* 81:5.

HIV Insite. 2006 (July 27). *Routine or opt-out counselling and testing: Findings from the 2006 PEPFAR meeting.* http://hivinsite.ucsf.edu/InSite?page=pa-hatip-71/ (accessed October 31, 2006).

Holzemer, W. L. 2002. HIV and AIDS: The symptom experience: What cell counts and viral loads won't tell you? *American Journal of Nursing* 102(4):48–52.

ICRW (International Center for Research on Women). 2005. *Towards achieving gender equality and empowering women.* Washington, DC: ICRW.

JLI (The Joint Learning Initiative on Human Resources for Health and Development). 2004. *Human resources for health: Overcoming the crisis.* Boston, MA: Harvard University.

Kaiser Family Foundation. 2006 (October 27). *Daily HIV/AIDS report: Botswana launches infant HIV testing program.* http://www.kaisertnetwork.org (accessed October 27, 2006).

Kalichman, S. 1995. *Understanding AIDS: A guide for mental health professionals.* Washington, DC: American Psychological Association.

Kemppainen, J. K., L. S. Eller, E. Bunch, M. J. Hamilton, P. Dole, W. Holzemer, K. Kirksey, P. K. Nicholas, I. B. Corless, C. Coleman, K. M. Nokes, N. Reynolds, L. Sefcik, D. Wantland, and Y.-F. Tsai. 2006. Strategies for self-management of HIV-related anxiety. *AIDS Care* 18(6):597–607.

Makoae, L. N., N. M. Seboni, K. Molosiwa, M. Moleko, S. Human, N. A. Sukati, and W. L. Holzemer. 2005. The symptom experience of people living with HIV/AIDS in Southern Africa. *Journal of the Association of Nurses in AIDS Care* 16(3):22–32.

Mermin, J. 2005 (May 26). *Community and home-based preventive care and ART.* Presentation at the PEPFAR Second Annual Field Meeting, Addis Ababa, Ethiopia.

Nicholas, P., J. K. Kemppainen, G. E. Canaval, I. B. Corless, E. F. Sefcik, K. M. Nokes, C. A. Bain, K. Kirksey, L. S. Eller, P. Dole, J. J. Hamilton, C. L. Coleman, W. L. Holzemer, N. Reynolds, C. J. Portillo, E. H. Bunch, D. J. Wantland, J. Voss, R. Phillips, Y.-F. Tsai, M. R. Mendez, T. Lindgren, S. M. Davis, and D. M. Gallagher. 2007. Symptom management and self-care for peripheral neuropathy in HIV/AIDS. *AIDS Care* 19(2):179–189.

OGAC (Office of the U.S. Global AIDS Coordinator). 2004. *The President's Emergency Plan for AIDS Relief: U.S. five-year global HIV/AIDS strategy.* Washington, DC: OGAC.

OGAC. 2005a. *PEPFAR first annual report to Congress.* Washington, DC: OGAC.

OGAC. 2005b. *The President's Emergency Plan for AIDS Relief: Indicators, reporting requirements, and guidelines for focus countries* (revised for FY2006 reporting). Washington, DC: OGAC.

OGAC. 2005c. *Final draft HIV/AIDS palliative care guidance #1: An overview of comprehensive HIV/AIDS care services in the President's Emergency Plan for AIDS Relief.* Washington, DC: OGAC.

OGAC. 2005d. *FY2005 Country Operational Plans.* Washington, DC: OGAC.

OGAC. 2006a. *FY2006 Country Operational Plans.* Washington, DC: OGAC.

OGAC. 2006b. *PEPFAR second annual report to Congress.* Washington, DC: OGAC.

OGAC. 2006c. *PEPFAR report on work force capacity and HIV/AIDS.* Washington, DC: OGAC.

OGAC. 2006d. *HIV/AIDS palliative care guidance #1: An overview of comprehensive HIV/AIDS care services in the President's Emergency Plan for AIDS Relief.* Washington, DC: OGAC.

OGAC. 2006e (June 12–15). *Building on successes: Ensuring long-term solutions.* Annotated version of rapporteur presentations at the President's Emergency Plan for AIDS Relief 2006 HIV/AIDS Implementers' Meeting, Durban, South Africa.

OGAC. 2006f. *Adult preventive care guidance.* Washington, DC: OGAC.

OGAC. 2006g. *Palliative care technical working group plan.* Washington, DC: OGAC.

OGAC. 2006h. *Responding to the needs of women and girls: Reproductive health and HIV/AIDS linkages* (PowerPoint Presentation). Washington, DC: OGAC.

OGAC. 2007a. *PEPFAR third annual report to Congress.* Washington, DC: OGAC.

OGAC. 2007b. Office of the Global AIDS Coordinator's Suggested Factual Changes to the PEPFAR Implementation: Progress and Promise Report. Email communication to IOM staff on March 29, 2007.

Peng, V. 2006 (June 2). *Challenge of integrated supervision of vertical health programs in Cambodia.* Presentation by USAID/URC Project for Health-Systems Strengthening, Phnom Penh, Cambodia.

Rehle, T., T. Saidel, S. Mills, and R. Magnani (eds.). 2000. *Evaluating programs for HIV/AIDS prevention and care in developing countries: A handbook for program managers and decision makers.* Arlington, VA: Family Health International.

Ro, M., H. Treadwell, and M. Northridge. 2003. *Community health workers and community voices: Promoting good health.* Battle Creek, MI: W. K. Kellogg Foundation.

UNAIDS (Joint United Nations Programme on HIV/AIDS) and UNICEF (United Nations Children's Fund). 2004. *The framework for the protection, care and support of orphans and vulnerable children living in a world with HIV and AIDS.* Geneva, Switzerland: UNAIDS.

UNICEF. 2006. *Africa's orphaned and vulnerable generations: Children affected by AIDS.* New York: UNICEF.

UNICEF and WHO (World Health Organization). 2006. *Management of sick children by community health programme workers: Intervention models and programme examples.* New York: UNICEF.

WHO (World Health Organization). 2004a. *Emergency scale-up of antiretroviral therapy in resource-limited settings: Technical and operational recommendations to achieve 3 by 5.* Geneva, Switzerland: WHO.

WHO. 2004b. *Guide to monitoring and evaluating HIV/AIDS care and support.* Geneva, Switzerland: WHO.

WHO. 2004c. *A community health approach to palliative care for HIV/AIDS and cancer patients in sub-Saharan Africa.* Geneva, Switzerland: WHO.

WHO. 2006. *Scaling up HIV/AIDS prevention, treatment and care: A report on WHO support to countries in implementing the "3 by 5" initiatives 2004–2005.* Geneva, Switzerland: WHO.

Yengi, W. 2005. *Expanding HIV care and treatment in the southern Highlands of Tanzania: Support of ART through home-based care outreach.* Presentation at the PEPFAR Second Annual Field Meeting, Addis Ababa, Ethiopia.

7

PEPFAR's Orphans and Other Vulnerable Children Category

Summary of Key Findings

- As of September 30, 2006, PEPFAR had provided services to more than 2 million orphans and other vulnerable children in the focus countries. There is no specific performance target for the number of orphans and other vulnerable children to be served, instead they are counted toward the overall care target.
- PEPFAR has adopted the international approach for core services for orphans and other vulnerable children and supported activities corresponding to those services. However, scale-up efforts for the provision of these services are hampered by several challenges, including a lack of social service systems to address the social and mental health support needs of children and a lack of systems with which countries can track and report vital statistics, such as birth registration, to facilitate determination of eligibility for both PEPFAR and non-PEPFAR services. PEPFAR is supporting efforts to develop such systems, and priority to social welfare and education workers in its workforce capacity-building efforts is greatly needed.
- The Office of the U.S. Global AIDS Coordinator (OGAC) and the U.S. Agency for International Development are collaborating to strengthen the collection and validity of strategic information needed by policy makers and program managers by revising the program-level indicator used to report data; providing clear guidance on how and when a child can be counted as served; standardizing services; and conducting targeted evaluations of service-related issues, including cost and program effectiveness.
- OGAC efforts to strengthen data could also include its adoption of some of the United Nations Children's Fund (UNICEF) program and outcome indicators, such as the number of girls enrolled in school and the grade levels they attain, to better position PEPFAR to evaluate the responsiveness and impact of PEPFAR-supported services. Adoption of these indicators could be undertaken with attention to continued harmony with one nationally integrated monitoring and evaluation system.

Recommendation Discussed in This Chapter

Recommendation 7-1: ***The needs of orphans and other children made vulnerable by AIDS cover a wide spectrum that cuts across all of PEPFAR's categories of prevention, treatment, and care and extends well beyond the health sector. It is essential for an HIV/AIDS response to address these needs adequately—not only to support these children in living healthy and productive lives, but also to protect them from becoming the next wave of the pandemic.*** **The U.S. Global AIDS Initiative should continue to support countries in the development of national plans that address the needs of orphans and other children made vulnerable by AIDS, as well as to support the priorities delineated in these plans. To ensure adequate focus on and accountability for addressing the needs of orphans and other vulnerable children, the U.S. Global AIDS Coordinator should work with Congress to set a distinct and meaningful performance target for this population. This target should be developed in a manner that both builds on the improvements PEPFAR has made in its indicator for children served and enhances its ability to support comprehensive and integrated HIV/AIDS programming.**

7

PEPFAR's Orphans and Other Vulnerable Children Category

CATEGORY, TARGET, AND RESULTS

Category

The Leadership Act treats orphans and vulnerable children as a fourth category for purposes of the President's Emergency Plan for AIDS Relief (PEPFAR) funding and reporting, although the services they receive—prevention, treatment, and care—cut across the other three categories. In PEPFAR's indicator guidance, an orphan is defined as a child under 18 who has lost either a mother or a father (OGAC, 2005f); in its second annual report, however, PEPFAR defined an orphan as a child under age 15 who has lost a mother, a father, or both (OGAC, 2006a). The Office of the U.S. Global AIDS Coordinator (OGAC) has previously defined vulnerable children as "those affected by HIV though the illness of a parent or principal caretaker" (OGAC, 2005f). New programmatic guidance addresses the conflicts created by varying definitions of those served under this category, which are discussed in detail in the section on issues and opportunities for improvement later in the chapter.

PEPFAR's activities targeting orphans and other vulnerable children fall into two subcategories: services to children and training for providers of those services.

Target

There is no quantified target for the number of orphans and other vulnerable children to be served by a specific deadline, as with the 2010 target for prevention and the 2008 target for treatment (OGAC, 2005c, 2006e. f). However, the Leadership Act mandates that no less than 10 percent of total PEPFAR funding allocated for prevention, treatment, and care be used to provide services to address the needs of orphans and other vulnerable children. Furthermore, the legislation prescribes that of that 10 percent, "at least 50 percent shall be provided through non-profit, nongovernmental organizations including faith-based organizations that implement programs at the community level" (p. 746). However, Country Teams, in collaboration with country governments, do set specific country targets for the number of orphans and other vulnerable children to be served by the program that count towards the 10 million people target for care.

Similar to the indicators for the other PEPFAR categories, this indicator counts the number of children provided PEPFAR-supported services (food/nutrition, shelter and care, protection, health care, psychosocial support, and education/vocational training), but does not allow determination of the quality or impact of those services (see Chapter 8 for a discussion of this issue). However, the evolution of PEPFAR's current indicator for the orphans and other vulnerable children category reflects one of OGAC's best efforts to strengthen the data provided by care indicators—potentially improving the quality of services, utilizing an approach to meet the individualized needs of children, and at the very least ensuring that recipients are receiving appropriate and standardized services and are being tracked over time.

In August 2006, OGAC informed the Country Teams through its *News to the Field* that the orphans and other vulnerable children indicator had been revised. The revision changes which children can be counted as served by an orphans and other vulnerable children program and how. Many of the PEPFAR targets, other than training, were defined as direct support (downstream) and indirect support (upstream). The corresponding indicators were the number served directly and the number served indirectly, disaggregated by gender. Although targets for the total number of orphans and other vulnerable children served directly for Country Operational Plans for fiscal year 2007 will be set as in previous years, use of the revised reporting indicator will be effective as of the fiscal year 2007 mid and annual reporting periods, with allowance made if the country's monitoring system is not yet able to provide the new breakdown (OGAC, 2006c,d). The new measure will be divided into two subcategories: orphans and other vulnerable children receiving *primary direct support* and those receiving *supplemental direct support.* Direct support is defined as follows: "direct recipients of support are orphans and vulnerable children who are regularly monitored in the six core areas (food/nutrition, shelter and care, protection, health care, psychosocial support, and education) and whose individual needs are addressed accordingly. Economic strengthening should be evaluated according to its benefit to the six core areas" (OGAC, 2006i, p. 10). Indirect support for orphans and other vulnerable children support is defined as follows: "indirect recipients of support are orphans and vulnerable children who are NOT individually monitored but who collectively benefit in some way from system strengthening or other interventions. For example, estimated number of orphans and vulnerable children benefiting from a policy change or improved system (i.e., birth registration, inheritance laws, or educational system or the estimated number of orphans and vulnerable children benefiting from the training or support for caregivers)" (OGAC, 2006i, p. 11). Reporting of primary direct support is defined as follows: "count orphans and other vulnerable children who are periodically monitored in all six core areas and who are receiving PEPFAR funded or leveraged support in three or more areas, in the relevant reporting period, that are appropriate for that child's needs and context" (OGAC, 2006i, p. 11). Reporting of supplemental direct support is defined as follows: "count orphans and other vulnerable children who are periodically monitored in all six core areas and who are receiving PEPFAR funded or leveraged support in one or two areas, in the relevant reporting period, that are appropriate for that child's needs and context" (OGAC, 2006i, p. 11). Total direct support is the sum of primary and supplemental support (OGAC, 2006i). The indicator guidance also states that the impact of services on children is not to be measured by routinely collected program indicators and references plans to collect national-level outcome and impact indicators periodically through population-based surveys and special studies (OGAC, 2005f).

Additionally, the announcement to the Country Teams states that an orphan or otherwise vulnerable child can be counted under only one category (not both direct and indirect) and that program-level monitoring will need to be done by core service area to provide the national-level breakdown between primary and supplemental direct support. OGAC also suggests that tracking this indicator by age group could be helpful for developing appropriate service strategies. The Orphans and Other Vulnerable Children Technical Working Group is available to assist countries that need to develop appropriate and necessary monitoring systems to report on the new indicator. The new definitions and other revisions may cause the numbers of orphans and other vulnerable children served to decrease from their previous annual levels. However, the benefit of measuring impact, measuring longitudinal benefit to orphans and other vulnerable children, and standardizing services to this population will improve the quality of the services provided and yield valuable data to inform future service planning and policy development or reform.

Results

Of the slightly more than 15 million children estimated to be orphaned or otherwise made vulnerable by HIV/AIDS, 7.4 million or 49 percent live in the focus countries (UNAIDS, 2006). Prior to fiscal year 2006, funding for services to orphans and other vulnerable children has been below the 10 percent required by the Leadership Act (see Chapter 3). According to OGAC's third annual report to Congress, however, the amount for fiscal year 2006 is approximately 12 percent of prevention, treatment, and care resources, but drops to 9 percent if amounts for pediatric AIDS are excluded (OGAC, 2007).

By the end of fiscal year 2006, OGAC reported that services had been provided to more than 2 million orphans and other vulnerable children. This is more than triple the children served in fiscal year 2004 (see Table 7-1). As for training in the same time period, OGAC trained six times the number of people to provide services to this population since fiscal year 2004. The number of service outlets ("programs providing care and support for orphans and vulnerable children" [OGAC, 2005a, p. 48]) to which PEPFAR provided technical support for the provision of services to orphans and other vulnerable children was only reported for fiscal year 2004, though OGAC reports it continues to provide technical assistance to an undisclosed number of service outlets as part if its capacity-building efforts.

BACKGROUND

Estimates of Numbers of Orphans and Other Vulnerable Children

In its *2006 Report on the Global AIDS Epidemic*, the Joint United Nations Programme on HIV/AIDS (UNAIDS) estimated the numbers of children orphaned as a result of HIV/AIDS by region and country, using age 18 as the delimiter. Countries were ranked 1–37 (1 being the highest) by the number of such children out of the global estimate of 15.2 million.

TABLE 7-1 PEPFAR Orphans and Other Vulnerable Children Results by Fiscal Year, 2004–2006

Category	Fiscal Year 2004	Fiscal Year 2005	Fiscal Year 2006
Total orphans and vulnerable children served	630,200	1,222,100	2,000,700
Total people trained as providers	22,600	74,800	143,000
Service outlets	700	Not available	Not available

SOURCE: OGAC, 2005a, 2006a, 2007.

TABLE 7-2 Estimates of Living Children Orphaned as a Result of HIV/AIDS in the PEPFAR Focus Countries and Country Population Totals, 2005–2006

Rank	Country	Number of Orphans due to AIDS (< 18 years)[a]	Percentage of Global Estimate	Country Total Population (2006)[b]	Number of Children in Country (0–14 yrs) (2005)[b]	Total OVC Index Score (0–100)[b]
	Global	15,200,000	100.0	N/A	N/A	N/A
1	South Africa	1,200,000	7.9	47,432,000	15,500,000	69
2	Kenya	1,100,000	7.2	34,256,000	14,700,000	N/A
2	Tanzania	1,100,000	7.2	38,329,000	16,300,000	55
3	Uganda	1,000,000	6.6	28,816,000	14,500,000	65
4	Nigeria	930,000	6.1	131,530,000	58,200,000	46
5	Zambia	710,000	4.7	11,668,000	5,300,000	29
8	Mozambique	510,000	3.4	19,792,000	8,700,000	41
9	Côte d'Ivoire	450,000	3.0	18,154,000	7,600,000	68
11	Rwanda	210,000	1.4	9,038,000	3,900,000	79
15	Botswana	120,000	0.8	1,765,000	660,000	N/A
20	Namibia	85,000	0.6	2,031,000	840,000	73
37	Ethiopia	N/A	N/A	77,431,100	34,500,000	57
37	Guyana	N/A	N/A	751,000	N/A	N/A
37	Haiti	N/A	N/A	8,528,000	N/A	N/A
37	Vietnam	N/A	N/A	84,238,000	N/A	N/A
	Total reported	7,415,000	48.9	513,759,100	180,700,000	

NOTE: All data are estimates. UNAIDS indicates that data are still preliminary for Canada, Ethiopia, and the United Kingdom. A child orphaned by AIDS is defined as any living child under the age of 18 who has lost one or both parents as a result of HIV/AIDS. N/A = not available.
SOURCE: Compiled from [a]UNAIDS, 2006, and Kaiser Family Foundation, 2007; [b]UNICEF, 2006a.

The rankings of the focus countries are shown in Table 7-2. As of 2005, South Africa, Kenya, Uganda, and Tanzania had each reported orphan populations of just over 1,000,000. Zambia, Nigeria, Mozambique, Côte d'Ivoire, Rwanda, and Botswana had reported orphan populations in the range of 120,000–930,000, with Botswana at the lowest end of the range and Nigeria at the highest. The estimate for Namibia was 85,000 orphans. The UNAIDS report noted that the data for Ethiopia were preliminary and not included in the table, and no data were reported for Vietnam, Haiti, or Guyana. It is important to note that these estimates do not include other vulnerable children; thus they are underestimates of the numbers of children who should be counted in the category of orphans and other vulnerable children and are in urgent need of services. Though estimates may appear low for some countries, the context of the magnitude of the problem is best understood by the proportion of the country's total population and total population of children the estimates represent.

Standards of Care

Global Approach to Addressing Needs of Orphans and Other Vulnerable Children

International events and efforts by international organizations, governments, and the civil sector led to the development of a normative approach for addressing the needs of children orphaned and otherwise made vulnerable by HIV/AIDS. Box 7-1 presents a summary of these key events. The United Nations Children's Fund (UNICEF) was instrumental in spearheading the formation of the Global Partners Forum for Children Affected by HIV/AIDS (GPFC) as a focal point for advocacy, dialogue, and prioritizing of action items. The result was a set of recommendations for global action in six key areas: (1) planning for national scale-up response; (2) ensuring that children have adequate legal protection; (3) expanding the role of community organizations in national responses; (4) improving access to education; (5) improving access to health care services for children and caregivers affected by HIV/AIDS, including pediatric treatment and prevention of mother-to-child transmission of HIV; and (6) supporting social welfare interventions.

The GPFC was initially convened in Geneva in 2003 by UNAIDS and UNICEF to mobilize action and monitor progress toward fulfilling the global commitments for children affected by HIV/AIDS set forth in the United Nations General Assembly's 2001 Declaration of Commitment on HIV/AIDS and the Millennium Development Goals (MDGs) (UNICEF, 2006b). The first meeting resulted in endorsement of *The Framework for the Protection, Care, and Support of Orphans and Vulnerable Children Living in a World with HIV and AIDS* ("The Framework"), which has become the normative approach for urgently addressing the needs of orphans and other vulnerable children (UNICEF, 2004). The GPFC's second convention, held by UNICEF and the World Bank in December 2004, resulted in acceleration of the abolishment of school fees and removal of other barriers to education in a joint effort with the Education for All Fast Tract initiative; the initiation of a system for reporting on care, with indictors to track donor and national government actions and resource commitments to children affected by HIV/AIDS; and the establishment and strengthening of global treatment targets for children with HIV/AIDS. The GPFC's third convention was held in England in 2006 by the Department for International Development (DFID), UNICEF, and UNAIDS with three major objectives: (1) to measure progress on the previous year's commitments at the GPFC;

BOX 7-1
Selected Events Leading to the Development of *The Framework for the Protection, Care, and Support of Orphans and Vulnerable Children Living in a World with HIV and AIDS*

1994: Lusaka Declaration adopted at a workshop in Zambia on support to children and families affected by HIV/AIDS. Issues reflected in the declaration include the need to assess the magnitude of the problem, the role of institutional care, the need for material and financial support for affected families, survival skills and vocational training for orphans and vulnerable children, and their right to basic education.

1998: United Nations held a General Discussion on "Children Living in a World with AIDS." The discussion stressed the relevance of the rights contained in the Convention on the Rights of the Child to prevention and care efforts, noting that HIV/AIDS was often seen primarily as a medical problem, whereas the holistic, rights-centered approach required to implement the convention was more appropriate to the much broader range of issues that must be addressed.

1998: Regional Children in Distress conference held in Pietermaritzburg, South Africa. Country representatives committed to establishing Orphans and Vulnerable Children Task Teams in their countries.

2000: First East and Southern African regional meeting on orphans and vulnerable children held in Lusaka, Zambia. Countries made commitments and plans to address the issue of the growing numbers of orphans and vulnerable children in their countries.

2001: United Nations General Assembly Special Session (UNGASS) met to review and address the problem of HIV/AIDS in all its aspects, as well as to secure a global commitment to enhancing coordination and intensifying efforts. The resulting Declaration of Commitment on HIV/AIDS includes a specific section and set of policy and strategy actions addressing orphans and other vulnerable children for signatory states.

2002: United Nations Special Session on Children resulted in the "World Fit for Children" declaration. This declaration reaffirmed the goals set by UNGASS in 2001.

2002: Regional workshop on orphans and other vulnerable children held in Yamoussoukro, Côte d'Ivoire, with representatives from 21 Central and West African countries, in the spirit of the Pietermaritzburg and Lusaka meetings. Country representatives committed to setting up task teams in their countries to develop action plans for ensuring achievement of the targets pertaining to orphans and other vulnerable children set forth in the 2001 UNGASS declaration.

2002: Africa Leadership Consultation entitled "Urgent Action for Children on the Brink" aimed at developing consensus on priorities for a scaled-up response to the orphans and vulnerable children crisis. Actions were proposed to mobilize the leadership, partnerships, and resources required to deliver on the UNGASS goals.

2002: Eastern and Southern Africa workshop on orphans and vulnerable children (with representation from 20 countries) held in Windhoek, Namibia, to assess the progress of countries toward meeting the UNGASS goals.

2003: UNAIDS and UNICEF convened the first Global Partners Forum in Geneva. *The Framework for the Protection, Care, and Support of Orphans and Vulnerable Children Living in a World with HIV and AIDS* was endorsed.

SOURCE: Adapted from Smart, 2003.

(2) to identify and remove constraints to expanding the response to children affected by HIV/AIDS; and (3) to enter into a global compact with an agreed-upon manageable and prioritized agenda aimed at expanding efforts to meet the needs and rights of children affected by HIV/AIDS on the basis of emerging evidence (DFID et al., 2006). The United Nations Convention on the Rights of the Child and other human rights instruments guide all actions in support of orphans and other vulnerable children (UNICEF and UNAIDS, 2004). While all eight goals of the United Nations' Millennium Declaration of 2000 can have an impact on the lives of children, one goal relates directly to HIV/AIDS (UNICEF, 2006c). While the authors of The Framework acknowledged that the response to the orphan crisis was growing, they maintained that the response lacked the "necessary urgency and remain[ed] unfocused and limited in scope." They also stated that "thousands of community-based programs have been implemented by faith-based and non-governmental organizations as well as communities themselves to ensure the well-being of orphans, but opportunities for significant expansion have not yet been grasped" (UNICEF and UNAIDS, 2004, p. 10). In addition, while more attention is being paid to the inclusion of the needs of these children in poverty reduction and other national development strategies, only two PEPFAR focus countries in sub-Saharan Africa identify orphans and other vulnerable children as "priority actions" in their full poverty reduction strategy papers,[1] but neither cites this area specifically in its poverty reduction strategy paper budgets (UNICEF, 2004). In addition, not all focus countries even have national strategies to address the needs of orphans and other vulnerable children.

Although OGAC representatives have participated in international efforts to address issues related to implementation of The Framework, OGAC delayed creating official program guidance for services to orphans and other vulnerable children until the late stages of PEPFAR and issued the guidance in final form in July 2006. A specific but limited care package for children living with AIDS was included as an appendix in OGAC's draft palliative care guidance issued early in 2005 before the issuance of its preventive care guidance for children in 2006. While palliative and preventive care guidance are important, they are not, however, equivalent to official guidance on meeting the needs of orphans and other vulnerable children who are HIV-negative or asymptomatic children living with HIV/AIDS, which was not disseminated until after the publication of OGAC's second annual

[1]According to the World Bank, poverty reduction strategy papers describe a country's macroeconomic, structural, and social policies and programs to promote growth and reduce poverty, as well as associated external financing needs. The papers are prepared by governments through a participatory process involving civil society and development partners, including the World Bank and the International Monetary Fund (World Bank, 2006).

report to Congress. OGAC also issued preventive care guidance for children in April 2006 (which is discussed further in this chapter), but this guidance did not comprehensively address the needs of orphans and other vulnerable children as described in The Framework. The sequencing of the various guidance documents issued for orphans and other vulnerable children may have contributed to the fragmented programming that the Committee heard about during its country visits.

The Framework

The Framework is a consensus document drafted jointly by the U.S. Agency for International Development (USAID), UNAIDS, UNICEF, and more than 90 other child advocacy organizations (UNICEF and UNAIDS, 2004). The five key strategies codified in The Framework evolved from those presented in "Urgent Action for Children on the Brink" in 2002 (UNAIDS et al., 2002):

- Strengthen the **capacity of families** to protect and care for orphans and vulnerable children by prolonging the lives of parents and providing economic, psychosocial, and other support.
- Mobilize and support **community-based responses**.
- Ensure access for orphans and vulnerable children to **essential services**, including education, health care, birth registration, and others.
- Ensure that **governments protect** the most vulnerable children through improved policy and legislation and channeling of resources to families and communities.
- Raise awareness at all levels through advocacy and social mobilization to create a **supportive environment** for children and families affected by HIV/AIDS (UNICEF and UNAIDS, 2004).

These strategies are detailed in Box 7-2. The Country Operational Plans provide examples of PEPFAR-supported activities aimed at meeting the needs of orphans and other vulnerable children. These examples are presented in the next section, organized according to the five key strategies listed above. As families and communities are the first line of response to HIV/AIDS, PEPFAR, through its collaboration with and funding to USAID, has adopted The Framework to address the needs of orphans and other vulnerable children through its community and family-based programs. Many organizations receive PEPFAR funds through grants and contracts from USAID, as it has primary responsibility for oversight and development of programming for orphans and other vulnerable children (OGAC, 2004). PEPFAR has not, however, adopted all of UNICEF's recommended core or additional indicators for measuring either the services provided or their impact on the lives of orphans and other vulnerable children and communities.

BOX 7-2
Key Strategies of UNICEF's *The Framework for the Protection, Care, and Support of Orphans and Vulnerable Children Living in a World with HIV and AIDS*

Strengthen the Capacity of Families

- Improve household economic capacity
- Provide psychosocial support to affected children and their caregivers
- Strengthen and support child care capacities
- Support succession planning
- Prolong the lives of parents
- Strengthen young people's life skills

Mobilize and Support Community-Based Responses

- Engage local leaders in responding to the needs of vulnerable community members
- Organize and support activities that enable community members to talk more openly about HIV/AIDS
- Organize cooperative support activities
- Promote and support community care for children without family support

Ensure Access to Essential Services

- Increase school enrollment and attendance
- Ensure birth registration for all children
- Provide basic health and nutrition services
- Improve access to safe water and sanitation
- Ensure that judicial systems protect vulnerable children
- Ensure placement services for family care for children
- Strengthen local planning and action

Ensure That Governments Protect the Most Vulnerable Children

- Adopt national policies, strategies, and action plans
- Enhance government capacity
- Ensure that resources reach communities
- Develop and enforce a supportive legislative framework
- Establish mechanisms for ensuring information exchange and collaborative efforts

Raise Awareness to Create a Supportive Environment

- Conduct a collaborative situation analysis
- Mobilize influential leaders to reduce stigma, silence, and discrimination
- Strengthen and support social mobilization activities at the community level

SOURCE: UNICEF and UNAIDS, 2004.

The Director of Program Services for OGAC participated in the third GPFC convention in London in February 2006. During the meeting, the OGAC representative shared the challenges faced by PEPFAR in providing services to orphans and other vulnerable children, including operationalizing a coordinated response across sectors that incorporates children into the Three Ones principles of harmonization (see Chapter 2), decentralizing to facilitate a scaled-up response and strengthen public systems while mobilizing and engaging communities, and tailoring approaches to the context created by the state of the epidemic and addressing gender- and age-specific needs. In addition, the GPFC identified the United States as only one of three donor countries that had actually provided a specific budget allocation (10 percent) for orphans and other vulnerable children, the United Kingdom and Ireland being the others (UNICEF, 2006b). Despite the difficulties encountered, the early success of PEPFAR in the planning and implementation of services for orphans and other vulnerable children, as discussed below, may be attributable in part to an existing international framework specific to the population and targeted to their needs that could inform programming, resource planning, and implementation.

REVIEW OF PROGRESS TO DATE

Strategies of the Framework

Strategy #1: Strengthen the Capacity of Families

Some of the strategies of The Framework prescribe specific services children need, while others describe the catalysts for action necessary in communities, governments, and legislative and judicial frameworks and institutions. Strategy #1 is aimed at strengthening the capacity of families to protect and care for orphans and other vulnerable children by prolonging the lives of parents and providing economic, psychosocial, and other support. If a mother or father loses a spouse to AIDS, the remaining parent is left to care for their children as a single parent and generally faces increased economic and child care responsibilities (UNICEF and UNAIDS, 2004). In many cases, the remaining parent may also be ill and face the prospect of his or her own eventual death, while also having to find adequate, appropriate, and permanent caregivers for his/her surviving children. Often, the role of caregiving for children and sick family members falls to adult women of the household. While shouldering these responsibilities, women may not be able to continue to give adequate attention to subsistence crop production. This in turn is likely to have an impact on both income generation and food security and availability for the entire household, including the children. Some research has shown that the impact of HIV/AIDS can reduce household income by as much as 60 percent (Donahue, 2005). Other studies have shown that families and households experience "distinct peaks of financial pressure" that correspond to the clinical stages experienced by ill family members (Donahue, 2005). For example, in the early stage after diagnosis, family members and caregivers may spare no expense for care and treatment.

In addition, women who bear the burden of caregiving for sick family members may become less able to care for their children (Donahue, 2005). The intergenerational transfer of knowledge and skills is also threatened by the extended illness and/or premature death of parents and other adults in the community (UNICEF and UNAIDS, 2004). Save the Children's (2004) report *Beyond the Targets: Ensuring Children Benefit from Expanded Access to HIV/AIDS Treatment* states that "children whose parent(s) are HIV-positive are at risk for losing their right to survival and development for a number of reasons" and that expanding access to care and treatment will likely help maintain a family unit and its livelihood. The result could be fewer children becoming orphaned because of HIV/AIDS, or if they do eventually become orphaned, perhaps when they are older and with less of an impact on their developmental and survival needs.

The PEPFAR strategy articulates support for a community-based, family-centered approach, especially for the care of orphans and other vulnerable children (OGAC, 2004). It also states that "best practices of community-support for these households will be identified and promulgated. Home-based care and support programs will be especially targeted to such families in order to do all that is possible to keep them intact and organizations with particular expertise in family care will be targeted for funding" (OGAC, 2004, p. 48). Based on the Committee's review of Country Operational Plans and documents from the Orphan and Vulnerable Children Technical Working Group, it appears that the majority of the allocation of PEPFAR funds for orphans and other vulnerable children services is mostly channeled through a limited number of agencies, mostly large, international non-profit, nongovernmental organizations.

The Committee examined Country Operational Plans from 2005 for examples of activities aimed at strengthening the capacity of families to provide care and support for orphans and other vulnerable children (see Box 7-3). The Committee's visits to the focus countries revealed that some of these programs were more advanced than others not only in their networks, but also in the extent to which they were supported by the community and integrated into overall HIV/AIDS service efforts, as well as in the scope and duration of services provided to meet the needs of children. These variations are likely due to differences in countries' efforts to develop and implement programs prior to PEPFAR. In the examples cited in Box 7-3, multiple partners and U.S. government agencies and programs (such as the

BOX 7-3
Selected Examples of PEPFAR-Supported Activities Intended to Strengthen the Capacity of Families for Care and Support of Orphans and Other Vulnerable Children

Côte d'Ivoire: home- and community-based counseling, psychosocial support, including counseling, play therapy, referrals, and education support and health and nutritional services

Mozambique: provision of basic income and shelter/housing needs with microfinancing and mobile banks

Ethiopia: training in business and financial skills for both adult women and older orphans and other vulnerable children who are heads of households, with increasing focus on those in rural areas

Kenya: provision of food and clothing including school uniforms and payment of school fees and other efforts to ensure school enrollment

Rwanda: increasing awareness of children's protection and rights

Tanzania: vocational training and life skills education to avoid more risky professions and activities

SOURCE: OGAC, 2005a,d, 2006b,g.

Peace Corps) were consistently involved. System-strengthening activities also characterized many of the programs, such as support for the development of a monitoring and evaluation system for programs and activities addressing orphan and other vulnerable children activities and programs. Other system-strengthening examples include facilitating collaborations among community-based organizations (including nongovernmental, community-based, and faith-based organizations); encouraging national and provincial coordination of services; cross-training providers of microfinance services in HIV/AIDS prevention, care, and treatment services; and facilitating collaboration with the civil sector to find sustainable alternatives to institutional care and support for these children (OGAC, 2005d).

Strategy #2: Mobilize and Support Community-Based Responses

As noted in Chapter 6, OGAC concurs with UNICEF's assessment that the community is the safety net after the family, and intends to provide direct support for building the capacity of community-based and nongovernmental organizations to support a greater number of community initiatives. According to UNICEF and UNAIDS (2004), the community can be instrumental in assisting the extended family in keeping family relationships intact when the nuclear family is struggling with caring for an increased number of dependent children. Activities should include engaging local leaders in responding to these needs; enabling communities to talk more openly about HIV/AIDS to combat stigma and discrimination; organizing cooperative support activities, such as providing respite care, communal gardens, and day care centers; and promoting and supporting community care for children without family support, such as foster care, adoption, and community monitoring of new caregivers to prevent neglect and abuse (UNICEF and UNAIDS, 2004). In addition, UNICEF and UNAIDS have stated that faith-based and nongovernmental organizations have an instrumental role in galvanizing and supporting community efforts (UNICEF and UNAIDS, 2004). Local leaders ranging from political and religious figures to journalists and teachers need to be made aware of the impact of HIV/AIDS on children and encouraged to take action to care for and protect the most vulnerable—particularly from the risks of sexual abuse and exploitative labor practices. In Africa, cultural values are often passed down through oral traditions, and traditional African culture reinforces the practice of caring for vulnerable children, while faith-based responses to orphans and other vulnerable children are widespread (Foster et al., 2005). A coordinated response will require partnerships among policy and resource organizations and the religious sector (Foster et al., 2005). Nonetheless, historical misunderstandings, a lack of appreciation of different perspectives, assumptions about the HIV status of children of HIV-positive or deceased parents, and difficulties in communicating because of differing organizational cultures and languages have all hampered coordinated and integrated efforts to respond to these children's needs.

Some of the literature has offered compelling arguments against providing institutional care for these children in orphanages and group homes. Ironically, the idea of institutional care was imported from the industrialized world, with the belief that its modernity would provide better care (Phiri and Tolfree, 2005). Institutional or residential care may have additional appeal because of its organizational convenience to social service professionals, its provision of a means to deal with large numbers of children when families and communities are overwhelmed with the children's needs, and the tangibility and visibility of the resources provided by donors (Phiri and Tolfree, 2005). Yet the literature also points to several disadvantages and negative impacts of institutional or residential care, including systematic exposure of children to malnutrition and exploitative behaviors; inadequate health care and hygiene; educational deprivation; harsh discipline; lack of stimulation, personal care, and attention; and institutional dependence. From a policy standpoint, institutional care yields poor results by serving small numbers at a high cost per child—estimated to be five to ten times higher than the cost of foster care provided by unrelated caregivers. There is evidence that community initiatives (with the help of external resources) can promote local solutions involving family- and community-based resources that achieve good results for large numbers at a low cost per child (Phiri and Tolfree, 2005). As noted, PEPFAR focuses most of its service provision for orphans and other vulnerable children in the context of community-based settings and as often as possible within a family (including extended family) unit. The program has, however, been criticized for a predominant emphasis on physical and material needs and a lack of attention to the psychosocial well-being of children (Huni, 2006). PEPFAR often uses linkages to antiretroviral therapy as a means to keep parents alive and keep family units intact to reduce the number of orphans and vulnerable status of children. In a few countries, however, PEPFAR, at the direction of the country leadership, is supporting institutional care in the form of orphanages.

Examples of activities in Country Operational Plans for fiscal years 2005 and 2006 designed to mobilize and support community-based responses for orphans and other vulnerable children are presented in Box 7-4. Several of these activities involved partnering with either U.S. government programs such as the Peace Corps or working closely with large interna-

BOX 7-4
Selected Examples of PEPFAR-Supported Activities Intended to Mobilize and Support Community-Based Responses for Orphans and Other Vulnerable Children

Botswana: support for selected community-based organizations for grant making and program promotion in the areas of volunteer management, equipment, materials development, service delivery, vocational training, and other income-generating projects to teach small-business skills for sustainable income

Kenya: technical support to conduct needs assessments, write proposals, manage programs, establish eligibility criteria, train community groups and providers to understand the rights and health needs of children, and develop training materials

Guyana: support for equity in access to educational, nutritional, and physical and social health opportunities for girls

Mozambique: collaboration with Peace Corps volunteers to support community mobilization and training to implement modest rehabilitation projects and support training for caregivers

Namibia: collaboration with national interfaith organizations to develop and sustain grassroots support programs focused on training providers, improving program management, mobilizing the involvement of community groups and their leaders, and providing small start-up grants for community projects

SOURCE: OGAC, 2005a,d, 2006b,g.

tional, nongovernmental organizations for institutional and community capacity building.

Strategy #3: Ensure Access to Essential Services

Essential services for orphans and other vulnerable children include education, health care, birth registration, and others. Article 65 of the Declaration of Commitment of the 2001 United Nations General Assembly Special Session (UNGASS) calls for increased access to such services and parity for orphans and other vulnerable children, with governments identified as critical actors in realizing this goal (UNICEF and UNAIDS, 2004). All sectors are called upon to develop innovative strategies and increase the resources available to meet the developmental needs of these children in an effective and sustainable way.

Of particular concern under this strategy are the issues of birth registration and education. One component of an effective national child welfare policy is a vital statistics program that registers births and deaths. The Millennium Development Initiative considers birth registration a basic vital statistic deemed important for countries to own, track, report, and record and is generally the responsibility of signatory governments to the Convention of the Rights of the Child (UNICEF and UNAIDS, 2004). It has many benefits, including enabling determination of service eligibility and inheritance, as well as permission for school attendance. Unfortunately, in several countries, particularly in rural areas, birth registration does not occur until a child approaches school age. An alternative to birth registration is sworn affidavits by parents, but this method places an undue burden on orphans. Of the 48 million children annually who are not registered at birth, 55 percent are born in sub-Saharan Africa, compared with only 2 percent in industrialized countries (Sharp, 2005). This situation has implications for gender equity in service eligibility and for efforts to decrease vulnerability to HIV/AIDS for young girls and women, especially if female children are born out of wedlock. Institutional, financial, and political constraints that affect the scaling-up of birth registration have a ripple effect on constraining the scale-up of interventions for orphans and other vulnerable children (Sharp, 2005).

Education can make a difference in the lives of orphans and other vulnerable children by providing information and skills that reduce their vulnerability to HIV exposure and infection. Moreover, schools can serve as important resource centers to meet broader community needs and can provide safe and structured environments although caution must be exercised to ensure that adolescent girls are safe from sexual harassment and coerced sexual behavior in school. Schools also provide emotional support and adult supervision (UNICEF and UNAIDS, 2004), which can serve as a daily respite to children whose homes are affected by HIV/AIDS. The introduction of school meals for children can provide relief in areas where food security is an issue. In-school meals combined with take-home rations (with the consultation of community leaders and donors to avoid dependency) may also improve food security for members of the child's household (UNICEF and UNAIDS, 2004). Despite these benefits, several studies have shown that sick and orphaned children have lower rates of school attendance than nonorphaned children, often exacerbated by high transaction costs associated with education, including school fees and transportation. Overburdened caregivers also contribute to missed opportunities for school attendance (UNICEF, 2006a).

BOX 7-5
Selected Examples of PEPFAR-Supported Activities Intended to Ensure Access to Essential Services for Orphans and Other Vulnerable Children

Ethiopia: linkage with USAID agricultural programs to improve food security by expanding the program coverage to focus on the needs of orphans and vulnerable children, with particular emphasis on female- and orphan-headed households. The focus is on the increased use of urban gardening systems to generate food for household consumption while decreasing water use, labor, and land requirements. Beneficiaries are linked to a network of nongovernmental organizations that are already running such programs and can facilitate market linkages for surplus income generation

Namibia: funding of a full-time position for a technical advisor to work with government ministries, focusing on the management of trust funds to serve orphans and other vulnerable children, as well as on aspects of database creation and management for the collection, tracking, and analysis of data related to these services

Tanzania: collaborations with regional and referral hospitals to facilitate development of caregiver capacity for patient care and monitoring adherence to antiretroviral therapy for HIV-positive orphans and other vulnerable children

Kenya: training of paraprofessional counselors and/or community members in HIV/AIDS awareness, child care and counseling, parenting skills, legal rights, and other topics necessary to the care of orphans and other vulnerable children and the provision of economic support or income generation

Côte d'Ivoire: monitoring and evaluation of the continued implementation of pilot programming to serve as a model for a network of linked social and health services through public–private partnerships that reinforce coordination and two-way referrals

SOURCE: OGAC, 2005d, 2006g.

Country Operational Plans for fiscal years 2005 and 2006 yield examples of a number of programs aimed at ensuring access to essential services for orphans and other vulnerable children (see Box 7-5). As with many of the other strategies, the Peace Corps is partnering with local organizations to implement and expand many of these activities. Some common characteristics of these initiatives include integration with existing PEPFAR-assisted health networks and home-based care programs, which may often be collocated or linked with existing prevention, treatment, and care programs. Other shared characteristics include integration with food security and nutrition programs, expansion of coverage to out-of-school youths and children in rural areas, and use of multiple agencies in local and regional partnerships to promote human and legal rights for orphans and other vulnerable children (OGAC, 2005d, 2006g).

Strategy #4: Ensure That Governments Protect the Most Vulnerable Children

Implementation of this strategy involves improving policy and legislation by channeling resources to families and communities. To meet their obligations under ratified human rights conventions, country governments must undertake and be supported in efforts to mobilize multisectoral responses. Most countries have policies and mechanisms to protect, care for, and support children, but these need to be reviewed to ascertain whether they reflect current international standards (UNICEF and UNAIDS, 2004; UNICEF, 2006a). Situational analyses conducted among and with a variety of key stakeholders can provide the data needed to inform the development and implementation of prioritized, costed, and evidence-based national strategic plans (UNICEF, 2006a).

There is great variability in national policies on child health, welfare, and education. Where these policies are most effective, they articulate the rights of children and provide a culturally appropriate background for the development of services for orphans and other vulnerable children. Challenges related to the provision of such services, identified at PEPFAR's third annual meeting, include the need for linkages to care and psychosocial support services for HIV-positive children, educational interventions, and linkages to child protective services—a particular challenge in countries with nascent or nonexistent social welfare systems. Other challenges identified include volunteer retention, targeting of the most vulnerable children, multiple displacements, support for elderly caregivers, and government leadership. OGAC reported some lessons learned, including the success of local child protection committees, the use of child-friendly national plans of action for orphans and other vulnerable children, the use of inheritance documents for children, and the provision of educational block grants (OGAC, 2006b).

Social security funded by national governments—including free access to health services for the poor, free basic education, and a package of social transfers to ensure a minimum standard of living (DFID et al., 2006)—has been shown to be a key tool for poverty reduction and growth. Yet one study (supported by the Nelson Mandela Children's Fund and Development Research Africa) involving a survey of 29,000 members of nearly 5,000 households in eight predominantly rural sites revealed that in countries where social security stipends are available for the elderly and for child support and dependency grants, eligible caregivers were not accessing the child-related grants for a variety of reasons. Less than one-third of eligible households reported that they were receiving child support, foster care, disability, and care dependency grants (Population Council, 2004).

As reported at PEPFAR's second annual meeting, small-scale interventions for orphans and other vulnerable children have been initiated in most focus countries. According to one presenter at the meeting, "It is easier for programs to focus on one marketable aspect that is easy to fund and get quick results; as well as to be clustered in accessible areas to reach a few children with duplicative services." At the same time, this presenter observed, "While many countries have expressed commitment by the development of national plans, there has been little legislative review for meeting the essential needs of children—particularly beyond policies that advocate free education for all" (Huni, 2006).

PEPFAR has funded projects in multiple countries to measure country efforts responding to the needs of orphans and other vulnerable children (see Box 7-6), including the joint development of the Orphans and Vulnerable Children Programme Index (UNICEF et al., 2004). The Index enabled country governments to conduct situational analyses of the state of orphans and vulnerable children. Its design built upon previous tools for measuring HIV/AIDS efforts, such as the AIDS Programme Effort Index, developed by USAID, UNAIDS, and the Policy Project, and the National Composite Policy Index, implemented by UNAIDS to measure progress toward specific UNGASS goals. The Index scores provide a profile of national and regional efforts, as well as measure the change in efforts over time. It provides a composite score (0–100, with 100 being the highest) based on an examination of eight components: national situation analysis, consultative process, coordinating mechanism, national action plans, policy, legislative review, monitoring and evaluation, and resources. In 2004, 36 countries in sub-Saharan Africa undertook application of the Index (UNICEF et al., 2004). See Table 7-2 for Index scores of the PEPFAR focus countries. According to the developers of the Index, their intent was not to rank or grade individual countries, but to provide useful data to international agencies and donors through profiles of regional and national efforts that have led to

BOX 7-6
Selected Examples of PEPFAR-Supported Activities Intended to Ensure That Governments Protect the Most Vulnerable Children

Botswana and Côte D'Ivoire: development and dissemination of national policy and planning documents to address the needs of children and development of in- and preservice training materials for social workers

Guyana: development and strengthening of referral networks among governments, nongovernmental organizations, social services, and care and support services, as well as support services for both in- and out-of-school children

Mozambique: assistance with capacity-building efforts for child advocacy staff in government ministries, including workshops on finance, coordination, and project oversight

Tanzania: support for programs that increase access to government benefits and building of the capacity of local government authorities, faith-based and nongovernmental organizations, and national organizations, and provision of resources for monitoring and evaluation

South Africa: support for the programs of the Department of Social Development to provide comprehensive services with special attention given to life skills education and training of community-based child and youth workers

SOURCE: OGAC, 2005a,d, 2006b,g.

improvements and identification of areas that may need greater emphasis in the future (UNICEF et al., 2004).

Strategy #5: Raise Awareness to Create a Supportive Environment

Implementation of this strategy for children and families affected by HIV/AIDS encompasses advocacy and social mobilization. Since the beginning of the pandemic, stigma and discrimination have been experienced by people with HIV and their family members, including orphans and other vulnerable children. It is thought that reducing stigma and discrimination may decrease the risk and opportunity of sexual and labor exploitation faced by many orphans and other vulnerable children as a result of their economic vulnerability and the failure to meet their basic needs in a safe and appropriate manner. Faith- and community-based organizations, the media, and nongovernmental organizations can play significant roles along with governmental organizations in raising awareness and promoting acceptance of community responsibility for caring for these children. Examples of PEPFAR-supported activities intended to create supportive environments for orphans and other vulnerable children are listed in Box 7-7.

BOX 7-7
Selected Examples of PEPFAR-Supported Activities Intended to Create a Supportive Environment for Children and Families Affected by HIV/AIDS

Botswana: technical support for monitoring and evaluation, geographic, mapping of services countrywide, training, development of materials on life skills, kids clubs, memory book development, child counseling, community mobilization and advocacy, and caring for caregivers. In a new initiative implemented by the Ministry of Education, it supported training of school administrators, school conveners, neighborhood agents, and social workers in all areas of support for orphans and other vulnerable children in pilot school-based programs, including addressing the psychosocial support needs of children by facilitating linkages among local networks to reintroduce children to school and ensure that they remain to realize their academic potential

South Africa: support for initiatives of local organizations to integrate services of the public and private sectors, improve multisectoral collaboration, strengthen existing and/or build new networks, increase access to foster care grants, develop materials and provide training to caregivers on psychosocial aspects of working with orphans and other vulnerable children that focus on their developmental needs and ways to eliminate stigma and discrimination

Côte d'Ivoire: targeted evaluation of programs and services that support adolescent girls in rebel-occupied zones, support for data collection, management, and analysis to develop an integrated national monitoring and evaluation system

Namibia: identification of significant concentrations of orphans and other vulnerable children, school attendance patterns, and reasons for nonattendance for service and program planning purposes

---

SOURCE: OGAC, 2005a,d, 2006b,g.

HIV Prevention

While many of PEPFAR's prevention activities target youths, it has been difficult to determine to what extent these programs are directed specifically at orphans and other vulnerable children. OGAC has made a number of procedural changes to both improve program linkages and provide more programmatic information on orphans and other vulnerable children, but it remains unclear how well PEPFAR is doing in reaching orphans and other vulnerable children with appropriate prevention messages. The fiscal year 2006 Country Operational Plans provide a number of examples of prevention interventions being funded by PEPFAR that target orphans and other vulnerable children, many of which are linked to other services being provided by PEPFAR (see Box 7-8).

BOX 7-8
Selected Examples of PEPFAR-Supported Prevention Activities Targeting Orphans and Other Vulnerable Children

In **Kenya,** a faith-based charity funded by PEPFAR trains young people to serve as volunteers in actively reaching out to their peers with targeted abstinence, be faithful, and other behavior change messages. The focus is on reducing the vulnerability of orphans and other vulnerable children to HIV infection through a community approach to prevention.

In **Namibia,** a faith-based organization's HIV youth prevention program aims to reduce the rate of HIV prevalence among youths aged 14–25, with a special focus on orphans and other vulnerable children, through delay of sexual debut, abstinence until marriage, and messages discouraging risk behaviors among sexually active youth. Another faith-based organization is working with its local congregations to offer abstinence and be faithful messages through community dramas as a component of a holistic program that also includes home-based care and counseling/referrals.

In **Uganda,** a community-based organization promotes HIV prevention beyond abstinence and being faithful by imparting comprehensive information and skills to the most at-risk populations and making environments safer for women, youths, and people living with HIV. A portion of the programs funding is used to work directly with older orphans and other vulnerable children to promote positive behaviors, such as delay in sexual debut and avoidance of early marriage and exchange of sex for money and gifts.

SOURCE: OGAC, 2006g.

PEPFAR's 2005 guidance for implementation of the ABC model (abstinence until marriage, being faithful, and using condoms), includes a number of programmatic directives related to young people that apply to orphans and other vulnerable children (OGAC, 2005e). Young people who have not had their sexual debut are to be encouraged to practice abstinence until they have established a lifetime monogamous relationship. For those youths who have initiated sexual activity, returning to abstinence is a primary message of PEPFAR's prevention programs. The guidance includes the following restrictions (OGAC, 2006c,d):

- PEPFAR funds may be used in schools to support programs that deliver age-appropriate AB information to young people aged 10 to 14.
- PEPFAR funds may be used in schools to support programs that deliver age-appropriate ABC information for young people above age 14.
- PEPFAR funds may be used to support integrated ABC programs

that include condom provision in out-of-school programs for youths identified as engaging in or at high risk of engaging in risky sexual behaviors.

- PEPFAR funds may not be used to distribute or otherwise provide condoms in school settings.
- PEPFAR funds may not be used in schools for marketing efforts to promote the use of condoms to youths.
- PEPFAR funds may not be used in any setting for marketing campaigns that target youths and encourage condom use as the primary intervention for HIV prevention.

These guidelines are reinforced in the draft work plans of the Technical Working Groups, which promote life skills and AIDS education programs delivered in school settings because these interventions have been shown to be effective, and which encourage programs targeting youth aged 10–14 to emphasize abstinence and the delay of sexual initiation. Given the reported early average age of sexual debut (and sometimes marriage) in many countries, however, PEPFAR may wish to re-examine its exclusive AB focus for younger adolescents.

A number of potential challenges to meeting the needs of orphans and other vulnerable children are associated with these funding restrictions and program considerations, in terms of both the location of programs (e.g., in versus out of school) and ages targeted. As discussed previously, the deteriorating health or death of parents or adult guardians forces many orphans and other vulnerable children to drop out of or interrupt school attendance because funds for tuition are lacking, or other obligations become the child's priority. Prevention programs in the school environment often will not reach this critical population. A number of out-of-school prevention programs exist in many of the focus countries, including community mobilization efforts that often include outreach to peers, adults, and out-of-school youths to expand access to prevention (OGAC, 2005d, 2006g). However, it is not possible to determine how many children are reached with prevention messages through these programs.

The age focus of prevention programs can also be limiting. Being orphaned and otherwise affected by HIV/AIDS can put children in situations in which they are vulnerable to becoming exposed to HIV. Prevention programs must also target these vulnerabilities, including sexual coercion by adults in exchange for food, money, housing, and educational/school opportunities. Such sexually predatory behavior can be committed by extended family members who may be caregivers, employers using an orphaned or vulnerable child's labor for domestic help, or school teachers promising better grades. Thus the risk of HIV exposure and infection may extend beyond the scope of age-specific interventions or school programs communicating abstinence and be faithful messages. While there are some examples of comprehensive prevention programs for children funded by PEPFAR, it is not clear how the Country Teams can ensure that prevention programs in the school environment will provide the range of prevention and care services needed given the current guidelines and planning and funding restrictions.

Preventive Care

Secondary preventive care services (including the administration of cotrimoxazole prophylaxis as early as possible for infants and children) have reduced mortality and morbidity not only for those living with HIV, but also for their family members and children (see Chapter 6). As discussed previously, OGAC released guidance for preventive care services for children aged 0–14 born to mothers who are HIV-positive, which was produced through the collaboration of several of the Technical Working Groups—Palliative Care, Food and Nutrition, and Orphans and Vulnerable Children. In recognition of the specific and age-dependent needs of children, the preventive care package for children varies from that for adults in significant ways. OGAC continues to encourage linkages of these services to other programs that support the basic health care and social service needs of children. Antiretroviral therapy and palliative care for children are addressed in additional guidance from OGAC.

In addition to the services identified in the adult preventive care guidance as outlined in Chapter 6, the guidance for children specifies direct funding for the following services (OGAC, 2006d):

- **Diagnosis of HIV infection in infants**, including purchase of reagents and equipment; establishment of laboratory programs needed to diagnose HIV infection in infants according to national guidelines; training of staff to perform testing; targeted evaluation of practical approaches for scaling up testing in infants; and follow-up and referral at the facility and community levels in accordance with PEPFAR's network model (see Chapter 6).
- **Childhood immunization**, including routine childhood immunizations and pneumococcal and influenza vaccines, referral and follow-up, linkages to routine immunization programs, and technical assistance to develop national policies and training programs for children living with HIV/AIDS. It should be noted that PEPFAR does not directly fund the purchase of *routine* vaccines for infants and children exposed to HIV, but does support the purchase of vaccines for pilot programs and targeted evaluations of new vaccines for children who are HIV-positive.
- **Prevention of serious infections**, including technical assistance for the development of national guidelines and training programs for preventing pneumonia, tuberculosis, malaria, and diarrheal disease in children who

have not been exposed to HIV or are HIV-positive, with recommended linkages to the President's Malaria Initiative and the Global Funds to Fight AIDS, Tuberculosis and Malaria.

- **Providing nutritional care,** including the provision of daily multiple micronutrient supplements for pregnant and lactating women, children, and especially infants weaned early and children under age 2; vitamin A and zinc supplementation according to national guidelines; and nutritional counseling linked to clinical and home-based care in areas where malnutrition is endemic.

Scale-up of PEPFAR's secondary preventive care services for both children and adults has the potential to help keep parents and families healthier longer, decrease the numbers of children who may become orphaned or otherwise made vulnerable as a result of HIV/AIDS, decrease stigma and discrimination against children and their family members, and improve a household's ability to positively cope with being affected by HIV/AIDS.

Progress in Addressing the Vulnerability of Young Girls

OGAC has articulated a commitment to focusing on the special vulnerability of girls to HIV/AIDS and its effects (OGAC, 2005a, 2006a). Many interventions are addressing the factors that make girls vulnerable, including efforts to increase their means of economic/social support, enable them to continue their education, and advocate an end to the practices of early marriage and transgenerational sex as solutions to what families may view as burdens created by orphaned girls (OGAC, 2006a). OGAC has reported that among the orphans and other vulnerable children served by PEPFAR activities, 52 percent have been girls (OGAC, 2006h). OGAC has also reported that PEPFAR is supporting 97 activities aimed at increasing the access of women and girls to income and productive resources (OGAC, 2006h). PEPFAR is also attempting to increase the focus of its programs on gender by working with community partners to reduce violence, including sexual coercion and rape, toward orphans and other vulnerable children, particularly adolescents (OGAC, 2006a).

ISSUES AND OPPORTUNITIES FOR IMPROVEMENT

Varying Definitions

Although the definition of an orphan can differ by country, the main variables are generally age and parental loss (USAID, 2003). International organizations and governments have variably used the under-15 or under-18 age groups to define a child as an orphan if one or both of the parents are deceased. USAID supports community definitions of orphans and does not specify a particular age to delimit childhood and adulthood; it also recognizes the international use of the term "child" as defined by the United Nations Convention on the Rights of the Child as any person under the age of 18 (USAID, 2002). The UNAIDS and UNICEF (2003) *Report on the Technical Consultation on Indicators Development for Children Orphaned and Made Vulnerable by HIV/AIDS* defined an orphan or otherwise vulnerable child as " a child below the age of 18 who has lost one or both parents or lives in a household with an adult death (age 18–59 years) in the past 12 months or is living outside of family care" (p. 4). In addition, "the concept of vulnerability is complex and may include children who are destitute from causes other than HIV/AIDS" (USAID, 2004, p. 1). The *Children on the Brink* series was issued in 2002 and 2004 (UNAIDS et al., 2002, 2004). The 2004 publication revised the age used to delimit childhood from under 15 to under 18 in recognition that "orphans and vulnerable children are not necessarily young children and that problems caused by orphaning extend well beyond the age of 15, [with] available data suggesting that adolescents make up the majority of orphans in all countries" (UNAIDS, 2004, p. 4).

The definition of an orphan in PEPFAR's second annual report as a child below age 15 who has lost one or both parents is consistent with that in the 2002 version of *Children on the Brink* (UNAIDS et al., 2002), but is inconsistent with the 2004 revision. This inconsistency between definitions raises concern about whether PEPFAR service outlets are providing and targeting services to the entire population eligible for those services, and whether the program is overlooking a population of children aged 16–18 who are often the heads of households after the death of a parent or are primary caregivers during the illness of a parent.

Another deviation from international definitions is PEPFAR's definition of vulnerable children as those affected by HIV through the illness of a parent or principal caretaker, which may limit the availability of services for those children who may be in greatest need and at greatest risk for exploitation and increased risk for exposure to HIV. The international community and premier child advocates generally have a more expansive definition of a child's vulnerability as being affected by any disease, including HIV/AIDS, that afflicts a parent/caregiver; living in a household that has taken in orphans; or living on the streets (UNAIDS, 2004). Vulnerability may also differ by community and intervention (Mahy, 2006). These misaligned definitions may also result in underserving child-headed households and many children who may become vulnerable when their households accept orphans.

USAID (2004) acknowledges that the concepts of orphans and other vulnerable children as social constructs have cultural variability, and that depending on their intended versus adopted use, the definitions can often be at odds with each other. For example, the terms may be used for collecting and reporting quantitative data, which would differ from their use for the development and implementation of programs and policies. USAID believes that making these distinctions is important and that "firewalls" should be built around the definitions to minimize the potential consequences of deviation from their original purposes. One of the most common misuses of the terms appears to be the use of quantitative definitions for program eligibility. USAID cautions that quantitative definitions must allow for absolute distinctions, whereas the definitions used in policy and program development and implementation must allow for the local variations that contribute to or cause vulnerability.

UNICEF has called for programs that address the needs of orphans and other vulnerable children living in a world with HIV/AIDS to serve all children who are orphans and are vulnerable regardless of the cause of their state. The primary reason for this position is that either referring to these children as "AIDS orphans" or limiting their eligibility for services to disease-specific vulnerability could further stigmatize them in their communities and families, which in turn could result in mistreatment and discrimination, alienation, or reluctance to access the very services intended to reduce their vulnerability and exposure to HIV infection and improve the quality of their lives. While PEPFAR remains focused on HIV/AIDS, it has put increasing emphasis on the provision of services to children in the context of other service programs and activities for all children in communities and states that "programs must implement effective measures to prevent gender inequity, avoid further degradation of family structures, reduce stigma, avoid marginalization, and that do not generate jealousy and conflict for beneficiaries. Services need to be designed to reduce stigma, not increase it" (OGAC, 2006i, p. 4).

After the publication of its second annual report to Congress and as the program evolved, OGAC disseminated its "Orphans and Other Vulnerable Children Programming Guidance for United States Government In-Country Staff and Implementing Partners." The guidance includes updated definitions for children orphaned or otherwise made vulnerable as a result of HIV/AIDS (OGAC, 2006i, p. 2):

> An orphan is a child, 0–17 years old, who has lost one or both parents to HIV/AIDS. A vulnerable child is a child, 0–17 years old, who is more vulnerable because of any or all of the following factors that result from HIV/AIDS:
>
> - Is HIV-positive
> - Lives without adequate adult support (e.g. in a household with chronically ill parents, a household that has experienced a recent death from a chronic illness, a household headed by a grandparent, and/or a household headed by child)

- Lives outside of family care (e.g. in residential care or on the streets), or
- Is marginalized, stigmatized, or discriminated against.

OGAC's adoption of definitions that are more closely aligned with the current international consensus (and the realities of the needs of children) eliminates some of the Committee's concerns about PEPFAR-supported programming, particularly for adolescents and child heads of household who may be in great need of support and services.

Establishment of Targets

If funding allocations and other budgetary constraints were removed, it would be appropriate for Country Teams, with the help of community-based service providers, to establish quantifiable targets for orphans and other vulnerable children to be served as has been done with PEPFAR's other categories. Even this target setting should be guided not only by the needs of children orphaned and otherwise made vulnerable by HIV/AIDS, but also by the needs of all children who have been orphaned or made vulnerable by any cause—not equivalently based on the estimated numbers of orphans in each country. Communities and countries would then have the flexibility to tailor their responses to all causes of orphanhood and vulnerability and integrate services for all children, while PEPFAR would be able to implement programs for these children in a community-based, family-centered context that would not increase stigma and discrimination due to HIV/AIDS.

Recommendation 7-1: *The needs of orphans and other children made vulnerable by AIDS cover a wide spectrum that cuts across all of PEPFAR's categories of prevention, treatment, and care and extends well beyond the health sector. It is essential for an HIV/AIDS response to address these needs adequately—not only to support these children in living healthy and productive lives, but also to protect them from becoming the next wave of the pandemic.* The U.S. Global AIDS Initiative should continue to support countries in the development of national plans that address the needs of orphans and other children made vulnerable by AIDS, as well as to support the priorities delineated in these plans. To ensure adequate focus on and accountability for addressing the needs of orphans and other vulnerable children, the U.S. Global AIDS Coordinator should work with Congress to set a distinct and meaningful performance target for this population. This target should be developed in a manner that both builds on the improvements PEPFAR has made in its indicator for children served and enhances its ability to support comprehensive and integrated HIV/AIDS programming.

Types and Quality of Services

The Committee had difficulty interpreting the reported results for this category and was left with the question of what it really means to have been served or received care as an orphan or otherwise vulnerable child. The Committee has expressed its concern throughout this report about the variability in types and quality of services, but this concern is most pressing with regard to orphans and other vulnerable children. It was difficult for the Committee to discern whether the current measure reflects how many children have received services or the number of times children have received services. Specific concerns relate to which services the children may have received as described in The Framework, whether the services met their changing needs or the intensity of those needs, and whether a child was counted as served each time if he or she received fewer than the core services from multiple providers. Additional concerns include the length of time over which services were provided and the coverage or reach of the program—especially to children in rural areas. The Committee strongly encourages attention to all of these concerns as OGAC collects data based on its revised indicator for orphans and other vulnerable children indicator. It should be noted that PEPFAR is supporting cost-effectiveness studies for orphans and other vulnerable children care as part of its pursuit of best practices for services to this population.

Workforce Issues

Capacity

Providers of health care services to orphans and other vulnerable children are suffering shortages similar to those discussed elsewhere in this report, which will not be repeated here. The multifaceted needs of children, however, require that other sectors, such as education and social welfare, receive more support for increased resources and technical assistance for development. Many countries, for example, have seen an increase in student enrollment with the abolition of fees to create universal access. As mentioned in Chapter 2, however, increasing deaths among teachers and parents or adult caregivers who can pay school fees have affected the quality of education (through interruptions in education; classroom overcrowding, which may be exacerbated by the desire to decrease the vulnerability of orphans and other vulnerable children by increasing school attendance; inadequate teacher training; and closures of schools). The numbers and characteristics of the school-age population have also been affected, as has the ability to attend school at all for children once they have been orphaned or otherwise made vulnerable as a result of HIV/AIDS (Africa Renewal, 1999, 2007; Earth Policy Institute, 2000; Bundy, 2003).

The U.S. Congressional Research Service (CRS, 2005) cites a study conducted by Hepburn (2001), who found that a teacher who is HIV-positive may lose 6 months of teaching time before dying from the disease. In 2006, Namibia—the country with the smallest reported percentage (0.6 percent) of the global estimate of children orphaned and otherwise made vulnerable because of AIDS—reported that since 2005, it had lost a significant number of teachers to AIDS-related illnesses. According to the Namibian Ministry of Basic Education, Sport, and Culture, roughly 550 teachers annually will die of AIDS-related complications by 2011—fueling teacher absenteeism and leading to a decline in productivity (Kaiser Daily HIV/AIDS Report, 2006). One potential consequence of the deaths of teachers and the interruptions in school enrollment and attendance in many countries is that the countries may not reach their Millennium Development Goals in the area of education. Bundy (2003) has summed it well with the "HIV/AIDS education paradox," in which "education is seen as the one of the most effective 'social vaccines' to prevent HIV/AIDS, but HIV/AIDS destroys education systems."

Child Welfare

In August 2006, UNICEF published a companion paper to The Framework entitled *Child Protection and Children Affected by AIDS,* with the primary purpose of articulating the need to recognize social welfare as a basic part of social services and identify strategies for strengthening this sector to better address vulnerability, abuse, and exploitation. These strategies also include creating legislative frameworks to enforce protective laws; improving the formal care system; supporting and monitoring the well-being of children in informal care; and involving other sectors, such as justice, education, and health, to protect the needs of vulnerable children (UNICEF, 2006c). As most nations have agreed to international conventions on human and children's rights, governments have a primary role of providing social services to vulnerable people and groups. Of particular importance, skilled staff in social service policy, strategic planning, and child welfare and coordination are critical to implementing any recommendation to provide social services. PEPFAR is strongly encouraged to ensure that social workers, child welfare workers, education leaders, law enforcement personnel, and teachers are accorded equal emphasis in human workforce development initiatives—both in in-service and preservice education efforts, and as part of partnerships between government and nongovernment organizations that may possess the expertise and skilled workers sufficiently and urgently needed to meet the needs of these children.

Training and Monitoring of Providers

While the Committee may have been able to ascertain the names of the implementing partners contracted to offer the training for providers of services to orphans and other vulnerable children from the Country Operational Plans, little information was available about the training facilitators or the curricula. Moreover, monitoring of the performance of these providers may have unique features. For some services, those trained may be facilitators or supervisors of others providing the actual service. For example, those trained do not provide educational services, but ensure that children are enrolled in school, have access to funds for educational fees if necessary, have the supplies needed, and participate actively in school. The training curricula may also vary considerably if caring for children involves awareness campaigns for birth registration; skills needed to navigate systems that provide or certify eligibility for services; and other issues related to child survival, such as immunizations and increased use of cotrimaxozole and other preventive care services. The Committee would also like to see more active monitoring of providers and services that include emotional and nutritional support for children.

CONCLUSION

The needs of children orphaned or otherwise made vulnerable by HIV/AIDS will continue to grow as the numbers of these children dramatically escalates as the pandemic continues. It is necessary for PEPFAR and other donors to continue to work with national leaders, families, communities, and organizations to focus their program and policy development efforts on ensuring the survival of these children—breaking the cycle of poverty, despair, disease, and death in which they have lived and seen loved ones die. Through these efforts, the U.S. Global AIDS Initiative can make positive and measurable contributions to the improved health, safety, vitality, and happiness of these children in the most appropriate environments for their development—families and communities.

REFERENCES

Africa Renewal (formerly Africa Recovery). 1999 (December). *AIDS saps Africa's educational system.* http://www.un.org/ecosocdev/geninfo/afrec/ (accessed January 3, 2007).

Africa Renewal (formerly Africa Recovery). 2007. Education in Africa: Africa Recovery special report. *Schools struggling with crises: Financial constraints hamper expansion of primary education in Africa.* http://www.un.org/ecosocdev/geninfo/afrec/ (accessed January 3, 2007).

Bundy. 2003. *Education and HIV/AIDS: Window of hope.* Washington, DC: World Bank.

CRS (Congressional Research Service). 2005. *AIDS orphans and vulnerable children (OVC): Problems, responses, and issues for Congress.* Washington, DC: Library of Congress.

DFID (Department for International Development), UNICEF (United Nations Children's Fund), and UNAIDS (Joint United Nations Programme on HIV/AIDS). 2006. *Technical consultation of global partners forum on children affected by HIV/AIDS. Improving outcomes for children affected by HIV and AIDS: Recapacitating social policy and the state in Africa.* London, England: DFID.

Donahue, J. 2005. Strengthening households and communities: The key to reducing the economic impacts of HIV/AIDS on children and families. In *A generation at risk: The global impact of HIV/AIDS on orphans and vulnerable children.* Edited by G. Foster, C. Levine, and J. Williamson. New York: Cambridge University Press. Pp. 37–65.

Earth Policy Institute. 2000 (July 18). *Africa is dying: It needs help.* http://www.earthpolicy.org (accessed January 3, 2007).

Foster, G., C. Levine, and J. Williamson. 2005. *A generation at risk: The global impact of HIV/AIDS on orphans and vulnerable children.* New York: Cambridge University Press.

Hepburn, A. 2001. *Primary education in eastern and southern Africa: Increasing access for orphans and vulnerable children in AIDS-affected areas.* Durham, NC: Duke University.

Huni, N. 2006. *Technical consultation on children affected by HIV and AIDS: Access to prevention, treatment, and care: Regional perspectives on successes and challenges: Africa (east and southern)* (PowerPoint Presentation). London, England: Regional Psychosocial Support Initiative.

Kaiser Daily HIV/AIDS Report. 2006 (October 24). *Significant number of teachers dying of AIDS-related complications in Namibia.* http://www.kaisernetowrk.org (accessed October, 24, 2006).

Kaiser Family Foundation. 2007. *Children orphaned by AIDS (<18 years old), 2005 global health fact sheet.* http://www.globalhealthfacts.org/topic.jsp?i=8 (accessed January 2, 2007).

Mahy, M. 2006 (February 7–8). *Monitoring and evaluating the response to children affected by HIV and AIDS.* Presentation provided at the Technical Consultation on Children Affected by HIV and AIDS. New York: UNICEF.

OGAC (Office of the U.S. Global AIDS Coordinator). 2004. *The President's Emergency Plan for AIDS Relief: U.S. five-year global HIV/AIDS strategy.* Washington, DC: OGAC.

OGAC. 2005a. *PEPFAR first annual report to Congress.* Washington, DC: OGAC.

OGAC. 2005b. *Final draft HIV/AIDS palliative care guidance #1: An overview of comprehensive HIV/AIDS care services in the President's Emergency Plan for AIDS Relief.* Washington, DC: OGAC.

OGAC. 2005c. *FY2005 funded targeted evaluation studies: Status update.* Washington, DC: OGAC.

OGAC. 2005d. *FY2005 Country Operational Plans.* Washington, DC: OGAC.

OGAC. 2005e. *PEPFAR ABC guidance.* Washington, DC: OGAC.

OGAC. 2005f. *The President's Emergency Plan for AIDS Relief: Indicators, reporting requirements, and guidelines for focus countries* (revised for FY2006 reporting). Washington, DC: OGAC.

OGAC. 2006a. *PEPFAR second annual report to Congress.* Washington, DC: OGAC.

OGAC. 2006b (June 12–15). *Building on successes: Ensuring long-term solutions.* Annotated version of rapporteur presentations at the President's Emergency Plan for AIDS Relief 2006 HIV/AIDS Implementers' Meeting, Durban, South Africa.

OGAC. 2006c. *Adult preventive care guidance.* Washington, DC: OGAC.

OGAC. 2006d. *Child preventive care guidance.* Washington, DC: OGAC.

OGAC. 2006e. *FY2006 funded targeted evaluation studies: Status update.* Washington, DC: OGAC.

OGAC. 2006f. *Centrally-funded targeted evaluation studies: Status update.* Washington, DC: OGAC.

OGAC. 2006g. *FY2006 Country Operational Plans.* Washington, DC: OGAC.

OGAC. 2006h. *PEPFAR report on gender-based violence and HIV/AIDS.* Washington, DC: OGAC.

OGAC. 2006i. *PEPFAR's orphans and vulnerable children programming guidance for United States government in-country staff and implementing partners.* Washington, DC: OGAC.

OGAC. 2007. *PEPFAR third annual report to Congress.* Washington, DC: OGAC.

Phiri, S. N., and D. Tolfree. 2005. Family- and community-based care for children affected by HIV/AIDS: Strengthening the front line response. In *A generation at risk: The global impact of HIV/AIDS on orphans and vulnerable children.* Edited by G. Foster, C. Levine, and J. Williamson. New York: Cambridge University Press. Pp. 11–36.

Population Council. 2004. *Challenges faced by households in caring for orphans and vulnerable children: Horizons research update.* Washington, DC: Population Council.

Save the Children. 2004. *Beyond the targets: Ensuring children benefit from expanded access to HIV/AIDS treatment.* London, England: Save the Children.

Sharp, N. 2005. *Birth registration: Technical consultation of global partners forum on children affected by HIV and AIDS.* Presentation at the PEPFAR Second Annual Field Meeting, Addis Ababa, Ethiopia.

Smart, R. 2003. *Policies for orphans and vulnerable children: A framework for moving ahead.* Washington, DC: The Policy Project.

UNAIDS (Joint United Nations Programme on HIV/AIDS). 2004. *"Three ones" key principles.* Conference paper 1, Washington consultation of April 4, 2004. Geneva, Switzerland: UNAIDS. http://www.unaids.org/NetTools/Misc/DocInfo.aspx?LANG=en&href=http://gva-doc-owl/WEBcontent/Documents/pub/UNA-docs/Three-Ones_KeyPrinciples_en.pdf (accessed September 20, 2006).

UNAIDS. 2006. *2006 report on the global AIDS epidemic.* Geneva, Switzerland: UNAIDS.

UNAIDS and UNICEF (United Nations Children's Fund). 2003. *Report on the technical consultation on indicators development for children orphaned and made vulnerable by HIV/AIDS.* Geneva, Switzerland and New York: UNAIDS and UNICEF.

UNAIDS, UNICEF, and USAID (U.S. Agency for International Development). 2002. *Children on the brink 2002: A joint report on orphan estimates and program strategies.* Geneva, Switzerland: UNAIDS.

UNAIDS, UNICEF, and USAID. 2004. *Children on the brink 2004: A joint report on orphan estimates and program strategies.* Geneva, Switzerland: UNAIDS.

UNICEF (United Nations Children's Fund). 2004. *Background and policy discussion oral report on the global challenge of orphans and vulnerable children.* New York: UNICEF.

UNICEF. 2006a. *Africa's orphaned and vulnerable generations: Children affected by AIDS.* New York: UNICEF.

UNICEF. 2006b. *Report on 3rd global partners forum for children affected by HIV/AIDS.* New York: UNICEF.

UNICEF. 2006c. *Child protection and children affected by AIDS: A companion paper to the framework for the protection, care and support of orphans and vulnerable children living in a world with HIV and AIDS.* New York: UNICEF.

UNICEF and UNAIDS. 2004. *The framework for the protection, care and support of orphans and vulnerable children living in a world with HIV and AIDS.* Geneva, Switzerland: UNAIDS.

UNICEF, UNAIDS, and Futures Group. 2004. *National response to orphans and vulnerable children in sub-Saharan Africa: The orphans and vulnerable children programme effort index.* New York: UNICEF.

USAID (United States Agency for International Development). 2002. *Expanded response to core indicators.* Washington, DC: USAID.

USAID. 2003. *Policies for orphans and vulnerable children: A framework for moving ahead: USAID policy initiative*. Washington, DC: USAID.

USAID. 2004. *Conducting a situational analysis of orphans and vulnerable children affected by HIV/AIDS: A framework and resource guide*. Washington, DC: USAID.

World Bank. 2006. *Poverty reduction strategies*. Washington, DC: World Bank. http://web.worldbank.org/WBSITE/EXTERNAL/TOPICS/EXTPOVERTY/EXTPRS/0,,menuPK:384207~pagePK:149018~piPK:149093~theSitePK:384201,00.html (accessed November 1, 2006).

Part III

Looking to the Future

8

Toward Sustainability

Summary of Key Findings

- In less than 2 years and under challenging circumstances, the U.S. Global AIDS Initiative has made progress toward meeting the 5-year targets of PEPFAR and has established a foundation for achieving the broader, longer-term goals of the Leadership Act.
- The continuing challenge for the U.S. Global AIDS Initiative is to simultaneously maintain the urgency and intensity that have allowed it to support a substantial expansion of HIV/AIDS services in a relatively short time while also placing greater emphasis on long-term strategic planning and increasing the attention and resources directed to capacity building for sustainability.
- Whether one is considering activities and programs within PEPFAR's categories of prevention, treatment, care or orphans and other vulnerable children—and often because of such categorization—similar challenges are evident. These include a need to improve the status of women and girls, the importance of capitalizing on opportunities for synergy by improving the integration of programs, the near exhaustion of existing capacity, and myriad questions that need to be addressed through evaluation and operations research.
- Despite the expanded availability of HIV/AIDS services supported by PEPFAR, the HIV/AIDS pandemic continues to devastate many countries and requires continued U.S. commitment.

Recommendations Discussed in This Chapter

Recommendation 8-1: The U.S. Global AIDS Coordinator should continue to focus on planning for the next decade of the U.S. Global AIDS Initiative, taking full advantage of the knowledge gained from the early years of PEPFAR about the focus countries' epidemics and how best to address them. The next strategy should squarely address the needs and challenges involved in supporting sustainable country HIV/AIDS programs, thereby transitioning from a focus on emergency relief.

Recommendation 8-2: The U.S. Global AIDS Initiative should continue to increase its focus on the factors that put women at greater risk of HIV/AIDS and to support improvements in the legal, economic, educational, and social status of women and girls.

Recommendation 8-3: To meet existing targets for prevention, treatment, and care, the U.S. Global AIDS Initiative should increase the support available to expand workforce capacity in heavily affected countries. These efforts should include education of new health care workers in addition to AIDS-related training for existing health care workers. Such support should be planned in conjunction with other donors to ensure that comparative advantages are maximized and be provided in the context of national human resource strategies that include relevant stakeholders, such as the ministries of health, labor, and education; other ministries; employers; regulatory bodies; professional associations; training institutions; and consumers.

Recommendation 8-4: The U.S. Global AIDS Initiative should increase its contribution to the global evidence base for HIV/AIDS interventions by better capitalizing on the opportunity PEPFAR represents to learn about and share what works. The U.S. Global AIDS Coordinator should further emphasize the importance of and provide additional support for operations research and program evaluation in particular—not as the primary aim but as an integral component of programs. All programs should include robust monitoring and evaluation that factors into decisions about whether and in what manner the programs are to continue. The initiative should maintain its appropriate openness to new and innovative approaches and programs, but unproven programs in particular should be required to have an evaluation component to determine their effectiveness.

8

Toward Sustainability

This chapter examines the President's Emergency Plan for AIDS Relief (PEPFAR) as a whole and focuses on themes that emerge across all four PEPFAR categories. The focus is on identifying improvements that would support the U.S. Global AIDS Initiative in making further progress toward its 5-year targets and the ultimate goal of the Leadership Act—U.S. leadership in addressing and controlling the HIV/AIDS pandemic.

COMMON THEMES

PEPFAR Has Supported Expanded Availability of HIV/AIDS Services

In the 15 focus countries, the U.S. Global AIDS Initiative has, as intended, supported HIV/AIDS activities and programs on a national scale, and the Office of the Global AIDS Coordinator (OGAC) reports substantial early progress toward its targets. In roughly 2 years, OGAC reports that PEPFAR has supported antiretroviral therapy (ART) for more than 800,000 adults and children; HIV testing and counseling for nearly 19 million people; services to prevent mother-to-child transmission of HIV to more than 6 million women, including preventive antiretroviral medications (ARVs) for more than half a million women found to be HIV-positive (estimated by OGAC to have resulted in the prevention of HIV infection in more than 100,000 infants); public education campaigns, school curricula, and other types of information and education community outreach that are estimated to have reached more than 140 million adults and children; care and support services for approximately 4.5 million adults, orphans, and other vulnerable children; training in HIV/AIDS care and support services for well over a million people, including physicians, nurses, clinical officers, pharmacists, laboratory workers, epidemiologists, community workers, teachers, midwives, birth attendants, and traditional healers; and expansion and strengthening of clinical laboratories, supply chain management systems, blood supply systems, safe medical practices, and monitoring and evaluation systems (OGAC, 2005a, 2006a, 2007). Although data are not yet available with which to determine the quality or impact of these services, the Committee believes this substantial expansion of services represents inroads into the HIV/AIDS epidemics in the focus countries. Although data are not yet available to determine the quality or impact of these services, the Committee believes that this substantial expansion of services represents significant inroads into the HIV/AIDS epidemics in the focus countries.

Transition from Emergency to Sustainability Is Critical for Success

In 2003, when the U.S. Congress passed the landmark Leadership Act, it was widely recognized that the HIV/AIDS pandemic in developing countries had reached crisis proportions and had to be addressed urgently. According to the Leadership Act:

> Congress recognizes that the alarming spread of HIV/AIDS in countries in sub-Saharan Africa, the Caribbean, and other developing countries is a major global health, national security, development, and humanitarian crisis. (p. 728)

A previous Institute of Medicine (IOM) committee that examined the issues surrounding scale-up of ART at the start of PEPFAR urged that "ART scale-up in resource-constrained settings worldwide must proceed immediately." The committee detailed the challenges involved, but stated:

> Recognizing these challenges, there remains an urgency to provide ART as rapidly as is feasible in order to extend the duration of as many lives as possible and reverse the course of social collapse in many countries heavily afflicted by HIV/AIDS. (IOM, 2005, p. 3)

In keeping with global consensus, congressional mandate, and expert opinion, OGAC characterized its strategy as an "emergency plan" and has implemented PEPFAR accordingly. A study by the Center for Strategic and International Studies issued shortly after publication of the PEPFAR strategy asserted that the ultimate success of PEPFAR would be judged in large part by the speed of its response; highlighted several "impressive, early, and accelerated steps taken to create and begin PEPFAR"; and made many recommendations for enhancing the capacity of the U.S. Global AIDS Coordinator (the Coordinator) to continue to implement the initiative rapidly and effectively (Nieburg et al., 2004, p. 3).

Hallmarks of PEPFAR have been its continued sense of urgency and the rapidity with which it has supported the implementation of programs and delivery of services—not only ART, but across the spectrum of HIV/AIDS care and support. As discussed in the preceding chapters, the speed with which PEPFAR has been implemented has drawn both praise and criticism and has had both positive and negative consequences.

Awareness of the 5-year life of the Leadership Act and the characterization of the strategy as a "Plan for Emergency Relief" has generated anxiety that the United States does not plan to be involved in the fight against HIV/AIDS for the long haul, as will be necessary to allow countries to develop sustainable programs. During the Committee's visits to the focus countries, it heard expressions of both deep appreciation and gratitude for U.S. leadership and generosity, and profound concern about whether and for how long the United States would sustain its commitment. Many of the people with whom the Committee met—officials of the host country governments, people working in community-based organizations of all varieties, people working in clinical facilities of all types, and people from all walks of life living with HIV/AIDS and its consequences—pointed to their organization, their facility, their personnel, their equipment, their supplies, or simply themselves and said they were there thanks to U.S. support. At the same time, however, they were already worried about what would happen after 5 years and asking: Could the country sustain these programs without continued support? What would happen to the people who were on ART? What about all the people waiting for programs to expand so they could be accommodated? Should people even start ART if there is a chance they would have to stop?

The understanding of the HIV/AIDS pandemic as an exceptional kind of long-term crisis requiring both an urgent as well as a sustained and sustainable response, and the thinking that the key to sustainability is country ownership and leadership and that the harmonization imperative is central to supporting countries all developed in concert (UN, 2003a,b; UNAIDS, 2004; Jooma, 2005). The Leadership Act highlighted the challenge of expanding "interventions from a pilot program basis to a national basis in a coherent and sustainable manner" (p. 714). The same IOM committee that urged the provision of ART as rapidly as feasible also made several recommendations for ensuring the sustainability of such initiatives (IOM, 2005). The same analysts from the Center for Strategic and International Studies who praised the urgency of PEPFAR's action also asserted that its ultimate success would be judged not only by the speed of its responses, but also by their sustainability (Nieburg et al., 2004). Increasingly, the approach advocated for addressing the HIV/AIDS crisis eschews the dichotomy between emergency relief and long-term development and favors instead a blending of "developmental relief" and "emergency development," while underscoring the importance of working within the framework of harmonization to promote country ownership and leadership for sustainability (UN, 2003a,b; UNAIDS, 2004, Jooma, 2005; Ooms, 2006). According to the United Nations:

> Both developmental relief—humanitarian assistance that contributes to sustainable development—and emergency development—urgent and accelerated assistance to aid nations in overcoming the long-term negative impact of AIDS, must be put into practice. Like traditional humanitarian assistance, the response must move quickly and draw on international human resources to complement in-country capacity; and like traditional development assistance, it must focus on capacity building, improving existing structures and sustainability. (2003b, p. 27)

Although PEPFAR is characterized as a plan for emergency relief, the Coordinator has also characterized harmonization as its central tenet and described "building capacity for sustainable, effective, and widespread HIV/AIDS responses" as one of the cornerstones of the PEPFAR strategy (OGAC, 2004, p. 4). From the outset, PEPFAR has sought to strengthen and expand the capacity of the focus countries to develop national HIV/AIDS programs and provide services. PEPFAR has provided substantial funding and technical assistance for many activities intended to be of lasting benefit—supporting focus country governments in the development of national plans and monitoring and evaluation systems; improving existing and building new facilities; developing curricula for and training a wide variety of health workers; strengthening and expanding laboratory, blood supply, and medical waste management systems; improving and expanding supply chains; and strengthening existing and fostering new community-based organizations (OGAC, 2005a,b, 2006a). PEPFAR's second annual report to Congress is titled *Action Today: A Foundation for Tomorrow* and evidences a continued commitment to harmonization and an increased emphasis on sustainability (OGAC, 2006a).

Recommendation 8-1: *The continuing challenge for the U.S. Global AIDS Initiative is to simultaneously maintain the urgency and intensity that have allowed it to support a substantial expansion of HIV/AIDS services in a relatively short time while also placing greater emphasis on long-term strategic planning and increasing the attention and resources directed to capacity building for sustainability.* The U.S. Global AIDS Coordinator should continue to focus on planning for the next decade of the U.S. Global AIDS Initiative, taking full advantage of the knowledge gained from the early years of PEPFAR about the focus countries' epidemics and how best to address them. The next strategy should squarely address the needs and challenges involved in supporting sustainable country HIV/AIDS programs, thereby transitioning from a focus on emergency relief.

The Committee's recommendations for improvement are premised on the assumption that Congress will reauthorize the U.S. Global AIDS Initiative and are directed toward helping PEPFAR continue the transition from emergency response to sustainability, and thus to make further progress toward both its 5-year performance targets and the ultimate goal of the Leadership Act. None of the issues raised by the Committee or its recommendations for enabling PEPFAR to progress more effectively should be construed as a lack of general support for the U.S. Global AIDS Initiative or its authorizing legislation.

Increasing Focus on Status of Women and Girls Is Key to Sustainability

The Leadership Act calls for a focus on women and girls and articulates the need to address their particular vulnerability if the response to the HIV/AIDS pandemic is to succeed. Specifically, the act requires that the PEPFAR strategy provide the following:

> • A description of the specific strategies developed to meet the unique needs of women, including the empowerment of women in interpersonal situations, young people and children, including those orphaned by HIV/AIDS and those who are victims of the sex trade, rape, sexual abuse, assault, and exploitation.
> • A description of the specific strategies developed to encourage men to be responsible in their sexual behavior, child rearing and to respect women including the reduction of sexual violence and coercion.
> • A description of the specific strategies developed to increase women's access to employment opportunities, income, productive resources, and microfinance programs. (p. 719)

The PEPFAR strategy is responsive to these mandates, and OGAC reports that PEPFAR is currently supporting numerous programs and services directed at reducing the risks faced by women and girls (see Table 8-1). Country Teams have categorized PEPFAR-supported activities according to whether they are focused in any of five areas: (1) increasing gender equity, (2) addressing male norms, (3) reducing violence and sexual coercion, (4) increasing income generation for both women and girls, and (5) ensuring legal protection and property rights (OGAC, 2004). However, no information is yet available with which to determine either the individual or collective impact of these activities on the status of and risks to women and girls.

To the extent possible with data collection systems that do not always identify the sex of the person receiving services, PEPFAR has been able to demonstrate that women and girls are receiving PEPFAR-supported prevention, treatment, and care services in proportions equal to or greater than

TABLE 8-1 Summary of PEPFAR Activities Responsive to Legislative Imperatives Concerning Women and Girls

Legislative Imperative	Number of Related Activities Identified as Responsive to Imperative in Fiscal Year 2006 Country Operational Plans
Increase gender equity	460
Address male norms and behavior	348
Reduce violence and coercion	243
Increase women's and girls' access to income and productive resources	97
Increase women's legal rights	80

SOURCE: OGAC, 2006h.

men and boys.[1] Table 8-2 summarizes the access of women and girls to PEPFAR-supported services.

Although it was formed relatively late,[2] OGAC has established a Technical Working Group on Gender. Its purpose is to support focus country programs in implementing "evidence-based, gendered approaches" in order to meet legislative requirements and PEPFAR goals (see Box 8-1). In June 2006, the Coordinator hosted a "Gender Consultation" and committed to acting on the recommendations developed as a result. The Committee urges the Coordinator to keep this commitment and implement the recommendations expeditiously.

> **Recommendation 8-2:** ***Most of the factors that contribute to the increased vulnerability of women and girls to HIV/AIDS cannot be readily addressed in the short term. The Leadership Act appropriately views these factors as priorities on the agenda for the fight against HIV/AIDS. In the transition from emergency response to sustainability, these factors will require increased emphasis and support, and the U.S. Global AIDS Initiative will need to keep gender issues at the core of its efforts.*** **The U.S. Global AIDS Initiative should continue to increase its focus on the factors that put women at greater risk of HIV/AIDS and to support improvements in the legal, economic, educational, and social status of women and girls.**

[1]For sites that PEPFAR supports directly, disaggregation of data by sex is possible, and the sex of more than 90 percent of clients is known. Disaggregation by sex of data on activities that PEPFAR supports indirectly is possible when enabled by national data collection systems.

[2]The Technical Working Group on Gender was established in September 2005, later than most of the other groups.

TABLE 8-2 Summary of Access to PEPFAR-Supported Services for Women and Girls

PEPFAR Category	Service	Access to Services
Prevention	Prevention of mother-to-child transmission	Accessed by women during 6 million pregnancies
Treatment	Antiretroviral treatment	Women 61% of recipients
Care	Voluntary counseling and testing	Women 70% of people served*
Orphans and Other Vulnerable Children	Services for orphans and other vulnerable children	Girls 51% of children receiving services

*Includes voluntary counseling and testing provided as part of services to prevent mother-to-child transmission.

SOURCE: OGAC, 2006h, 2007.

BOX 8-1
Objectives of the Gender Technical Working Group

At the country level:

- Provide targeted technical assistance to country programs to ensure that they meet PEPFAR legislative requirements related to gender issues.
- Assist country programs in designing and implementing evidence-based approaches and best practices addressing gender issues.
- Assess the progress of all country programs in addressing gender issues, and strengthen their capacity to monitor and report on this progress.
- Conduct technical reviews of country program plans and strategies to help ensure that gender-related legislative requirements are being addressed and that best practices for addressing gender issues are being incorporated into programs.

At the central level:

- Provide technical guidance to other Technical Working Groups to promote integration of gender-sensitive approaches into their programmatic guidance and oversight.
- Provide program and policy guidance and support OGAC in responding to PEPFAR legislative requirements and requests related to gender issues, women, and girls.
- Organize forums (globally and regionally) to exchange technical information on gender issues and promote networking.
- Identify areas for and facilitate development of targeted evaluations for program improvement.

SOURCE: OGAC, 2006d.

The Committee believes these improvements are necessary to create conditions that will facilitate the access of women and girls to HIV/AIDS services; support them in changing behaviors that put them at risk for HIV transmission; allow them to better care for themselves, their families, and their communities; and enhance their ability to lead and be part of their country's response to its HIV/AIDS epidemic (WHO, 2007).

Expanded Capacity Is Necessary to Meet Current and Future Needs

The impact of capacity constraints on the implementation of PEPFAR is a common theme of this report. PEPFAR's initial emergency approach was to rely heavily on U.S.- and country-based contractors who had existing operations that could be scaled up relatively quickly with an infusion of resources and to strengthen the existing capacity in the focus countries. Through this approach, the initiative has supported the delivery of counseling and testing, ART, prevention of mother-to-child transmission, and other HIV/AIDS services to millions of people; the renovation and equipping of hundreds of counseling and testing, treatment, pharmacy, information technology, laboratory, and other facilities; and the training of thousands of clinicians, pharmacists, laboratory technologists, epidemiologists, information technology specialists, and other health care workers (OGAC, 2005a, 2006a, 2007). OGAC reported that to date PEPFAR has provided nearly \$350 million for capacity building including training and the development of networks, human resources, and local organizations (OGAC, 2007). However, the growing consensus is that existing capacity for HIV/AIDS services is nearing exhaustion, and donors need to focus more on helping to expand capacity. During its visits to the focus countries, the Committee saw many programs of all varieties, but particularly those providing ART, that were overflowing their capacity, had long waiting lists, and had insufficient numbers of staff who were highly stressed. The shortage of health care workers of all kinds was particularly acute. To be successful over the long term, the U.S. Global AIDS Initiative will need to continue to help increase the capacity of the focus countries to sustain and expand their gains against the epidemic, both directly by investing in capacity building and indirectly by implementing PEPFAR in a way that strengthens and does not undermine existing public health systems. "Capacity" needs to be conceptualized broadly and will need to be expanded at all levels: individual, family/household, community, and country.

Initially, the Leadership Act assumed that the primary challenge of the U.S. Global AIDS Initiative would be to afford and provide ARVs—hence the budget allocation of 55 percent of total PEPFAR funding for treatment, 75 percent of this for ARVs. As implementation has progressed, that challenge has remained, while many other challenges to providing ART and other services have come to the fore. These include prevailing conditions such as poverty and malnutrition; generally weak public health infrastructures; other prevalent diseases, such as malaria and tuberculosis; nascent civil society sectors; and severe human resource shortages. Because PEPFAR both is disease-specific and works in parallel with rather than through partner governments, these challenges are especially compelling, requiring PEPFAR to be particularly vigilant to ensure that its implementation does not have unintended negative consequences for overall public health in the focus countries.

Facilities

In the focus countries, facilities for delivering HIV/AIDS services are generally limited in number, geographic distribution, and capacity. The Committee visited areas that had no facilities of certain types, sites that were the only facility of their kind in large catchment areas requiring lengthy travel for the people who needed to use them, and facilities that appeared to be very small relative to the numbers of people they were intended to serve. PEPFAR is supporting a range of activities to address these limitations, from mobile testing and treatment programs to construction projects. During its visits to the focus countries, the Committee saw many examples of PEPFAR-supported renovations of facilities and a few examples of PEPFAR-supported new construction, and some of the Country Teams reported being able to support the construction of new facilities through various mechanisms. However, the Country Teams expressed to the Committee a great deal of confusion about the differing regulations of the many PEPFAR implementing agencies concerning new construction. OGAC reported that it recently issued a report clarifying these regulations and the capabilities of the implementing agencies and that it encourages Country Teams to support new construction where necessary and appropriate. This report was issued after the Committee had completed its visits to the focus countries, and thus the Committee was not able to confirm its effect with the Country Teams.

Community-Based Organizations

Although PEPFAR initially relied heavily on existing U.S.- and country-based contractors and large contracts, it has several mechanisms in place to strengthen the civil sectors of the focus countries by increasing the number and capacity of indigenous, particularly community-based organizations (OGAC, 2005a, 2006a). Country Teams are evaluated on the basis of the number of new and indigenous partners they are bringing into the program, and OGAC has policies in place to limit the proportion of a Country Team's budget that can go to any one partner, which has decreased over time (OGAC, 2005c, 2006d,e). Early in the program, OGAC utilized an innovative mechanism for "umbrella" organizations that would help to develop and strengthen small, local organizations capable of obtaining and managing PEPFAR funds (OGAC, 2005a, 2006a). Overseeing and being accountable for numerous small and fledgling organizations is considerably more challenging for Country Teams than managing fewer, larger, more experienced contractors, however, and the Country Teams expressed to the Committee their need to be able to spend more time with these organizations and in the field. OGAC and the ambassadors need to ensure that Country Teams have adequate resources for this critical capacity-building effort.

Supply Chain

Many aspects of the supply chain for public health commodities require strengthening in all of the focus countries, and PEPFAR supports the development of this crucial component of the public health infrastructure. The recently established Partnership for Supply Chain Management will contribute to the sustainability of focus country infrastructure only to the extent that it effectively supports the development of indigenous capacity in all aspects of the supply chain, from manufacturing, to management, to distribution. The partnership has not been in existence long enough for the Committee to evaluate its effectiveness, but its ultimate success needs to be measured in these terms. For a fuller discussion of the partnership see Chapter 5.

Coordination

Effective coordination among both U.S. foreign aid programs and other donors and effective leadership by the host country governments are especially critical for a program that is disease-specific and works in parallel with country governments. The U.S. ambassadors to the focus countries need to continue to coordinate PEPFAR with other U.S. aid programs, such as those addressing food and nutrition, reproductive health, and child welfare, to achieve effective integration of services and maximize the synergy among these programs. It is also necessary for the Coordinator to continue to participate in global efforts to coordinate and capitalize on the relative strengths of the various HIV/AIDS, health, and development donors. See Chapter 3 for a fuller discussion of coordination.

Evaluation

Many activities supported by PEPFAR can have benefits for the larger public health system and the civil sector of the host countries. For example, programs to strengthen laboratory capacity, ensure safe blood supplies, promote safe medical practices and proper handling and disposal of medical waste, strengthen supply chain management, empower communities, strengthen information systems, promote registration of births and orphans, and change inheritance laws (OGAC, 2005a, 2006a,b,c,f,g) have benefits that are not exclusive to the HIV/AIDS response. However, any such benefits and any unintended negative consequences will not be fully appreciated if the initiative is evaluated only with respect to HIV/AIDS targets. To be certain that PEPFAR is strengthening and not undermining existing public health systems, accountability for its impact on public health and public health systems overall is critical. Measures of this impact need to include workforce and infrastructure, as well as other health outcomes, such as infant mortality and all-cause mortality (WHO et al., 2004). Implementation of these measures in turn will require continued PEPFAR support for strengthening national public health monitoring and evaluation systems.

Human Resources

ART is a complex intervention that is being expanded in areas already short of personnel (IOM, 2005). It is widely acknowledged that the lack of trained health workers is a major challenge to further scaling up of AIDS services, particularly ART (IOM, 2005; Gilks et al., 2006; UNAIDS, 2006). The UNAIDS Global Steering Committee, for example, has ranked this as one of the major obstacles to scaling up the HIV/AIDS response (UNAIDS, 2006). Likewise, policy makers and field staff in some of the most affected countries cite the lack of human resources for health as the single most serious obstacle to scaling up treatment. While there are no estimates available of the additional health personnel needed to respond to the global HIV/AIDS crisis, the World Health Organization (WHO) had estimated it would be necessary to train an extra 100,000 health workers just to meet its "3 by 5" program target of treating 3 million people by 2005 (WHO, 2004a).

Plans for ART scale-up developed by some host countries and in progress in others include specific efforts to increase the health care workforce, with an emphasis on numbers of nurses, clinical officers, and pharmacists, among others (Kober and Van Damme, 2004; UNAIDS, 2006). Conceptually, there are three approaches to addressing the shortage of human resources:

- Train more personnel.
- Retain the personnel already in place.
- Increase the efficiency of existing personnel by providing training in ART and shifting responsibilities from the scarcest groups to others.

To date, PEPFAR's strategy has focused on the second and third approaches. Its policy is

> to provide support, within national plans and priorities and the principles of the "3 ones", for policy reform to promote task-shifting from physicians and nurses to community health workers; development of information systems; human resources assessments; training support for health workers, including community health workers; retention strategies; and twinning partnerships. (OGAC, 2006c, p. 7)

Retention strategies Shortages of health care personnel for ART are a problem in all focus countries, but the nature of the problem varies greatly, both qualitatively and quantitatively, among countries. Some countries with well-established medical and nursing schools that meet foreign standards are particularly subject to "brain drain" to Europe, Canada, and the United States. Moreover, the presence of donors and nongovernmental organizations in the country can offer a number of attractive, better-paid alternatives for physicians and nurses relative to direct patient care, with the result that brain drain is internal as well as external. The problem of retention has plagued sub-Saharan Africa for many years and is far more acute now that ART is under way (Chankova, 2006; Huber, 2006; Wonodi, 2006).

Appropriate distribution of health care workers is difficult to accomplish, as it has been in the developed world. Many health care workers prefer not to work in rural areas, to which transportation is limited and erratic, and where professional communication is constrained and housing is poor. Physicians, clinical officers, and nurses that the Committee encountered in such settings often expressed to the Committee a desire to return to a large city once their term of rural service was over.

PEPFAR is supporting a number of activities focused on retention of health workers (OGAC, 2006c). In the process, Country Teams are increasingly able to identify techniques that work and can be shared across countries. In Zambia, for example, the Country Team is collaborating with the Ministry of Health to support a physician retention scheme that provides incentives to 30–35 physicians who serve in rural areas throughout the country, such as housing, hardship allowance, transportation, and educational stipends for their children. PEPFAR estimates that this initiative will result in an additional 5,000 people receiving ART services. In Namibia, the Ministry of Health provides a package of benefits, including medical benefits, housing support, paid maternity leave, a "13th cheque" on workers' birthdays, and competitive salaries. A nongovernmental organization in Uganda retains lay health workers who provide ART follow-up care in remote areas by providing, along with a supportive work environment, field and transportation allowances, refunds for medical expenses, and salary increments for good performance (OGAC, 2006c).

One aspect of retention that is not emphasized in PEPFAR's workforce strategy is the need to protect health workers from exposure to HIV and to identify and treat those who are exposed or infected. Postexposure prophylaxis is established policy in many countries but does not appear to be used frequently. There are few specific counseling and testing campaigns for health workers, some of whom express concern about being tested because of the lack of privacy. All of the relevant policies are currently present in PEPFAR's prevention and treatment strategy but are not consolidated in a manner that would enable the development of an effective approach for health workers. This important issue requires greater emphasis since in some countries, as many as 25 percent of all workers may be presumed to be infected, and losses to HIV are increasingly frequent.

Improvements in efficiency through task shifting A mainstay of PEPFAR policy, also endorsed by WHO, is task shifting from scarce workers to those who are more generally available (Gilks et al., 2006). The term is somewhat confusing in that it covers everything from the full delegation of responsibility for treatment to clinical officers and/or nurses to the training of lay counselors to offer counseling and testing and of community workers to support adherence. One approach is WHO's integrated management of adult, adolescent, and childhood illness, which promotes the shifting of responsibility for follow-up of stable patients to clinical teams at primary care facilities (WHO, 2004b). These teams are expected to be able to treat nonsevere opportunistic infections, manage ART, undertake simple clinical decision making, and promote prevention of transmission in areas where the HIV burden is high (Gilks et al., 2006). In many settings, such responsibilities can be assumed without changes in existing standards for the practice of nurses or clinical officers.

Another, more radical approach has been demonstrated in Zambia and Malawi (Harries et al., 2006; Stringer et al., 2006), where specially trained clinical officers and nurses are responsible for the complete management of ART. Other areas in which adaptation of practice rules and shifting of tasks are needed include requirements that only pharmacists or pharmacy technicians may dispense ARVs.

Recently, the Ministry of Health in Mozambique removed the requirement that only physicians may prescribe ARVs, so that prescribing may be done by other health professionals with appropriate, targeted training. Similarly, Kenya and Ethiopia now allow clinical officers to prescribe ARVs. Rwanda has adopted a pilot program that allows nurses to prescribe ARVs and now permits trained nurses to provide follow-up to patients on ART. In Uganda, lay people, many of them people living with HIV/AIDS, have been trained to provide basic nursing care; supply refills of medications for ART, tuberculosis, and opportunistic infections; and monitor adherence (OGAC, 2006c).

PEPFAR's support of ministries of health in making such changes and its dissemination of information on their success are important elements of the development of an efficient cadre of workers to carry out treatment (OGAC, 2006c). While task shifting is an important step toward addressing the shortage of health care workers, however, there are also a number of ways in which existing personnel can improve efficiency without practice rules being altered. These include changes in protocols to reduce the number of repeat visits made by stable patients, reductions in the requirements for what must take place during a visit, and improvements in record keeping and the efficiency with which facilities operate. In this area as well, PEPFAR's emphasis on identifying and sharing the most successful innovations is particularly important.

Improvements in efficiency through training Since the beginning of the program, PEPFAR has supported training of more than 100,000 service providers in ART. Also, the program supported more than 1,900 sites for ART in the 15 focus countries (OGAC, 2005a, 2006c, 2007). As of July 2006, OGAC estimated that $140 million had been committed to training (OGAC, 2006c).

Twinning, which pairs educational institutions to build cooperation in development, was proposed by WHO as an attractive approach to policy reform in sub-Saharan Africa as early as 1997. Twinning between industrialized and developing countries, across developing countries, and between institutions within a country has been a mainstay of PEPFAR policy (WHO, 2001; OGAC, 2005a, 2006a,c). Support in this area includes curriculum development that integrates HIV/AIDS care into nursing and medical school curricula.

Training of more personnel As described, PEPFAR's initial emergency approach to personnel was to focus on HIV-specific training of existing clinicians and other health care workers. Contributions to expansion of the general workforce have been very limited, even when such expansion has been an explicit part of the country's AIDS plan and the effort has been endorsed and supported by other donors. As noted earlier, during its visits to the focus countries, the Committee saw many programs of all varieties—particularly ART programs—in need of additional staff. Some Country Teams expressed concern that they were not allowed to fund activities unless they were specifically part of the HIV/AIDS effort and thus could not support, for example, the training of new clinical officers, who in some countries are the mainstay of the treatment effort.

Recommendation 8-3: To meet existing targets for prevention, treatment, and care, the U.S. Global AIDS Initiative should increase the support available to expand workforce capacity in heavily affected countries. These efforts should include education of new health care workers in addition to AIDS-related training for existing health care workers. Such support should be planned in conjunction with other donors to ensure that comparative advantages are maximized and be provided in the context of national human resource strategies that include relevant stakeholders, such as the ministries of health, labor, and education; other ministries; employers; regulatory bodies; professional associations; training institutions; and consumers.

It is important to keep in mind that a large portion of the workforce for HIV/AIDS in resource-constrained countries is not professional and is often uncompensated. Many programs that PEPFAR is supporting, particularly those in its care category, rely heavily on volunteers. These volunteers are usually familial caregivers—most often women, young girls, and elderly grandmothers, who are often as vulnerable and in as great a need of assistance as the people for whom they are caring—and they may be unable to continue in this role for long. Little is known about the extent to which volunteers receive any form of compensation or the potential effect this would have on the management and sustainability of community and country programs. Further exploration of these workforce and caregiver issues is critical to the sustainability of community- and home-based services and could be a focus of PEPFAR's targeted evaluation efforts.

Comprehensiveness and Integration of Services Need to Be Improved

The need for comprehensive, integrated HIV/AIDS programs is a common theme throughout this report. One of the Committee's greatest concerns is that the current management of PEPFAR, in its attempt to design budgeting, planning, and reporting mechanisms responsive to the congressional budget allocations, actively works against integration. In countries that have undertaken integrated planning, Country Teams have reported struggling to provide responsive support. Optimal integration is critical not only for the success of individual interventions or services, but also to achievement of the additional benefits that derive from the synergy among them (Salomon et al., 2005).

The Committee finds that PEPFAR is responsive to the Leadership Act's call for integration in its strategy and guidance, but may be falling short of doing so in practice. According to the strategy, PEPFAR is based on an integrated HIV/AIDS prevention, treatment, and care model that is the "established best practice of providing a continuum of care consisting of a full range of integrated HIV/AIDS services. The availability of each of the continuum's activities—prevention, treatment, and care—strengthens and reinforces the effect of each intervention" (OGAC, 2004, p. 17). The importance of networks, linkages, and referrals—to "integrate medical and non-medical services to care for the whole person and the family at the community level" (Dybul, 2005)—is emphasized throughout PEPFAR's strategy and guidance documents (OGAC, 2004, 2006d,e), as well as supporting materials for the Country Teams provided by the Technical Working Groups (OGAC, 2006d,e). Improving integration is the subject of a number of PEPFAR's current targeted evaluations and a priority for future ones.

Although PEPFAR's annual and other reports have highlighted some successes with integration (OGAC, 2005a, 2006a), OGAC is not systematically evaluating whether it is succeeding at supporting integrated programs and services. Thus the Committee was unable to determine whether the initiative has improved in the area of integration overall. During its visits to the focus countries, the Committee observed several positive examples of integration among PEPFAR-supported programs—of systems for referral from counseling and testing programs to ART programs, of linkages between ART services and home-based care services, and of integration of HIV and tuberculosis testing and treatment. But the Committee also observed many missed opportunities for improving the comprehensiveness and effectiveness of services through better integration—for example, between programs aimed at prevention of mother-to-child transmission and infant feeding programs; between counseling and testing services and further counseling services, ART, and other treatment; between counseling and testing and clinics addressing sexually transmitted infections and reproductive health; between HIV and tuberculosis testing and treatment services; among multisectoral services for orphans and other vulnerable children; and between HIV/AIDS and food aid programs.

Faith-based organizations play an important role in the fight against HIV/AIDS and have a broad reach into communities in all the focus countries (WHO, 2004c; GHC, 2005; EPN, 2006). PEPFAR is partnering with a wide range of such organizations (OGAC, 2005d). However, the Committee is concerned that exemptions for faith-based organizations could contribute to a lack of comprehensive services available at the community level and of routine integration of prevention into all programs. Specifically, the Leadership Act underscores the importance of involving faith-based organizations in the initiative and states that "[a]n organization that is otherwise eligible to receive assistance . . . to prevent, treat, or monitor HIV/AIDS shall not be required, as a condition of receiving the assistance, to endorse or utilize a multisectoral approach to combating HIV/AIDS, or to endorse, utilize, or participate in a prevention method or treatment program to which the organization has a religious or moral objection" (p. 733). In practical terms, this means that organizations with a religious or moral objection are exempt from having to promote and provide condoms, even when doing so is necessary to address the needs of the population with which they are working. For example a faith-based organization with an objection to condoms could be operating a counseling and testing program, ART program, or prevention program and not be providing information about condoms or condoms themselves.

During its country visits, the Committee was told by some faith-based organization partners that when individual clients requested access to or information about condoms, they were referred to a service outlet that could give them what they wanted, and that this process would ensure that all individuals who needed condoms would get them. During the country visits, however, the Committee heard concerns about the extent to which these referrals were routine and consistent. Conversely, the Committee did not observe or hear about organizations that had sought an exemption from providing abstinence/be faithful information and programming.

It is critical that prevention succeed, and thus PEPFAR needs to have strong mechanisms for ensuring that all proven prevention interventions are available where needed. Even as defined by PEPFAR, nearly everyone is a high-risk person in a generalized epidemic with high prevalence; thus most people need information about and access to all preventive methods, including condoms. PEPFAR's own definition highlights the need to ensure at a minimum that faith-based organizations that do not themselves provide proven interventions are consistently facilitating access to those interventions elsewhere. Ideally, PEPFAR would actively link these faith-based organizations with partners that would provide these interventions and ensure that such linkages were successfully addressing all prevention needs of their clients.

Increased Knowledge About What Works Against the AIDS Pandemic Is Needed

Because of its magnitude and reach, the U.S. Global AIDS Initiative represents a golden opportunity to learn about what works best in addressing the pandemic. The Leadership Act emphasizes the importance of both basic and applied research, and requires that research be an integral part of PEPFAR. In addition, because of the many gaps in the knowledge base for addressing HIV/AIDS, the initiative has an obligation to "learn by doing" (IOM, 2005). In doing so, the initiative can help the global community learn not only about what approaches are cost-effective for preventing infection and caring for people affected by HIV/AIDS and its consequences, but also about how to scale up effective programs, how to implement programs in a manner that builds capacity and strengthens health systems overall, how best to manage such global initiatives, and how to work most effectively within the framework of harmonization to empower countries to own and lead the fight against their HIV/AIDS epidemics.

Functioning as a Learning Organization

Beginning with its strategy, PEPFAR has been committed to learning, and the program has displayed many of the characteristics of a successful learning organization. The PEPFAR strategy envisioned OGAC as a "small organization focused on leadership, coordination, learning, and oversight" that would "strive to remain flexible and innovative in its approaches" (OGAC, 2004, p. 67). The Committee has seen many examples of OGAC's success in realizing this vision and encourages OGAC to continue in this vein. Chapter 3 provides greater detail about the evolution of OGAC and its management practices.

The Committee was also impressed by the energy, commitment, creativity, and agility of the Country Teams and is concerned about whether they are adequately supported to sustain these qualities. At the time of the Committee's visits to the focus countries, rapid scale-up of activities had to be managed largely with existing staff. Heavy demands for plans and reports from OGAC, other agencies, and Congress, as well as the imperative to coordinate with numerous entities both within the U.S. government and in the country at large, were creating a tremendous strain on the Country Teams. Although the Country Teams indicated that the situation had improved somewhat since the program's inception and that OGAC's management was continuing to evolve, the possibility of stagnation or "burnout" or of insufficient resources for oversight to maintain quality continues to be of concern. Improvements in and regularization of planning and reporting requirements, increased resources for the coordination function—including the recently identified best practice of a PEPFAR Country Team coordinator—and increased technical support for Country Teams are all promising developments.

The Committee encourages OGAC to continuously solicit input from and be fully responsive to the Country Teams and to increasingly have the program directed from the field upward, particularly as the Country Teams continue to gain knowledge and understanding of effective implementation. Of particular concern are two frustrations the Country Teams commonly expressed to the Committee: that heavy demands from OGAC reduce the time available to spend with implementing partners in supporting and overseeing their programs, and that inflexibility in central policies reduces their ability to tailor programming to the specific needs of the country and thus to be as harmonized with country strategies and plans as is appropriate.

Currently OGAC does not formally evaluate or provide systematic information about its performance on critical aspects of program management such as coordination, both internally and externally; harmonization; communications; transparency; comprehensive and integrated programming; continuous improvement; and contributions to the evidence base. The initiative would benefit from fuller and more formal evaluation of these aspects. Such evaluations would need to incorporate the concepts of "downward accountability" and "horizontal accountability," thus including solicitation of feedback from program participants at all levels—partners, other donors, host country governments, and particularly people in the focus countries.

Research

The PEPFAR strategy commits to building the evidence base on what works against HIV/AIDS and fostering innovation (OGAC, 2004), and the initiative is indeed helping to expand knowledge about the implementation of HIV/AIDS programs and services in resource-constrained countries. The U.S. Global AIDS Initiative supports global AIDS research through several entities: the National Institutes of Health (NIH), the Centers for Disease Control and Prevention (CDC), the U.S. Agency for International Development (USAID), and OGAC. NIH and CDC support basic, clinical, social science, translational, and clinical operations research on therapeutic and preventive regimens, microbicides, and vaccines (NIH, 2005). USAID supports applied and operations research focused on addressing the needs for program implementation in resource-limited countries. USAID's HIV/AIDS research agenda includes studies of ART, prevention of mother-to-child transmission, ABC (abstinence/be faithful/use condoms), male circumcision, injection safety, nutrition, psychosocial issues for orphans and other vulnerable children, microbicides, and vaccines. Although significant, these NIH, CDC, and USAID research activities generally are not funded through PEPFAR or controlled by the Coordinator, and thus were not a focus of the Committee's work. Instead, the Committee focused on the research OGAC controls and supports directly.

OGAC is currently supporting about $22 million worth of targeted evaluations, primarily in the focus countries, to support the programs and policies of the initiative. These evaluations cover a wide range of topics as summarized in Table 8-3.

Although OGAC has not yet articulated an overall strategy for research, it recently issued a "Blueprint for Public Health Evaluations in PEPFAR." The blueprint describes the underlying strategy for a broadened conception of targeted evaluations and outlines a new management structure for such evaluations, including roles and responsibilities and the process for the review and approval of evaluation proposals (OGAC, 2006i). As part of the

TABLE 8-3 Summary of PEPFAR Targeted Evaluations

	Number of Targeted Evaluations[a]	Total Budget by Program Area[b]
Abstinence/Be Faithful	5	4,025,000
Condoms and Other Prevention	1	275,000
Prevention of Mother-to-Child Transmission	14	4,945,000
HIV/AIDS Treatment/Antiretroviral Drugs	2	1,200,000
HIV/AIDS Treatment/ART Services	15	4,140,000
Palliative Care/Basic Health Care and Support	4	1,812,000
Orphans and Other Vulnerable Children	6	4,175,000
Counseling and Testing	3	620,000
Palliative Care for Tuberculosis and HIV	6	376,000
Strategic Information	8	1,247,000
Total	64	$22,815,000

[a]OGAC documents list two targeted evaluations with no information on the program area, budget, or agency.

[b]There is no budget information for 12 of the 64 evaluations.

materials provided to support the development of annual country operational plans, OGAC has also given the Country Teams a list of priorities for targeted evaluations (OGAC, 2006d,e). The list is extensive and includes priorities for prevention, treatment, and care and other cross-cutting issues, such as gender and orphans and other vulnerable children.

Additional research needs are a common theme across the chapters on PEPFAR's prevention, treatment, care, and orphans and other vulnerable children categories. The Committee encourages OGAC to target (or continue to target) evaluations to the following issues:

Evaluation of prevention programs is especially important for two reasons. First, although there is good evidence and general agreement that behavior changes—including those represented by ABC—are effective in reducing the spread of HIV/AIDS, there is less evidence and agreement about the effectiveness of specific approaches and programs for changing behavior. Second, PEPFAR's target of preventing 7 million new infections by 2010 will be measured at the country level using modeling techniques that reflect the state of the art and have been developed in conjunction with global health partners such as the Joint United Nations Programme on HIV/AIDS (UNAIDS). PEPFAR's approach and estimates will thus be consistent with other global estimates, and the estimates will also be made jointly with the Global Fund. Because these will be country-level estimates, however, it will not be possible to learn from them which approaches and programs have had the greatest and most cost-effective impact on preventing infections. Hence there is a particular need for evaluation of prevention programs at the program level.

There are still more questions than answers about how best to provide ART under conditions like those found in the PEPFAR focus countries. The International Epidemiologic Databases to Evaluate AIDS Consortium, which is supported by U.S. Global AIDS Initiative funds, provides a rich resource for exploring these questions in clinical research settings. PEPFAR support for operations research in all ART programs would serve to expand the global knowledge base for addressing critical questions, including how to provide high-quality, cost-effective ART; how to scale up ART to the national level; and how to sustain ART and avoid the development of widespread resistance. In particular, focused analysis is required to address logistical and process obstacles that have arisen as a result of the rapid emergency scale-up, including treatment of children, nutritional support, how to optimize care delivery, resistance monitoring, adherence, down referral, sources of treatment failure, and optimal approaches to the treatment of HIV/AIDS and tuberculosis in children.

Evaluation of care programs is particularly important for appropriate decision making about the scaling up of programs that are truly effective in terms of both desired outcome and costs. Currently, little is known about how care services are affecting the health status and quality of life of people living with and affected by HIV/AIDS or their communities. Focused analysis of the following topics could improve the provision of care services and their ultimate impact:

- Optimal approaches to providing family-centered, community-based care services that are well-linked to PEPFAR's network model.
- Understanding and reducing stigma and discrimination through culturally appropriate and culturally specific interventions.
- The appropriate use of volunteers and familial caregivers for complex and long-term caregiving tasks as part of PEPFAR's home-based care services, including examination of factors that contribute to burnout and fatigue, appropriate training for the skills needed, potential types of compensation, and programmatic contributions that can bolster the physical and mental health of these caregivers.
- Optimal approaches for integrating care services with prevention and treatment to create a continuum of services that can best meet the needs of families and communities.

Little is known about the effectiveness and impact of programs for orphans and other vulnerable children. The global community has only recently defined the basic package of services that should be provided to these children, and there is much to learn about the relative effectiveness of the specific strategies and programs for providing those services (UNAIDS and UNICEF, 2004). Unlike its prevention target, PEPFAR's target for providing care to 10 million people affected by HIV/AIDS is measured very early in the process and in terms of individual people. At this point, the care target counts the number of people who receive services. Eventually, as with prevention, it will be necessary to know about the impact of those services on the health status and social well-being of a country's population of children. Thus it will be critical to have program-level information about the relative effectiveness of programs for children.

To promote quality and sustainability, all programs need to be supported in managing their own quality assurance and quality improvement processes. Initially, PEPFAR's emphasis was on supporting programs in having data systems to allow for self-assessment. Like other donors that have demanded attribution of results, PEPFAR has too often created parallel data collection and reporting systems that have burdened program sites and not necessarily given them the ability to use the data for their own quality assurance and improvement purposes. PEPFAR can address this need by continuing to provide strong support for the development of country monitoring and evaluation systems and participating fully in the Third One of harmonization—one national monitoring and evaluation system. In addition, PEPFAR has supported some quality improvement projects using a model originally developed by USAID (USAID, 2006). OGAC is currently seeking to expand its quality improvement activities, including increasing the number of quality improvement projects and providing related training to all headquarters staff.

Recommendation 8-4: The U.S. Global AIDS Initiative should increase its contribution to the global evidence base for HIV/AIDS interventions by better capitalizing on the opportunity PEPFAR represents to learn about and share what works. The U.S. Global AIDS Coordinator should further emphasize the importance of and provide additional support for operations research and program evaluation in particular—not as the primary aim but as an integral component of programs. All programs should include robust monitoring and evaluation that factors into decisions about whether and in what manner the programs are to continue. The initiative should maintain its appropriate openness to new and innovative approaches and programs, but unproven programs in particular should be required to have an evaluation component to determine their effectiveness.

Dissemination

Sharing of knowledge and outside scrutiny are essential to expanding the knowledge base. Creation of the PEPFAR ExtraNet and broadening of participation in PEPFAR's annual meeting (see Chapter 3) are promising developments. The initiative will need to continue to expand its avenues for sharing knowledge gained through the implementation of PEPFAR.

Measuring Success

Key to understanding what works against the HIV/AIDS pandemic is to learn whether PEPFAR has succeeded—that is, to understand the outcomes and impact of the effort. Although it would be premature to judge success in these terms at this time, OGAC is supporting the structures and processes necessary to evaluate the outcomes and impact of PEPFAR. OGAC's outcome and impact indicators were developed as part of the global effort to harmonize monitoring and evaluation efforts, and thus are referenced to and largely consistent with those of other organizations such as Global Fund, UNAIDS, UNICEF, and WHO (OGAC, 2004, 2005c; WHO et al., 2004). Further efforts to harmonize monitoring and evaluation are ongoing, and PEPFAR's continued commitment and active participation will be required if they are to be successful (GIST, 2006).

To measure what really matters—reductions in disability, disease, and death from HIV/AIDS; increases in the capacity of partner countries to sustain and expand HIV/AIDS programs without setbacks in other aspects of their public health systems; and improvements in the lives of the people living in these countries—the United States and other donors will be heavily dependent on the capabilities of the partner countries. To understand whether these ultimate goals are being achieved and what contributions the U.S. Global AIDS Initiative is making to their achievement, it will be necessary to study national trends, such as rates of new HIV and other infections; rates of survival from HIV/AIDS and other diseases; child survival, development, and well-being; and the general health status of the population and key subpopulations. Particularly within the agreed framework of harmonization, the data and analyses necessary to study these trends will have to come primarily from the partner countries themselves (UN, 2003a,b; UNAIDS, 2004; OGAC, 2005b). Thus the United States, in conjunction with other donors, will need to continue to place priority on helping to strengthen the monitoring and evaluation systems of the partner countries.

CONCLUSION

The Committee found that the U.S. Global AIDS Initiative has made a strong start, is progressing toward its 5-year targets, and is increasingly well positioned to support countries in controlling their epidemics. At the same time, however, PEPFAR has not yet reached the half-way mark for any of its targets, each focus country still faces an enormous challenge in controlling its epidemic, and the HIV/AIDS pandemic continues to grow. The Joint United Nations Programme on HIV/AIDS has estimated that more than 4 million people worldwide became newly infected with HIV in 2006, and unless prevention efforts are highly successful, millions more will become infected every year (UNAIDS, 2006). Of the nearly 7 million people in low- and middle-income countries now estimated to need ART or to face an early death, fewer than one-quarter are receiving the therapy (WHO, 2006), and millions more of those already infected with HIV will eventually need it. Fewer than 1 in 10 pregnant women infected with HIV in low- and middle-income countries are benefiting from ARVs to prevent transmission to their babies, and at most 12 percent of the children born to these women who require ART are receiving it (WHO, 2006). With ART and appropriate care, AIDS is a chronic disease—it can be managed but not cured—and people receiving ART will need to be on it for the rest of their lives. Only a fraction of the legions of devastated families and orphaned children are currently receiving the support services they need, and the number of children orphaned by AIDS globally is projected to exceed 20 million by 2010 (UNICEF, 2006).

The Committee believes that continued commitment by the United States, along with all other donors, to supporting the fight against the HIV/AIDS pandemic will be required until countries have developed sustainable programs, and that continued U.S. leadership is necessary to prevent complacency and battle fatigue and to bring the virus under control. In sustaining this commitment and this leadership, the United States will continue to answer the call from the global community:

> AIDS is exceptional and the response to AIDS must be equally exceptional. It requires ongoing leadership on both the national and international levels. Twenty-five years into the epidemic, the global response to AIDS must be transformed from an episodic, crisis-management approach to a strategic response that recognizes the need for long-term commitment and capacity-building, using evidence-informed strategies that address the structural drivers of the epidemic. (UNAIDS, 2006, p. 17)

REFERENCES

Chankova, S. 2006. *Evidence-based planning of human resources for health: Examples from sub-Saharan Africa.* Global Health Council Presentation, October 2006. Bethesda, MD: Abt Associates, Inc.

Dybul, M. 2005 (May 24). *Integrated prevention, treatment and care: Network systems.* Presentation at the PEPFAR Second Annual Field Meeting, Addis Ababa, Ethiopia.

EPN (Ecumenical Pharmaceutical Network). 2006. *Annual report, 2005.* Kenya: EPN Publications.

GHC (Global Health Council). 2005. *Faith in action: Examining the role of faith-based organizations in addressing HIV/AIDS: A multi-country, key informant survey.* Washington, DC: GHC.

Gilks, C. F., S. Crowley, R. Ekpini, S. Gove, J. Perriens, Y. Souteyrand, D. Sutherland, M. Vitoria, T. Guerma, and K. De Cock. 2006. The WHO public-health approach to antiretroviral treatment against HIV in resource-limited settings. *The Lancet* 368(9534):505–510.

GIST (Global Implementation Support Team). 2006. *Fact sheet: The Global Implementation Support Team: Coordinating UN action and provision of technical support for accelerating HIV/AIDS responses in countries.* http://data.unaids.org/pub/BrochurePamphlet/2006/2006_gist_en.pdf (accessed January 12, 2007).

Harries, A. D., E. J. Shouten, and E. Libamba. 2006. Scaling up antiretroviral therapy in resource-poor settings. *The Lancet* 367:1870–1872.

Huber, S. C. 2006. *Empowering communities to address their health challenges.* Global Health Council Presentation, October 2006. Boston, MA: Management Sciences for Health.

IOM (Institute of Medicine). 2005. *Scaling up treatment for the global AIDS pandemic: Challenges and opportunities.* Washington, DC: The National Academies Press.

Jooma, M. B. 2005. Southern Africa assessment: Food security and HIV/AIDS. *African Security Review* 14(1).

Kober, K., and W. Van Damme. 2004. Scaling up access to antiretroviral treatment in southern Africa: Who will do the job? *The Lancet* 364(9428):103–107.

Nieburg, P., J. Kates, and J. S. Morrison. 2004. *Enhancing the rapid response capacity of the U.S. global AIDS coordinator: Lessons from other U.S. emergency responses. A report of the CSIS HIV/AIDS Task Force in collaboration with the Kaiser Family Foundation.* Washington, DC: Center for Strategic and International Studies.

NIH (National Institutes of Health). 2005. *FY 2005 international project listing.* Rockville, MD: NIH.

OGAC (Office of the U.S. Global AIDS Coordinator). 2004. *The President's Emergency Plan for AIDS Relief: U.S. five-year global HIV/AIDS strategy.* Washington, DC: OGAC.

OGAC. 2005a. *PEPFAR first annual report to Congress.* Washington, DC: OGAC.

OGAC. 2005b. *The President's Emergency Plan for AIDS Relief: Defining U.S. support for national strategies* (PowerPoint Presentation, July 2005). Washington, DC: OGAC.

OGAC. 2005c. *The President's Emergency Plan for AIDS Relief: Indicators, reporting requirements, and guidelines for focus countries* (revised for FY2006 reporting). Washington, DC: OGAC.

OGAC. 2005d. *PEPFAR: Community and faith-based organizations.* Report to Congress mandated by report 108-599, accompanying H.R. 4818. Washington, DC: U.S. Department of State.

OGAC. 2006a. *PEPFAR second annual report to Congress.* Washington, DC: OGAC.

OGAC. 2006b. *PEPFAR report on food and nutrition for people living with HIV/AIDS.* Washington, DC: OGAC.

OGAC. 2006c. *PEPFAR report on work force capacity and HIV/AIDS.* Washington, DC: OGAC.

OGAC. 2006d. *PEPFAR: Technical considerations for the FY2007 Country Operational Plans.* Washington, DC: OGAC.

OGAC. 2006e. *PEPFAR FY2007 COP resource guide.* Washington, DC: OGAC.

OGAC. 2006f. *Report on education: The President's Emergency Plan for AIDS Relief.* Washington, DC: OGAC.

OGAC. 2006g. *Report on refugees and internally displaced persons: The President's Emergency Plan for AIDS Relief.* Washington, DC: OGAC.

OGAC. 2006h. *The President's Emergency Plan for AIDS Relief report on gender-based violence and HIV/AIDS.* Washington, DC: OGAC.

OGAC. 2006i. *A blueprint for public health evaluations in the President's Emergency Plan for AIDS Relief.* Washington, DC: OGAC.

OGAC. 2007. *PEPFAR third annual report to Congress.* Washington, DC: OGAC

Ooms, G. 2006. Health development versus medical relief: The illusion versus the irrelevance of sustainability. *PLoS Medicine* 3(8):e345.

Salomon, J., D. Hogan, J. Stover, K. Stanecki, N. Walker, P. D. Ghys, and B. Schwartlander. 2005. Integrating HIV prevention and treatment: From slogans to impact. *PLoS Medicine* 2(1):e16.

Stringer J., I. Zulu, J. Levy, E. M. Stringer, A. Mwango, B. H. Chi, V. Mtonga, S. Reid, R. A. Cantrell, M. Bulterys, M. S. Saag, R. G. Marlink, A. Mwinga, T. V. Ellerbrock, and M. Sinkala. 2006. Rapid scale-up of antiretroviral therapy at primary care sites in Zambia: Feasibility and early outcomes. *The Journal of the American Medical Association* 296:782–793.

UN (United Nations). 2003a. *Monterrey Consensus of the International Conference on Financing for Development: The final text of agreements and commitments adopted at the International Conference on Financing for Development, Monterrey, Mexico, 18–22 March 2002.* Geneva, Switzerland: UN.

UN. 2003b. *Organizing the UN response to the triple threat of food insecurity, weakened capacity for governance and AIDS, particularly in Southern and Eastern Africa: Document discussed at the UN High-Level Committee on Programmes, 6th session, Rome, Italy, 18–19 September 2003.* Geneva, Switzerland: UN.

UNAIDS (Joint United Nations Programme on HIV/AIDS). 2004. *"Three ones" key principles.* Conference paper 1, Washington consultation of April 4, 2004. Geneva, Switzerland: UNAIDS. http://www.unaids.org/NetTools/Misc/DocInfo.aspx?LANG=en&href=http://gva-doc-owl/WEBcontent/Documents/pub/UNA-docs/Three-Ones_KeyPrinciples_en.pdf (accessed September 20, 2006).

UNAIDS. 2006. *2006 report on the global AIDS epidemic.* Geneva, Switzerland: UNAIDS.

UNAIDS and UNICEF. 2004. *The framework for the protection, care and support of orphans and vulnerable children living in a world with HIV and AIDS.* Geneva, Switzerland: UNAIDS.

UNICEF (United Nations Children's Fund). 2006. *Africa's orphaned and vulnerable generations: Children affected by AIDS.* New York: UNICEF.

USAID (U.S. Agency for International Development). 2006. *Quality assurance and workforce development project: Year four annual report: Performance period, July 1, 2005–June 30, 2006, July 31, 2006.* Washington, DC: USAID.

WHO (World Health Organization). 2001. *What do we know about capacity building? An overview of existing knowledge and good practice.* Geneva, Switzerland: WHO.

WHO. 2004a. *Emergency scale-up of antiretroviral therapy in resource-limited settings: Technical and operational recommendations to achieve 3 by 5.* Geneva, Switzerland: WHO.

WHO. 2004b. *Acute care—Integrated management of adolescent and adult illness: Interim guidelines for first-level facility health workers.* Geneva, Switzerland: WHO.

WHO. 2004c. *World health report 2004.* Geneva: WHO.

WHO. 2006. *Fact sheet: Progress in scaling up access to HIV treatment in low- and middle-income countries.* Geneva, Switzerland: WHO.

WHO. 2007. *Statement by Dr. Margaret Chan, WHO Director-General, on occasion of International Women's Day.* http://www.who.int/mediacentre/news/statements/2007/s05/en/ (accessed March 8, 2007).

WHO, UNAIDS, The Global Fund to Fight AIDS, Tuberculosis and Malaria, USAID, U.S. Department of State, U.S. Department of Health and Human Services, Centers for Disease Control and Prevention, UNICEF, and the World Bank. 2004. *Monitoring and evaluation toolkit HIV/AIDS, tuberculosis and malaria.* Geneva, Switzerland: WHO.

Wonodi, C. 2006. *Healthcare worker crisis, the worker's angle* (Global Health Council PowerPoint Presentation, October 2006). Baltimore, MD: Johns Hopkins School of Public Health and Rivers State, Nigeria: Ministry of Health.

APPENDIX A

Acknowledgments

The Committee would like to acknowledge and thank all of the people who were generous with their time and expertise and presented at one of our meetings or made themselves available for extended discussions. We would especially like to thank the people in the focus countries for graciously using their very limited time to host us and show us their programs.

Speakers at Open Meetings, Officials and Organizations the Committee Held Discussions with:

Christine Abrams, Office of the U.S. Global AIDS Coordinator
Aspen Pharmacare
Andrew Ball, World Health Organization
Ties Boerma, World Health Organization
Constance Carrino, U.S. Agency for International Development
Ambassador Johnnie Carson, National Intelligence Council
Helen Cornman, PACT
Paul DeLay, Joint United Nations Program on HIV/AIDS
Madhuvanti Deshmukh, CARE International
Bill Dilday, Office of the U.S. Global AIDS Coordinator
Nobayeni Dladla, Embassy of South Africa
Mark Dybul, Office of the U.S. Global AIDS Coordinator
Nina Ferencic, World Health Organization
Julian Fleet, Joint United Nations Programme on HIV/AIDS
Peter Ghys, Joint United Nations Programme on HIV/AIDS

Charlie Gilkes, Joint United Nations Programme on HIV/AIDS
Global Health Council—Global AIDS Roundtable
Thurma Goldman, Health Resources and Services Administration
Teguest Guerma, World Health Organization
Geeta Rao Gupta, International Center for Research on Women
Shannon Hader, Centers for Disease Control and Prevention, Zimbabwe
Karen Hawkins-Reed, Centers for Disease Control and Prevention, Democratic Republic of Congo
Ini Huijts, World Health Organization
Ambassador Cameron Hume, U.S. Department of State
InterAction—PEPFAR Implementer Roundtable
David Jamieson, Supply Chain Management System
Sarah Kambou, International Center for Research on Women
Phyllis J. Kanki, Harvard PEPFAR
Peter Kilmarx, Centers for Disease Control and Prevention, Botswana
Ambassador Jimmy Kolker, Office of the AIDS Coordinator
Peter Lamptey, Family Health International
Madeleine Leloup, World Health Organization
Daniel Low-Beer, Global Fund
Ambassador Princeton Lyman, Africa Policy Studies Council on Foreign Relations
Purnima Mane, Joint United Nations Programme on HIV/AIDS
Kathy Marconi, Office of the U.S. Global AIDS Coordinator
Tim Mastro, Centers for Disease Control and Prevention, Atlanta
Michael McGunnigle, Supply Chain Management System
Jonathan Mermin, Centers for Disease Control and Prevention, Uganda
Michele Moloney-Kitts, Office of the U.S. Global AIDS Coordinator
Allen Moore, Center for Strategic and International Studies
J. Stephen Morrison, Center for Strategic and International Studies
Paul Nunn, World Health Organization
Okey Nwanyanwu, Centers for Disease Control and Prevention, South Africa
Laura Nyblade, International Center for Research on Women
Joseph F. O'Neill, Office of the U.S. Global AIDS Coordinator
Rich Owens, Supply Chain Management System
Sara Pacque-Margolis, formerly of the Office of the U.S. Global AIDS Coordinator
Jean W. Pape, Haitian Group for the Study of Kaposi's Sarcoma and Opportunistic Infections
Joseph Perriens, World Health Organization
Peter Piot, Joint United Nations Programme on HIV/AIDS
Susan Purdin, International Rescue Committee
Patrick Purtell, Office of the U.S. Global AIDS Coordinator

Karina Rapposelli, Office of the U.S. Global AIDS Coordinator
Mario Raviglione, World Health Organization
Stacy Rhodes, Save the Children
Alex Ross, World Health Organization
Deborah Rugg, Centers for Disease Control and Prevention, Atlanta
Carolyn Ryan, Office of the U.S. Global AIDS Coordinator
Manuel Tomas Schick, World Health Organization
Kenneth Schofield, U.S. Department of State
Bernhard Schwartländer, Global Fund
Richard A. Shaffer, U.S. Department of Defense
John Sheptor, Supply Chain Management System
Michele Sidibe, Joint United Nations Programme on HIV/AIDS
Yves Souteyrand, World Health Organization
Carl C. Stecker, Catholic Relief Services
Bill Steiger, U.S. Department of Health and Human Services
Nancy Stetson, Senate Foreign Relations Committee
Jeffrey Stringer, Centre for Infectious Disease Research in Zambia
Ambassador Randall Tobias, U.S. Agency for International Development
Joseph Valadez, World Bank
Diana Weil, World Health Organization
Cathy Wilfert, Elizabeth Glaser Pediatric AIDS Foundation
Mitch Wolfe, Centers for Disease Control and Prevention, Vietnam
Lee Yerkes, Elizabeth Glaser Pediatric AIDS Foundation

Focus Country Meetings

PEPFAR Core Team Leads

Dana DeRuiter: Ethiopia, Uganda, Tanzania
Reuben Granich: Nigeria, Kenya
Daniela Ligiero: Guyana, Haiti
Nithya Mani: Côte D'Ivoire, Rwanda, Vietnam
Elizabeth Onjoro-Meassick: Zambia, Namibia
Karina Rapposelli: Botswana, South Africa, Mozambique

U.S. Government Agencies

Department of Defense
Department of Health and Human Services
- Centers for Disease Control and Prevention
- Food and Drug Administration
- Health Resources and Services Administration
- National Institutes of Health

Department of Labor

Department of State
Peace Corps
U.S. Agency for International Development

Botswana

U.S. Embassy
Ambassador Katherine H. Canavan
Ted Pierce, PEPFAR Coordinator

Organizations

Academy for Educational Development
The African Comprehensive HIV/AIDS Partnerships
Athlone Hospital Antiretroviral Clinic
Bana Ba Keletso Orphan Daycare Center, Molepolole
Baylor Center of Excellence
Botswana Business Coalition on HIV/AIDS
Botswana Christian AIDS Intervention Program
Botswana-Harvard AIDS Institute Partnership Laboratory
Botswana Network of AIDS Services
Botswana Network on Ethics, Law and HIV/AIDS
BOTUSA-Francistown Prevention of Mother-to-Child Transmission of HIV Project
Central Medical Stores
Harvard School of Public Health AIDS Initiative
Humana People to People
Infectious Diseases Care Clinic Francistown
Infectious Diseases Care Clinic PEPFAR Gaborone
Institute of Development Management
John Snow Incorporated, Francistown
Jubilee HIV Laboratory, Francistown
Makgabaneng Project
Ministry of Education
Ministry of Health
National AIDS Coordinating Agency
Orphans and Vulnerable Children Grantee Project, Francistown
PACT/Botswana Council of Churches Grantee Project, Francistown
Pathfinder
Regional Psychosocial Support Initiative
Tebelopele Voluntary Counseling and Testing Centres
Technical Support Services
United Nations Development Program
Youth Health Organization

Côte d'Ivoire

U.S. Embassy
Ambassador Aubrey Hooks
Monica Nolan, PEPFAR Coordinator

Ethiopia

U.S. Embassy
Ambassador Vicki Huddleston
Catherine Avery, PEPFAR Coordinator

Organizations

Adama Hospital
Adama Hospital, Antiretroviral Therapy Treatment Services
AIDS Resource Center
Armed Forces General Hospital
Department for International Development
Development Cooperation Ireland
Drug Administration and Control Authority
Ethiopian Health and Nutrition Research Institute
Ethiopian Muslim Development Agency
Ethiopian Orthodox Church and Inter Church Aid Commission
Felegehiwot Hospital
Global Fund
Health Communication Partnership
High Risk Corridor Initiative
HIV/AIDS Prevention and Control Office
International Center for AIDS Care and Treatment Programs/Columbia University
International Orthodox Christian Charities
International Training and Education Center on HIV
IntraHealth International
Italian Development Cooperation
JHPIEGO
John Snow Incorporated/Making Medical Injections Safer
Joint United Nations Programme on HIV/AIDS
Management Sciences for Health/Rational Pharmaceutical Management
Ministry of Defense
Ministry of Health
Ministry of Youth, Sports and Culture
PACT
Pharmaceutical Administration and Supply Services

Pharmaceuticals and Medical Supplies Import and Whole Sale Share Company
Save the Children/United States
Woreta Health Center, Prevention of Mother-to-Child Transmission of HIV Program
World Health Organization

Guyana

U.S. Embassy
Ambassador Roland Bullen
Julia Rehwinkel, PEPFAR Coordinator

Organizations

Catholic Relief Services
Francois Xavier Bagnoud Guyana
Genito Urinary Medicine Clinic
Guyana HIV/AIDS Reduction and Prevention Project
Guyana Responsible Parenthood Association
Linden Care Foundation
Maurice Solomon Accounting
Mercy Hospital
Ministry of Health
National Blood Transfusion Service
Pan American Health Organization
Red Cross
United Nations Children's Fund
United Nations Development Programme

Haiti

U.S. Embassy
Ambassador Janet Sanderson
Chris Barratt, PEPFAR Coordinator

Organizations

Haitian Group for the Study of Kaposi's Sarcoma and Opportunistic Infections
Promoteurs Objectif ZeroSida

Kenya

U.S. Embassy
Ambassador William Bellamy
Warren (Buck) Buckingham, PEPFAR Coordinator

Organizations

Academic Model for Prevention and Treatment of HIV/AIDS
ARC Tivoli
The Association of People with AIDS in Kenya
Baptist AIDS Response Agency
Bomu Clinic
Coast Provincial General Hospital
Coptic Hospital
Department of Defense HIV/Prevention and Treatment Program
The Eastern Deanery AIDS Relief Program
Joint United Nations Programme on HIV/AIDS
Kenya Medical Supplies Agency
Kenya Network of Positive Teachers
Kenya Treatment Access Movement
Kenyatta National Hospital
Kericho District Hospital
Kericho Youth Center
Live With Hope Center
Ministry of Health
Mission of Essential Drugs and Supplies
Moi Teaching and Referral Hospital
Mosoriot District Health Clinic
National AIDS Control Council
National HIV/AIDS and Sexually-Transmitted Disease Control Program of Kenya
Network of African People Living with HIV/AIDS
Nyanza Provincial General Hospital
Voluntary Counseling and Testing for the Deaf
Walter Reed Medical Research Unit
Women Fighting AIDS in Kenya

Mozambique

U.S. Embassy
Ambassador Helen LaLime
Linda Lou Kelley, PEPFAR Coordinator

Organizations

Agence Française de Développement
Business Against AIDS Association
Canadian International Development Agency
Central de Medicamentos e Artigos Médicos
Clinton Foundation

Columbia University
Conselho Nacional de Combate ao HIV/SIDA
DELIVER Project
Department for International Development
Development Cooperation Ireland
European Commission
Family Health International
Foundation for Community Development
Habitat for Humanity
Health Alliance International
HIV/AIDS Taskforce
HIV/AIDS Working Groups
International Center for AIDS Care and Treatment Programs Columbia University
John Snow Incorporated
Joint United Nations Programme on HIV/AIDS
Milhorho—Song and Dance Association
Military Hospital
Ministry of Defense
Ministry of Health
Ministry of Women and Social Action
Multisectoral Technical Group
National AIDS Council
Peace Corp
Prevention of Mother-to-Child Transmission of HIV Jose Macamo
Policy Project
Population Services International
Project Hope
Royal Netherlands Embassy
Samaritan's Purse
United Nations Children's Fund
United Nations Population Fund
World Food Program
World Relief
World Vision

Namibia

U.S. Embassy
Ambassador Joyce Barr
Aaron Daviet, PEPFAR Coordinator

Organizations

Catholic Aids Action
Council of Churches
European Union
Evangelical Lutheran Church in Namibia Center
Family Health International
German Agency for Technical Cooperation
Global Fund
International Training and Education Center on HIV
Johns Hopkins University
Katutura Hospital
LifeLine
Management Sciences for Health
Ministry of Health and Social Services
Namibia Institute of Pathology
National Health Training Center
Okahao Hospital
Onandjokwe Treatment Center
Oshakati Hospital
Oshakati Tonateni Voluntary Counseling and Testing Center
Oshikuku Catholic Health Service
Population Services International
POTENTIA
Project Hope
Tonateni Voluntary Counseling and Testing Center
United Nations Theme Group
University Research Corporation

Nigeria

U.S. Embassy
Ambassador John Campbell
Nina M. Wadhwa, PEPFAR Coordinator

Organizations

Catholic Relief Services
Enabling HIV/AIDS + TB and Social Sector Environment
Faith Alive Support and Treatment Center
Family Health International/Global HIV/AIDS Initiative
Gwagdalada Treatment Hospital
Harvard School of Public Health
John Snow Incorporated—DELIVER

Joint United Nations Programme on HIV/AIDS
Jos University Teaching Hospital HIV/AIDS Treatment Center
Ministry of Defense
Ministry of Health
National Action Committee on AIDS
Network of People Living with HIV/AIDS
Our Lady of Apostle Hospital—Harvard supported Prevention of Mother-to-Child Transmission of HIV Project
Sacred Heart for Gwagwalada Specialist Hospital
SBAF Project
Society for Family Health
United Nations Children's Fund
University of Maryland/AIDS Care and Treatment in Nigeria
World Bank
Wuse General Hospital

Rwanda

U.S. Embassy
Janet Wilgus, Deputy Chief of Mission
Regan Whitworth, PEPFAR Coordinator

Organizations

AIDSRelief
CARE
Catholic Relief Services
Central Purchasing of Essential Medicines in Rwanda
Community HIV/AIDS Mobilization Project
Family Health International/ Project Implementing AIDS Prevention and Care
Global Fund
IntraHealth
Kigeme Hospital
Kirambi Health Center
Management Sciences for Health/Rational Pharmaceutical Management Plus
Ministry of Health
Ministry of State for HIV/AIDS
National AIDS Commission
National Blood Transfusion Program
National Reference Laboratory
National University of Rwanda/Tulane University
Ntoma Health Center

Rwanda Network of People Living with HIV/AIDS The Capacity Project Rwanda
Treatment and Research AIDS Center
World Bank
World Relief

South Africa

U.S. Embassy
Don Teitelbaum, Chargé d'Affaire
Gray Handley, Health Attaché
Karen Kelley, PEPFAR Coordinator

Organizations

Academy Educational Development
Addington Hospital
Catholic Diocese of Rustenburg
Catholic Relief Services
Columbia University
Department for International Development
EngenderHealth, Men as Partners, Newtown
European Commission
European Union
Foundation for Professional Development
Health Systems Trust
Helen Joseph Hospital
Higher Education HIV/AIDS Projects
HIV/AIDS Task Force
HIV/AIDS Working Groups
John Snow Incorporated
Johns Hopkins University Centre for Communication Programs
Kalafong Provincial Hospital
KwaZulu-Natal Department of Health
Mindset
National Department of Correctional Services
National Department of Health
National Department of Social Development
National Institute for Communicable Diseases
Ndlovu Medical Centre
Nurturing Orphans of AIDS for Humanity
PACT
Prince Mshyeni Hospital
Rational Pharmaceutical Management Plus

Reproductive Health and HIV Research Unit
Rietvlei Hospital
Right to Care
Salvation Army, Soweto
Sizanani Village
Solidarity Centre
Soul City
South African Government
South African National Blood Service
South African National Defense Force
South African National Treasury
Southern Africa Catholics Bishop's Conference
St. Mary's Hospital, Mariannhill
St. Patrick's Hospital

Tanzania

U.S. Embassy
Ambassador Michael L. Retzer
D. Purnell Delly, Deputy Chief of Mission
Elise Jensen, PEPFAR Coordinator

Organizations

Canadian International Development Agency
CARE Tumaini Project/CARE International
Catholic Relief Services
Clinton Foundation
Columbia University International Center for AIDS Care and Treatment
Deloitte Tanzania
Elizabeth Glaser Pediatric AIDS Foundation
Engender Health
Family Health International
German Development Cooperation
John Snow Incorporated—DELIVER Project
Kilimanjaro Christian Medical Center
Management Sciences for Health
Ministry of Health
Mount Meru Hospital
Muhumbili University College of Health Sciences
National AIDS Control Programme
National AIDS Council
National Blood Transfusion Services and Laboratory Services
Same District Hospital

Selian Lutheran Hospital
Tanzania AIDS Society
Tanzania Commission on AIDS
Tanzanian German Programme to Support Health
United Nations Children's Fund
United Nations World Food Programme
Women against AIDS in Kilmanjaro (Kiwakkuki)
World Health Organization
World Vision

Uganda

U.S. Embassy
William Fitzgerald, Chargé d'Affaire
Julia Henn, PEPFAR Coordinator

Organizations

The AIDS Support Organization
Basic Education and Policy Support Activity
Business Preventing AIDS and Accelerating Access to Anti-retroviral Treatment Project
Care International
Core Initiative
Creative Associates International
Department for International Development
Elizabeth Glaser Pediatric AIDS Foundation
Embassy of Norway
Embassy of Sweden
Ernst and Young
European Commission
European Union
German Technical Cooperation
Health Communication Partnership
Home-Based AIDS Care
Inter Religious Council of Uganda
Ireland Development Agency
John Snow Incorporated—AIDS/HIV Integrated District Model Program
John Snow Incorporated—DELIVER Project
Johns Hopkins University/Communication for Development Foundation Uganda
Joint Clinical Research Center
Joint Medical Stores
Joint United Nations Programme on HIV/AIDS

Makerere University
Mbale Regional Laboratory
Meeting Point
The Mildmay Centre
Ministry of Education and Sports
Ministry of Finance Planning and Economic Development
Ministry of Gender, Labor and Social Development
Ministry of Health
Mulago-Mbarara Teaching Hospitals' Joint AIDS Program
National Medical Stores
Nile Brewery
Partners Ireland
Pediatric Infectious Diseases Clinic, Mulago
PEPFAR Advisory Board
Population Services International Uganda
Reach Out
Safety Stop Program
Straight Talk Foundation
Swedish International Development Agency
Tororo District Hospital
Uganda AIDS Commission
Ugandan Women's Efforts to Save Orphans
Uphold
U.S. National Institutes of Health
World Bank
World Health Organization
World Vision
The Young Empowered and Healthy Initiative

Vietnam

U.S. Embassy
Ambassador Michael W. Marine
Nahoko Nakayama, PEPFAR Coordinator

Organizations

Academy Educational Development
Bach Mai Hospital
Binh Thanh Out-Patient Clinic
Blue Sky Club, Ho Chi Minh City
Buddhist Association
Care International

Cua Bac Pagoda
Center for Community Health and Development
Central Pharmacy Company #1
Committee of Concerned Partners
Department for International Development
District 4 Out-Patient Clinic, Ho Chi Minh City
District 6 Out-Patient Clinic, Ho Chi Minh City
Drug Administration Department
Family Health International
The Futures Group
Government of Vietnam Secretariat for HIV/AIDS
Hai Au Club—Injection Drug User Center, Hai Phong
Hai Phong Department of Health
Hanoi School of Public Health
Ho Chi Minh City Provincial AIDS Committee
Institute for Social Development Studies
Joint United Nations Programme on HIV/AIDS
Life-Gap Project
Management Sciences for Health
Médecins du Monde
Military Institute of Hygiene and Epidemiology
Ministry of Health
National Institute for Clinical Research and Tropical Medicine
National Institute of Hygiene and Epidemiology
Office of Ho Chi Minh City Sub-Department of Social Evils Prevention
PACT
Population Council
Population Services International
Provincial AIDS Committee
Red Flame Women Club, Hai Phong
Save the Children
Sexually Transmitted Infections/HIV/AIDS Prevention Centre
SMARTWorks Project
Tam Binh Orphanage
United Nations
Viet Tiep Hospital, Hai Phong
Vietnam Administration for AIDS Control
Vietnam POLICY Project
World Health Organization
World Vision
World Wide Orphans Foundation

Zambia

U.S. Embassy
Andrew A. Passen, Chargé d'Affaire
M. Cristina F. Garces, PEPFAR Coordinator

Organizations

Africare
Arthur Davidson Hospital
Bwafwano Orphans and Vulnerable Children Program
Catholic Relief Services
Central Statistics Office
Chipokota Myamba Rural Health Clinic
Company Clinic
Corpmed Medical Centre
Corridors of Hope
Embassy of the Kingdom of the Netherlands
Family Health International/Zambia Prevention Care and Treatment Project
Global Development Alliance
Health Services and Systems Program
JHPIEGO
John Snow Incorporated—DELIVER Project
John Snow Incorporated/Support to the HIV/AIDS Response in Zambia Project
Joint United Nations Programme on HIV/AIDS
Konkola Copper Mines
Ministry of Education
Ministry of Health
Munali High School
Nangongwe District Clinic
National AIDS Council
Netherlands Embassy
Palliative Care Association of Zambia
Project Concern International
Reaching HIV/AIDS Affected People with Integrated Development and Support Consortium
St. Theresa Mission Hospital
Tropical Diseases Research Centre
University Teaching Hospital, Department of Pediatrics
Zambia Medical Injection Safety Project
Zambia National AIDS Network

APPENDIX B

Methods

INTRODUCTION

This study was carried out by the Institute of Medicine (IOM) Committee on the President's Emergency Plan for AIDS Relief (PEPFAR) Implementation Evaluation, three subcommittees, several consultants, and staff, all of whom are listed in the front matter. Short biographies for each person can be found in Appendix G. The Committee is composed of 13 members. Committee members were selected for their international experience in low- and middle-income countries, as well as their individual expertise in the following areas relevant to the Committee's charge: behavioral science, bioethics, biostatistics, community nursing, community development, economics, epidemiology, infectious disease (adult), informatics, maternal and child health, modeling, monitoring and evaluation, operations research, professional training/education, public health program management, quality of care, and social services. Three advisory subcommittees comprised of six to seven members each, are focused on prevention, treatment, and care, including orphans and other vulnerable children. Additional members who serve only on the subcommittees provide expanded expertise in the following areas: child psychology/psychiatry, child welfare/services, demography, health communication, health education, infectious disease (pediatric), laboratory quality, logistics, palliative care, and pharmaceutical care.

The Committee began its work on this report in February of 2005 with its initial meeting and concluded in February of 2007 with finalization of this report in response to review. The Committee employed a wide range of methods, including information-gathering and deliberative meetings; review of the scientific and other literature; review of PEPFAR and other documentation; analysis of PEPFAR budget and performance data; discussions with a wide range of PEPFAR staff, participants, and stakeholders; and visits to the PEPFAR focus countries. Some Committee members and staff participated in both PEPFAR annual meetings—in Ethiopia in May of 2005 and in South Africa in June of 2006—including the U.S. government–only sessions, as well as the Office of the U.S. Global AIDS Coordinator's (OGAC) monthly outreach meetings, relevant Congressional hearings, meetings of the Center for Strategic and International Studies Task Force on HIV/AIDS, the Partnership for Supply Chain Management launch meeting on May 24, 2006, in Washington, DC—"Delivering HIV/AIDS Commodities to Customers Insights and Partnerships for Seamless Supply Chains"—and the PEPFAR Gender and HIV/AIDS Consultation on June 1, 2006, also in Washington, DC.

EVALUATION PLAN

On October 31, 2005, the Committee published its plan for carrying out this short-term evaluation of PEPFAR. The plan outlined the Committee's evaluation questions and approach to the study (IOM, 2005). This report is included as Appendix C and is also available free of charge at the following web address: http://www.nap.edu/catalog/11472.html.

Evaluating Within the Framework of Harmonization

Figure 1-1 in Chapter 1 summarizes the Committee's evaluation plan, and shows the focus countries and "harmonization" at the center of the plan. In April 2004, the Joint United Nations Programme on HIV/AIDS (UNAIDS), the United Kingdom, and the United States co-hosted a high-level meeting at which donors reaffirmed their commitment to harmonization—that is, to strengthening national AIDS responses to be led by the affected countries themselves. They endorsed the "Three Ones" as guiding principles to improve the country-level response (UN, 2003; UNAIDS, 2004; OGAC, 2005):

- One agreed upon HIV/AIDS Action Framework that provides the basis for coordinating the work of all partners.
- One National AIDS Coordinating Authority, with a broad-based multisectoral mandate.
- One agreed upon country-level Monitoring and Evaluation System (UNAIDS, 2004).

PEPFAR is fully committed to harmonization and the Three Ones principles (OGAC, 2005). Although these principles were not formally in place at the time of the passage of the Act, the legislation calls for the United States to be coordinated with other donors, and this commitment is consistent with the legislation, as well as other U.S. policy (UN, 2003). All of the PEPFAR focus countries have national AIDS authorities, and thus with this commitment, harmonization became the centerpiece of the structure of PEPFAR (OGAC, 2005). As such, it is central to the structure of the IOM evaluation. The imperative to operate within the framework of harmonization adds complexity to both the implementation of PEPFAR and the evaluation of it—it requires that PEPFAR implementation be judged primarily in terms of how effectively it is working through, with, and in support of countries and whether, in the final analysis, countries are becoming more effective at addressing their HIV/AIDS epidemics. Figure B-1 illustrates an example of this complexity and how the Committee approached the analysis. Examples of the challenges at the nexus of PEPFAR's imperatives to meet its targets, be harmonized, evidence-based, and in compliance with U.S. law and policy are discussed throughout the report.

MEETINGS

The Committee held a total of six meetings, three of which were partly for the purpose of information gathering and thus these portions of the meetings were open to the public. All three of the meetings with open sessions were held in 2005 and involved the full committee. A brief description of each open meeting follows, and the agendas are in Appendix G. Available slide presentations can be viewed on the project website at www.iom.edu/pepfar.

Meeting #1

The first meeting was held in Baltimore, MD, with open sessions on February 23 and 24, 2005. The Committee heard from officials from the Office of the U.S. Global AIDS Coordinator, as well as some of the implementing agencies, including the Office of Global Health Affairs at the Department of Health and Human Services, the Global Health Bureau at the U.S. Agency for International Development, the Global AIDS Program at the U.S. Centers for Disease Control and Prevention (CDC), and the HIV/AIDS Prevention Program at the U.S. Department of Defense. The Health Attaché from the Embassy of South Africa (one of the PEPFAR focus countries) and the Senior Program Director and Chief of Party from Catholic Relief Services (one of the initial PEPFAR implementing partners), also addressed the Committee. In addition, the Committee heard from

		Country Plan and Programs Based on Best Available Science?	
		Yes	**No**
PEPFAR Harmonized with Country Plan and Programs?	**Yes**	**Ideal State** Country is pursuing sound plans and programs and PEPFAR is supporting them Demonstrates successful harmonization	**Problem State** Country is pursuing unsound plans and programs and yet PEPFAR is supporting them PEPFARs commitment to harmonization poses a problem unless there are signs that its support is improving country practices
	No	**Problem State** Country is pursuing sound plans and programs, but PEPFAR is not supporting them Demonstrates the challenge of harmonization for PEPFAR's policies and practice	**Less than Ideal State** Country is pursuing unsound plans and programs, but PEPFAR is not supporting them Not characterized as ideal because we would prefer to see countries engaging in sound practice But from the perspective of evaluating PEPFAR, this is OK — at least PEPFAR is not supporting unsound practice

FIGURE B-1 Nexus of evidence base and harmonization.
NOTE: The schematic has been oversimplified to make a general point—the responses would not be "Yes/No" but rather a matter of degrees.

senior officials from the monitoring and evaluation units of the World Bank (in person), the Global Fund, the World Health Organization (WHO), and UNAIDS (all by phone).

Meeting #2

The second meeting was held in Washington, DC, with open sessions on April 19 and 21, 2005. During these sessions, the U.S. Global AIDS Coordinator and other OGAC officials gave presentations to the Committee, as did officials from six of PEPFAR's implementing partners: the Centre for Infectious Disease Research in Zambia (CIDRZ), the Elizabeth Glaser Pediatric AIDS Foundation, Family Health International, Haitian Group for the Study of Kaposi's Sarcoma and Opportunistic Infections (GHESKIO), Harvard PEPFAR, and Save the Children. A panel of Chiefs of Party from the Global AIDS Program at the U.S. Centers for Disease Control and Prevention—representing the programs in Botswana, Democratic Republic of Congo, Uganda, Vietnam, and Zimbabwe—addressed the Committee via videoconference.

Meeting #4

The fourth meeting was held in Washington, DC, with an open session on September 15, 2005. The Committee heard from two people who were senior Congressional staff involved in the initial development of the legislation that was eventually passed as the United States Leadership against HIV/AIDS, Tuberculosis, and Malaria Act of 2003 and from several OGAC officials. The meeting included a panel of ambassadors with experience in one or more of the PEPFAR focus countries—including Kenya, Nigeria, South Africa, and Uganda—with additional perspective from the Executive Director, Task Force on HIV/AIDS and Director of the Africa Program at the Center for Strategic and International Studies, who had led delegations to several of the PEPFAR countries. The Committee also heard from a panel of three PEPFAR implementing partners—Pact, CARE, and the International Rescue Committee.

LITERATURE AND DOCUMENTATION

The Committee searched widely for literature relevant to the standards for and implementation of programs to address HIV/AIDS epidemics. The Committee searched and retrieved references primarily from the PubMed and Cochrane bibliographic databases, as well as the websites of key organizations such as WHO, UNAIDS, the United Nations Children's Fund (UNICEF), World Bank, Global Fund, the Kaiser Family Foundation, the Global Health Council, the Center for Global Development, and the Center for Strategic and International Studies. The Committee reviewed extensive documentation of PEPFAR implementation including the authorizing legislation—the United States Leadership against HIV/AIDS, Tuberculosis, and Malaria Act of 2003—and its legislative history; the websites of OGAC, CDC, the U.S. Agency for International Development (USAID), implementing partners, the U.S. embassies in the focus countries, and the focus country governments and/or lead HIV/AIDS entities; the PEPFAR strategy, operational plans, and first and second annual reports; the 2005 and 2006 Country Operational Plans for all of the focus countries as well as the guidance and technical considerations for developing these plans; the work plans and technical considerations of all of the Technical Working Groups; the HIV/AIDS strategies and operational plans for all of the focus countries when available; all guidance, reports, and other documents published by OGAC as well as those directly relevant to PEPFAR published by implementing agencies such as CDC and USAID; all of the abstracts and presentations from the 2005 and 2006 PEPFAR Annual Meetings; presentations and Congressional testimony given by PEPFAR officials; and documentation provided by implementing partners and other interested parties.

BUDGET AND PERFORMANCE DATA

With the intention of respecting global efforts at harmonization of monitoring and evaluation—in which PEPFAR is a participant (Rugg et al., 2004; OGAC, 2005)—the Committee relied on existing indicators and data sources to the greatest extent possible. The Committee reviewed and analyzed all publicly available PEPFAR budget data and performance data, as well as information about HIV/AIDS funding, epidemiology, and activities in the focus countries. The primary sources for PEPFAR data were PEPFAR Congressional Notifications, Country Operational Plans, Annual Reports and other interim reports, and analyses of the Country Operational Plan Reporting System provided by OGAC. The primary sources of data on the focus countries were their own websites and publications, OGAC, UNAIDS, WHO, the World Bank, and Kaiser Family Foundation. The Committee did not audit or independently verify these data; however it did some checks for internal consistency as well as congruence with external sources. The Committee did not audit any aspect of the program and thus is unable to address issues such as contract compliance, diversion of funds, or corruption.

DISCUSSIONS WITH PARTICIPANTS AND STAKEHOLDERS

Especially because many of the aspects of program implementation that the Committee reviewed had a significant qualitative component, the Committee sought to have discussions with as many relevant participants and stakeholders as possible. For example, with respect to coordination, in addition to examining whether there were structures and processes in place to facilitate coordination, the Committee also solicited the perspectives of all the major parties that were intended to be coordinated.

Throughout the process—during the development of the evaluation plan, in response to the publication of the plan, in preparation for the visits to the PEPFAR focus countries, and after the visits—the Committee had discussions with a wide variety of people, in Washington, DC, and Geneva, Switzerland, both in person and by phone, including

- OGAC and implementing agency officials
- Staff of the U.S. Congress
- Groups of implementing partners and other stakeholders organized by the PEPFAR Implementer Roundtable of InterAction and the Global AIDS Roundtable of the Global Health Council
- Officials of the Global Fund, UNAIDS, WHO, and the World Bank

In order to encourage the participants in these discussions to speak candidly, the Committee members assured them that they would not attribute statements made in these discussions to individuals by name, organization, or country. The people and organizations with whom the Committee had discussions are listed in Appendix A. Discussions were grouped as follows and summarized across the various perspectives provided:

- OGAC and implementing agency officials
- Miscellaneous implementers and stakeholders
- Other HIV/AIDS donors and programs
- Focus country visits (see below for description of process and analysis)

In order to facilitate consistency across discussions, the Committee developed generic guides for each type of meeting or site visit to be conducted. These guides were based on the questions outlined in the evaluation plan, identified a standard set of issues to be addressed, and also allowed for additional issues to be explored depending on the circumstance. These guides were tailored to the extent possible based on what the Committee was able to learn in advance about the particular people or program involved.

FOCUS COUNTRY VISITS

As a result of PEPFAR's structure and commitment to harmonization, the majority of implementation activities are occurring in the focus countries. Thus, visits to the focus countries to directly observe implementation activities were a critical part of the Committee's evaluation plan. The Committee anticipated that these country visits would provide insight into the programmatic successes and challenges through concrete examples and first-hand accounts of how PEPFAR was working on the ground, and found that they did.

In recognition of the unique nature of the HIV/AIDS epidemic and the country response to it in each of the 15 focus countries, PEPFAR has been designed to support national leadership and to adapt to the specific needs of each country. The Committee therefore thought it important to observe how the conditions prevailing in each focus country were affecting the implementation of PEPFAR. The Committee—in small delegations of four to seven people—visited 13 of the 15 focus countries between late October of 2005 and late February of 2006. The Committee cancelled a planned visit to Côte d'Ivoire and was unable to plan a visit to Haiti, both due to security concerns. In lieu of a visit, the Committee conducted several conference calls with the Country Teams and implementing partners in Côte d'Ivoire and Haiti. Because the delegations could not be large enough to include all areas of expertise required, all delegation members were expected to familiarize themselves with all of the discussion guides and to serve as "generalists" during the visit. Each country visit lasted for 1 week, giving the Committee a total of 13 weeks in the focus countries. Most of the delegations were split for part of the agenda in order to be able to visit more sites. Of a total of 27 Committee members, consultants, and liaisons, 20 participated in country visits together with five staff. The majority of

BOX B-1
Generic Agenda for Focus Country Visits

Day 1—Monday

Purpose: Understand PEPFAR Mission staff's perspective on program implementation (especially coordination and harmonization)

- Morning: Introductory Meeting with U.S. Ambassador and PEPFAR leadership team
- Afternoon: Meetings with PEPFAR Mission Staff—focused on prevention, treatment, care, and management
- Evening: Debrief and work on visit report

Day 2—Tuesday

Purpose: Understand perspective of country officials, other donors, and partners on PEPFAR implementation (especially coordination and harmonization)

- Morning: Meeting with National AIDS leadership and staff (for example, Ministry of Health)
- Meeting with National AIDS coordinating entity
- Afternoon: Meeting with National monitoring and evaluation authority
- Meeting with Other Donors and Partner Organizations
- Evening: Debrief and work on visit report

Day 3—Wednesday

Purpose: Examine PEPFAR-supported prevention, treatment, and care programs

- Morning and Afternoon: IOM Team breaks into two groups for program visits

people participated in more than one country visit, resulting in a total of 68 person-weeks of observation in the focus countries.

Agendas for the Country Visits

The Committee developed a generic 1-week agenda for the country visits that was intended to provide as comprehensive an overview of PEPFAR implementation as possible in a short time (see Box B-1). The Committee tailored the agenda to the particular circumstances of each focus country in concert with PEPFAR staff, PEPFAR implementing partners, national officials, other donors, community leaders, and others. The agendas included some discussions that were consistent across all countries—such as with the U.S. Country Team and focus country government HIV/AIDS officials, and some that varied widely depending on the country. The Committee selected a purposive sample of sites to both illustrate the breadth of the program in that country and exemplify PEPFAR's successes and challenges there. The

- Team 1: For example, visit different types of prevention programs
- Team 2: For example, visit different types of treatment programs
- Evening: Dinner with local community representatives (people living with HIV [PLWH] groups, community leaders, partner nongovernmental organizations, other nongovernmental organizations)
- Debrief and work on visit report

Day 4—Thursday

Purpose: Examine PEPFAR-supported prevention, treatment, and care programs

- Morning and Afternoon: IOM Team breaks into two groups for program visits
- Team 1: For example, visit different types of care programs
- Team 2: For example, visit different types of orphan programs
- Evening: Debrief and work on visit report

Day 5—Friday

Purpose: Examine PEPFAR-supported capacity-building efforts

- Morning and Afternoon: IOM Team breaks into two groups for program visits
- Team 1: For example, visit to offices responsible for national supply chain management, blood bank, information technology program, etc.
- Team 2: For example, visit training and workforce development programs, medical records program, laboratories, etc.
- Exit meeting with U.S. ambassador and PEPFAR Mission staff to request additional information, clarifications, etc.
- Evening: Debrief and work on visit report

Committee approached the country visits as a continuous learning process, and attempted to leave some flexibility in the agendas to allow the visiting teams to adapt to what they learned as the visit progressed. In practice, because the agendas were ambitious and logistic challenges were numerous, there was little flexibility to be exercised.

Country Visit Process

Prior to each visit, the Committee sent letters to all parties with whom they were scheduled to meet to confirm the appointment, to provide information about the study and the delegation members who would be coming, and to outline the major topics of discussion.

The Committee endeavored to create an environment in which people felt free to speak frankly and thus—in addition to assuring participants that the Committee would not attribute remarks to individuals, organizations, or countries—requested of OGAC that no OGAC staff be present during discussions with the PEPFAR Country Teams and that no PEPFAR staff be present during visits to sites that PEPFAR was supporting. PEPFAR staff honored this request. In a few instances, it was necessary for diplomatic purposes to be introduced by PEPFAR staff, but they left after the introductions had been made.

The Committee explained at every meeting that all materials given to the delegation would have to be made available in the public domain, that is, in our public access file. After each visit was completed, the Committee also sent follow-up letters to every party with whom it had met to thank them and to reiterate that any documents they had given to the delegation would be available in the public domain.

Especially for the first several trips, each delegation was expected to produce a brief report on Thursday night to go to the next delegation on Friday before its visit started. The purpose of the report was to highlight any major considerations or lessons learned with respect to logistics, diplomacy, or the substance of the discussions. In practice, no major unanticipated issues were identified and later delegations did not produce these reports.

Analyses of Country Visit Information

Pre-Visit Analysis

To guide the development and conduct of each country visit, the Committee reviewed and analyzed information available about the country's demography and general and AIDS-specific epidemiology, as well as national AIDS strategies and plans, PEPFAR focus country profiles, and PEPFAR Country Operational Plans for fiscal year 2005.

Individual Country Visit Analysis

By the end of the visit, each delegation was expected to develop a summary of its consensus on the key observations, findings, and conclusions about the implementation of PEPFAR in that particular country, by synthesizing the information from the many meetings and site visits. For example, after having discussed harmonization with a range of parties with whom PEPFAR is involved, the delegation endeavored to "triangulate" among the various sources to reach a conclusion about how well PEPFAR was harmonizing in that country (see Figures B-1 and B-2). Most teams continued to work on these analyses after the visit was completed.

Cross-Country Visit Analysis

To reach conclusions across the focus countries, the Committee conducted several types of analyses. First, the Committee compiled all of the summary reports by topic or issue. For example, findings related to coordination were pulled from each of the summary reports to provide a view

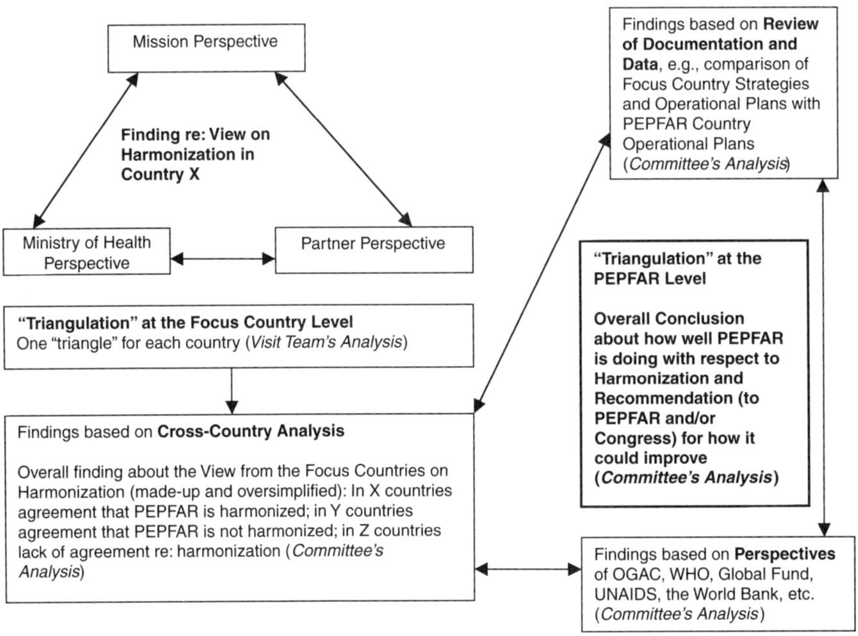

FIGURE B-2 Showing examples of "triangulation" at two levels: (1) analyzing focus country visit data, and (2) integrating it with other data to reach conclusions and develop recommendations.

of PEPFAR's coordination efforts across all of the focus countries. Second, several committee members who served on more than one country visit developed individual cross-country conclusions based on the unique set of countries that they had visited. Third, the Committee synthesized all of the other analyses as well as notes from all of the visits to produce a set of findings and conclusions about the overall perspective from the focus countries on PEPFAR. Finally, the Committee "triangulated" this synthesis of information from the focus countries with other sources of information—including documentation and other interviews—to reach conclusions about key aspects of PEPFAR implementation such as harmonization (see Figure B-2).

A great deal of information about the focus countries is a matter of public record—for example, information about the nature of their HIV/AIDS epidemics, their national AIDS strategies and sometimes their operational plans, and their PEPFAR Country Operational Plans. When discussing this kind of information in the report, the Committee identifies specific countries by name. However, when discussing information that is based on discussions had in the focus countries, the Committee avoids attribution of comments even by country. As discussed earlier, the Committee assured all parties with whom it spoke that it would not attribute comments and believes that this assurance helped to facilitate candid discussions.

LIMITATIONS

The focus country visits were not designed to allow the Committee to go deeply into and reach definitive conclusions about any one focus country, program, or aspect of implementation—with perhaps the exception of overall PEPFAR management, coordination, and harmonization. Thus, the Committee did not attempt to reach conclusions about specific countries or programs and has not based conclusions about any aspect of PEPFAR solely on the visits. However, the Committee believes that the cumulative information from all of the visits—effectively 13 weeks on the ground in PEPFAR focus countries, discussions with hundreds of people, and visits to dozens of sites—gave it a comprehensive and detailed picture of PEPFAR implementation overall as viewed from the focus countries.

The Committee provides examples of PEPFAR-supported programs throughout the report. The Committee selected these examples from the Country Operational Plans simply to illustrate the types of activities included in the various PEPFAR categories. The Committee neither visited or reviewed the details of all of the programs described in the examples provided nor evaluated any of them.

Given the nature of the enterprise and the kinds of information collected—comprehensive but not exhaustive looks at each country, discussions with people who were not required to provide documentation of their assertions, site visits that did not necessarily permit the delegations to get "behind the scenes" and were largely dependent on collective personal impressions, a great many compelling sights and people—the Committee endeavored to remain cognizant of its limitations and avoid going beyond these. The Committee sought to grapple with and synthesize the entirety of the information and to guard against the natural human tendency to let one example, or anecdote, or personality carry too much weight in the final analysis. Information from the country visits that is cited in the report relates to points where there was the greatest commonality of observation and agreement across countries and among Committee members.

In compliance with the Federal Advisory Committee Act Amendments of 1997 (P.L. 105-153), all materials presented to the Committee must be publicly available via our public access file. Because OGAC determined that some portions of the Country Operational Plans are procurement sensitive and therefore could not be in the public domain, they provided the Committee with redacted versions of the full Country Operational Plans, in addition to the Country Operational Plan information that is available on the OGAC website. Because the Committee's interest was not in appreciating the finest level of detail in the Country Operational Plans, it accepted OGAC's assertion that the missing material would have little effect on the Committee's ability to develop a general understanding of the programming in a country or its alignment with national plans and priorities. Further, because OGAC considers some draft guidance and other documents to be sensitive until finalized, the Committee has only reviewed those that OGAC will allow into the public domain and thus has not been privy to the guidance development process or guidance which has yet to be finalized.

REFERENCES

IOM (Institute of Medicine). 2005. *Plan for a short-term evaluation of PEPFAR implementation.* Washington, DC: The National Academies Press.

OGAC (Office of the U.S. Global AIDS Coordinator). 2005. *The President's Emergency Plan for AIDS Relief: Defining US support for national strategies* (PowerPoint Presentation, July 2005). Washington, DC: OGAC.

Rugg, D., G. Peersman, and M. Carael. 2004. *Global advances in HIV/AIDS monitoring and evaluation.* Minneapolis, MN: Wiley Periodicals, Inc.

UN (United Nations). 2003. *Monterrey Consensus of the International Conference on Financing for Development: The final text of agreements and commitments adopted at the International Conference on Financing for Development, Monterrey, Mexico, 18–22 March 2002.* Geneva, Switzerland: UN.

UNAIDS (Joint United Nations Programme on HIV/AIDS). 2004. *"Three ones" key principles.* Conference paper 1, Washington consultation of April 4, 2004. Geneva, Switzerland: UNAIDS. http://www.unaids.org/NetTools/Misc/DocInfo.aspx?LANG=en&href=http://gva-doc-owl/WEBcontent/Documents/pub/UNA-docs/Three-Ones_KeyPrinciples_en.pdf (accessed September 20, 2006).

APPENDIX
C

Plan for a Short-term Evaluation of PEPFAR Implementation

Letter Report # 1

Committee on the President's Emergency Plan for AIDS Relief (PEPFAR) Implementation Evaluation

Board on Global Health
Board on Children, Youth, and Families

INSTITUTE OF MEDICINE
OF THE NATIONAL ACADEMIES

THE NATIONAL ACADEMIES PRESS
Washington, D.C.
www.nap.edu

THE NATIONAL ACADEMIES PRESS 500 Fifth Street, N.W. Washington, DC 20001

NOTICE: The project that is the subject of this report was approved by the Governing Board of the National Research Council, whose members are drawn from the councils of the National Academy of Sciences, the National Academy of Engineering, and the Institute of Medicine. The members of the committee responsible for the report were chosen for their special competences and with regard for appropriate balance.

This study was supported by Contract No. SAQMPD04C1166 between the National Academy of Sciences and the U.S. Department of State. Any opinions, findings, conclusions, or recommendations expressed in this publication are those of the author(s) and do not necessarily reflect the view of the organizations or agencies that provided support for this project.

Additional copies of this report are available in limited quantities from the Committee for the Evaluation of PEPFAR Implementation, Board on Global Health, Institute of Medicine, 500 Fifth Street, N.W., Washington, DC 20001. The full text is available online at http://www.nap.edu.

For more information about the Institute of Medicine, visit the IOM home page at: **www.iom.edu.**

Printed in the United States of America.

The serpent has been a symbol of long life, healing, and knowledge among almost all cultures and religions since the beginning of recorded history. The serpent adopted as a logotype by the Institute of Medicine is a relief carving from ancient Greece, now held by the Staatliche Museen in Berlin.

"Knowing is not enough; we must apply.
Willing is not enough; we must do."
—Goethe

INSTITUTE OF MEDICINE
OF THE NATIONAL ACADEMIES

Advising the Nation. Improving Health.

THE NATIONAL ACADEMIES

Advisers to the Nation on Science, Engineering, and Medicine

The **National Academy of Sciences** is a private, nonprofit, self-perpetuating society of distinguished scholars engaged in scientific and engineering research, dedicated to the furtherance of science and technology and to their use for the general welfare. Upon the authority of the charter granted to it by the Congress in 1863, the Academy has a mandate that requires it to advise the federal government on scientific and technical matters. Dr. Ralph J. Cicerone is president of the National Academy of Sciences.

The **National Academy of Engineering** was established in 1964, under the charter of the National Academy of Sciences, as a parallel organization of outstanding engineers. It is autonomous in its administration and in the selection of its members, sharing with the National Academy of Sciences the responsibility for advising the federal government. The National Academy of Engineering also sponsors engineering programs aimed at meeting national needs, encourages education and research, and recognizes the superior achievements of engineers. Dr. Wm. A. Wulf is president of the National Academy of Engineering.

The **Institute of Medicine** was established in 1970 by the National Academy of Sciences to secure the services of eminent members of appropriate professions in the examination of policy matters pertaining to the health of the public. The Institute acts under the responsibility given to the National Academy of Sciences by its congressional charter to be an adviser to the federal government and, upon its own initiative, to identify issues of medical care, research, and education. Dr. Harvey V. Fineberg is president of the Institute of Medicine.

The **National Research Council** was organized by the National Academy of Sciences in 1916 to associate the broad community of science and technology with the Academy's purposes of furthering knowledge and advising the federal government. Functioning in accordance with general policies determined by the Academy, the Council has become the principal operating agency of both the National Academy of Sciences and the National Academy of Engineering in providing services to the government, the public, and the scientific and engineering communities. The Council is administered jointly by both Academies and the Institute of Medicine. Dr. Ralph J. Cicerone, and Dr. Wm. A. Wulf are chair and vice chair, respectively, of the National Research Council.

www.national-academies.org

COMMITTEE FOR THE EVALUATION OF PEPFAR IMPLEMENTATION

JAIME SEPÜLVEDA AMOR *(Chair)*, Director General, National Institutes of Health, Mexico

HELEN SMITS *(Vice Chair)*, Former Faculty of Medicine, Eduardo Mondlane University, Mozambique

CHARLES CARPENTER *(Treatment Subcommittee Chair)*, Professor of Medicine, Bio Med Medicine, Miriam Hospital, Brown University, Providence, Rhode Island

JAMES CURRAN *(Prevention Subcommittee Chair)*, Dean, Professor of Epidemiology, Rollins School of Public Health, Emory University, Atlanta, Georgia

WILLIAM L. HOLZEMER *(Care Subcommittee Chair)*, Professor of Nursing and Associate Dean, International Programs, School of Nursing, University of California, San Francisco

STEFANO BERTOZZI, Director of Health Economics, National Institutes of Health, Mexico

GEOFF GARNETT, Professor of Microparasite Epidemiology, Faculty of Medicine, Imperial College, London, United Kingdom

RUTH MACKLIN, Head, Division of Philosophy and History of Medicine, Department of Epidemiology and Population Health, Albert Einstein College of Medicine, New York

AFFETTE McCAW-BINNS, Professor, Reproductive Health Epidemiology, Section of Community Health, University of the West Indies, Jamaica

A. DAVID PALTIEL, Associate Professor and Head, Division of Health Policy and Administration, Yale University, New Haven, Connecticut

PRISCILLA REDDY, Director, Health Promotion Research and Development, National Health Promotion & Behavioural Intervention Research Unit, Medical Research Council of South Africa

DAVID ROSS, Director, Public Health Informatics Institute, Decatur, Georgia

HEATHER WEISS, Director, Harvard Family Research Project, Harvard University, Boston, Massachusetts

Subcommittee Members, Liaisons, and Study Consultants

MAUREEN BLACK, John A. Scholl Professor of Pediatrics, University of Maryland School of Medicine, Baltimore

HOOSEN COOVADIA, Victor Daitz Professor of HIV/AIDS Research, Centre for the AIDS Programme of Research, South Africa

HENRY FOMUNDAM, Acting Director, National HIV and AIDS Programme, MEDUNSA Pharmacovigilance Centre, South Africa
PAUL GERTLER, Chief Economist, Human Development Network, World Bank, Washington, D.C.
CARL LATKIN, Professor, Department of Health, Behavior, and Society, Johns Hopkins University Bloomberg School of Public Health, Baltimore, Maryland
JAMES NTOZI, Professor, Department of Population Studies, Makerere University, Uganda
JAMES SHERRY, Vice President, Policy, Research and Advocacy, Global Health Council, Washington, D.C.
OLAITAN SOYANNWO, Professor of Anesthesia and Consultant Anesthetist, College of Medicine, University of Ibadan and University College Hospital, Ibadan, Nigeria
BURTON WILCKE, Jr., Chair and Associate Professor, Department of Biomedical Technologies, University of Vermont, Burlington
MICHAEL MERSON, *(Board on Global Health Liaison)*, Anna M. R. Lauder Professor of Public Health, Yale School of Medicine, New Haven, Connecticut
ELENA O. NIGHTINGALE *(Board on Children, Youth, and Families Liaison),* Scholar-in-Residence, Institute of Medicine, The National Academies, Washington, D.C.
JULIA COFFMAN (*Consultant*), Independent Evaluation Consultant, Alexandria, Virginia
THOMAS N. DENNY *(Consultant),* Associate Professor Pathology, Laboratory Medicine, Associate Professor of Pediatrics, Associate Professor of Preventive Medicine and Community Health and Assistant Dean for Research in Health Policy UMD—New Jersey Medical School, New Jersey
FLORENCIA ZULBERTI *(Consultant),* Assistant Director for Global Health, National Institutes of Health, Mexico

Staff

PATRICK KELLEY, Director, Board on Global Health
ROSEMARY CHALK, Director, Board on Children, Youth, and Families
MICHELE ORZA, Study Director
ALICIA GABLE, Senior Program Officer (until June 2005)
KIMBERLY SCOTT, Senior Program Officer (from September 2005)
HEATHER COLVIN, Program Officer (until July 2005)
J. ALICE NIXON, Program Officer (from July 2005)
WEZI MUNTHALI, Research Associate (until October 2005)
ALYSON SCHWABER, Research Associate (until September 2005)

DIANNE STARE, Research Assistant (until September 2005)
ANGELA MENSAH, Senior Program Assistant (from June 2005)
KIMBERLY WEINGARTEN, Senior Program Assistant
ELIZABETH SHARP, Science and Technology Policy Fellow (January 2005 through April 2005)
SHARLENE BAGGA, Science and Technology Policy Fellow (June 2005 through August 2005)
CLAUDIA GROSSMAN, Science and Technology Policy Fellow (June 2005 through August 2005)

Reviewers

This report has been reviewed in draft form by individuals chosen for their diverse perspectives and technical expertise, in accordance with procedures approved by the NRC's Report Review Committee. The purpose of this independent review is to provide candid and critical comments that will assist the institution in making its published report as sound as possible and to ensure that the report meets institutional standards for objectivity, evidence, and responsiveness to the study charge. The review comments and draft manuscript remain confidential to protect the integrity of the deliberative process. We wish to thank the following individuals for their review of this report:

Solomon R. Benatar, Professor of Medicine and Director, Bioethics Centre, Department of Medicine, Faculty of Health Sciences, University of Cape Town, Cape Town, Republic of South Africa
Thomas J. Coates, Professor, Department of Medicine, Division of Infectious Diseases, Prevention and Policy Research, David Geffen School of Medicine, University of California, Los Angeles, Los Angeles
Nils Daulaire, President and CEO, Global Health Council, White River Junction, Vermont
Anne Mills, Professor of Health Economics and Policy, London School of Hygiene and Tropical Medicine, London, United Kingdom
Philip Onyebujoh, Special Programme for Research and Training in Tropical Diseases, World Health Organization, Geneva, Switzerland

Mauro Schechter, Professor of Infectious Diseases, and Head, AIDS Research Laboratory, Hospital Universitario Clementino Fraga Filho Universidade, Rio de Janeiro, Brazil

Although the reviewers listed above have provided many constructive comments and suggestions, they were not asked to endorse the conclusions or recommendations nor did they see the final draft of the report before its release. The review of this report was overseen by **Neal A. Vanselow**. Appointed by the National Research Council and Institute of Medicine, he was responsible for making certain that an independent examination of this report was carried out in accordance with institutional procedures and that all review comments were carefully considered. Responsibility for the final content of this report rests entirely with the authoring committee and the institution.

Preface

Concern for the over 40 million people infected with HIV and others at risk of infection or otherwise affected through the impact on their families and communities moved the U.S. Congress on behalf of the American people to pass in May 2003 an unprecedented $15 billion international public health initiative—the U.S. Leadership against HIV/AIDS, Tuberculosis, and Malaria Act. With so much at stake from both a human and a fiscal perspective, Congress mandated that the Institute of Medicine review the groundbreaking initiative created by the legislation—the President's Emergency Plan for AIDS Relief (PEPFAR). An independent, rigorous, multidisciplinary expert review of PEPFAR is in the best interests of the taxpayer, the scientific community, program implementers, and—most importantly—the people whose lives are in the balance.

The IOM's legislative mandate to conduct an evaluation of PEPFAR is a complex challenge, in part because PEPFAR is effectively many programs in one. PEPFAR seeks to prevent seven million HIV infections, provide two million HIV-infected people with antiretroviral therapy, and care for ten million people affected by HIV/AIDS. These people live in fifteen different "focus countries," most with limited health care system capacity for scale-up of HIV/AIDS-related services. Thus, our evaluation is of a multiplicity of programs that assume the characteristics and complexities of each of the focus countries.

The legislative mandate calls for our study of PEPFAR to be delivered at the three-year mark and in time to inform reauthorization discussions. This report outlines our plan for the mandated study, to be published next fall.

Due to delays between passage of the legislation, appropriation of funds, and initiation of programs, we are required to evaluate PEPFAR very early in its implementation when many of its programs are relatively immature. Our short-term evaluation can provide insights into whether PEPFAR is making reasonable progress toward its goals and can suggest ways in which the program can be improved to ensure that it ultimately meets its goals. However, it cannot adequately measure what matters most—the impact on the lives of the people the legislation seeks to serve. In recognition of this, in addition to providing the short-term evaluation that will be responsive to the legislative mandate, the IOM Committee was charged to plan a long-term evaluation to determine whether PEPFAR has ultimately succeeded in improving the lives of the people in the focus countries by preventing infections, treating patients, and caring for people. We plan to publish the plan for a long-term study shortly after publication of the mandated report.

Our collective responsibility in caring for those in need around the world demands that the challenge of the global HIV/AIDS pandemic be met in a way that is ethically, scientifically, and fiscally sound. We have been humbled by the myriad of questions raised by this global pandemic about how to most effectively prevent the spread of this disease and care for those affected by it. Given limited resources, there is an obligation to match the will to help others with the will to learn how best to help them. This international IOM committee has taken on the challenge of evaluating PEPFAR with determination and humility and is passionately committed to contributing to the effectiveness of PEPFAR in confronting the HIV/AIDS pandemic. We appreciate the help received from so many to date in developing this plan and look forward to a collaborative process of learning together as it is implemented.

Jaime Sepúlveda Amor, MD, Dr.Sc.
Chair

INTRODUCTION

HIV/AIDS has evolved into the world's greatest public health crisis. Forty million people are estimated to be living with HIV/AIDS, 64 percent of them in sub-Saharan Africa (UNAIDS, 2004a). HIV prevalence among adults 15-49 years of age now exceeds 15 percent in many countries and has approached nearly 30 percent in Botswana, Lesotho, Swaziland, and Zimbabwe. In 2004 alone, almost 5 million people are thought to have become infected with HIV, including 2 million women and 800,000 children. UNAIDS estimated that 3.1 million people died of AIDS worldwide in 2004, and that AIDS has reversed the gains in life expectancy that had been achieved by Africa over the past 50 years (UNAIDS, 2004a).

By 2003, an estimated 12 million children had been orphaned in sub-Saharan Africa as a result of HIV/AIDS, half of whom are between the ages of 10 and 14 (UNAIDS, 2004a). Girls and women are especially vulnerable to HIV, and now account for 50 percent of people living with HIV worldwide and 57 percent of those in sub-Saharan Africa (UNAIDS, 2004a). In addition, HIV/AIDS has severely strained national economies and contributed to political instability in many of the countries experiencing an epidemic.

The U.S. Leadership against HIV/AIDS, Tuberculosis, and Malaria Act

Global funding in response to HIV/AIDS has increased dramatically since 2001. On May 27, 2003, the U.S. Congress passed Public Law 108-25: the United States Leadership against HIV/AIDS, Tuberculosis, and Malaria Act of 2003 (the Act). Provisions of this legislation 1) required the President to establish a comprehensive, integrated 5-year strategy to combat global HIV/AIDS, including specific objectives, strategies, and approaches related to HIV/AIDS prevention, treatment, and care; 2) assigned priorities for relevant executive branch agencies; 3) required improved coordination among such agencies; and 4) projected general levels of resources needed to achieve the stated goals. The legislation emphasized the establishment of programs that focus on national HIV/AIDS strategies of recipient countries, women and children, strengthening of health care infrastructure and workforce, and effective monitoring and evaluation to assess programmatic success. This legislation also required the President to establish the Office of the Global AIDS Coordinator (OGAC) within the U.S. Department of State, which would have primary responsibility for oversight and coordination of all U.S. international activities to combat the HIV/AIDS pandemic. On October 6, 2003, Randall Tobias was sworn in as the first Global AIDS Coordinator, with the rank of Ambassador. On February 23, 2004,

Ambassador Tobias presented the U.S. 5-year Global HIV/AIDS Strategy to Congress.

President's Emergency Plan for AIDS Relief (PEPFAR)

The initiative is commonly known by the title given to the U.S. 5-year Global HIV/AIDS Strategy: "The President's Emergency Plan for AIDS Relief", or PEPFAR. In order to measure the progress of the initiative, the PEPFAR strategy establishes three overarching goals:

- To encourage bold leadership at every level to fight HIV/AIDS;
- To apply best practices within bilateral HIV/AIDS prevention, treatment, and care programs, in concert with the objectives and policies of host governments' national HIV/AIDS strategies; and
- To encourage partners, including multilateral organizations and other host governments, to coordinate at all levels to strengthen response efforts, to embrace best practices, to adhere to principles of sound management, and to harmonize monitoring and evaluation efforts to ensure the most effective and efficient use of resources (OGAC, 2004).

The PEPFAR strategy also describes the principles according to which it will achieve its mission and goals, including responding with urgency to the crisis; seeking new approaches; coordinating the U.S. Government oversight and direction of PEPFAR activities; drawing on the scientific evidence base in developing interventions; establishing measurable goals for programs; harmonizing program development and implementation with the host countries; integrating prevention, treatment and care programs; building national capacity; encouraging national leadership; and coordinating with other partners (OGAC, 2004).

PEPFAR, while encompassing activities in over 120 countries, is focused on the development of comprehensive and integrated prevention, treatment, and care programs in 15 countries selected largely because they are heavily affected by HIV/AIDS (OGAC, 2005b). With regard to funding, $10 billion of the $15 billion authorized under the Act is to be allocated to efforts in these 15 countries over five years (OGAC, 2005b). Currently, the 15 PEPFAR focus countries are Botswana, Cote d'Ivoire, Ethiopia, Guyana, Haiti, Kenya, Mozambique, Namibia, Nigeria, Rwanda, South Africa, Tanzania, Uganda, Zambia, and Vietnam. PEPFAR has established additional goals for its prevention, treatment and care programs in these countries, specifically: to support prevention of 7 million new HIV infections, treatment of

2 million HIV-infected people with antiretroviral therapy (ART), and care of 10 million people infected and affected by HIV/AIDS.[1]

OGAC is responsible for maintaining the focus of PEPFAR by leading policy development, program oversight, and coordination both among U.S. government departments and agencies and with other donors and governments. Additionally, OGAC is responsible for the allocation of funds which are distributed through a number of U.S. government departments and agencies including the Departments of State, Defense (DoD), Commerce, Labor (DoL), and Health and Human Services (HHS); the U.S. Agency for International Development (USAID); and the Peace Corps (OGAC, 2005a). The two largest implementing entities are USAID and HHS which includes the Centers for Disease Control and Prevention (CDC), Food and Drug Administration, National Institute of Health (NIH), and Health Resources and Services Administration (HRSA). Within OGAC, staffing is organized into several groups, all of which include OGAC staff as well as representatives from the other U.S. government departments and agencies coordinated by OGAC. These groups include the Policy Group, incorporating representation from USAID, HHS, the White House and the National Security Council; the Deputy Principals Group, handling program management and logistics with representation from agencies including the Peace Corps, HHS, USAID, DoD and DoL; and a Scientific Steering Committee, consisting of representatives from CDC, NIH, USAID, and DoD (Moloney-Kitts, 2005). Finally, Core and Technical Teams, whose members are drawn from a wide range of U.S. government agencies, are responsible for supporting programs in PEPFAR countries with specific technical and implementation issues.

Each of the focus countries has a U.S. Government Mission team that is intended to provide a unified strategy and voice and is responsible for coordination of PEPFAR-sponsored programs in the country. The team is led by the U.S. ambassador and includes representatives from all of the implementing departments and agencies. It is supported by a core team based in OGAC which serves as a liaison between the field and headquarters. In many countries, high-level PEPFAR advisory committees have been formed to ensure a close working relationship between the U.S. government and host-country counterparts (OGAC, 2005a). In an effort to create self-sustaining, lasting systems to address HIV/AIDS, PEPFAR emphasizes the development of national leadership, human resources, and other capacities through collaboration of Mission teams with existing country partners, as well as with other donors.

---

[1]For purposes of this goal, PEPFAR defines "treatment" as antiretroviral therapy (ART) and categorizes other types of treatment—such as therapy for opportunistic infections or for pain management—under "care."

Study Goals and Approach

The Act mandates that the Institute of Medicine (IOM) evaluate PEPFAR and directs the President to consider IOM's findings. Specifically Sec. 101 (c) (1) of the Act states:

> *"Not later than 3 years after the date of the enactment of this Act, the Institute of Medicine shall publish findings comparing the success rates of the various programs and methods used under the [PEPFAR] strategy.*
>
> *In prioritizing the distribution of resources under the [PEPFAR] strategy, the President shall consider the findings published by the Institute of Medicine under this subsection."*

Thus, the current task of the IOM is to be responsive to this mandate and provide to Congress in time for reauthorization discussions an assessment of PEPFAR implementation at the three-year mark. The IOM has undertaken an independent, expert consensus committee process to plan, conduct, and report on this short-term evaluation, the scope of which is limited to the implementation of PEPFAR in the focus countries and does not include the U.S. contribution to the Global Fund to Fight AIDS, Tuberculosis, and Malaria (Global Fund) which is also coordinated by OGAC. The IOM Committee for the Evaluation of PEPFAR Implementation (the Committee) has three advisory Subcommittees focused on prevention, treatment, and care (see Appendix 1). This letter report outlines the Committee's plan for the short-term evaluation.

In addition to the size and complexity of PEPFAR, two additional features make the Committee's task an especially challenging one: PEPFAR is of necessity a dynamic, evolving program and it is still relatively early in its implementation.

As its name implies, OGAC has implemented PEPFAR on an emergency basis and, as the Act acknowledged, has had to "maintain sufficient flexibility and remain responsive to the ever-changing nature of the HIV/AIDS pandemic." Thus PEPFAR is a rapidly-moving, continuously-evolving target for evaluation. The Committee is prepared to find considerable changes in PEPFAR throughout its evaluation, and has developed an approach to the evaluation that will allow it to adapt not only to changes in PEPFAR implementation, but also to what the Committee learns as the evaluation proceeds. The Committee's evaluation plan should be viewed as a work-in-progress that will be modified to reflect both the dynamic nature of PEPFAR and what the Committee learns—particularly as it visits the PEPFAR focus countries to directly observe implementation activities.

Ultimately the "success" of PEPFAR will be judged by whether it has achieved its near-term goals of effectively supporting the prevention of 7 million HIV infections, treatment for 2 million people with HIV/AIDS with ART, and care of 10 million people infected with and affected by HIV/AIDS, as well as its longer-term goal of sustainable gains against the HIV/AIDS epidemics in the focus countries. However, although the Act was passed in May 2003, funds were not appropriated until January 2004, and the majority of the first year's funding was not obligated until September 2004 (see Appendix 2). Thus, at the time of the Committee's evaluation, PEPFAR will have been supporting the implementation of prevention, treatment and care programs in the focus countries for less than two years—less time than perhaps Congress had envisioned when they wrote the mandate for the IOM study. It would not be reasonable or feasible to evaluate PEPFAR solely against these goals so early in implementation, and therefore in this short-term evaluation the Committee plans instead to evaluate how PEPFAR is progressing toward 1) achieving these goals and 2) building the monitoring and evaluation capacity to demonstrate that it has achieved them.

The short-term evaluation can provide insights into whether PEPFAR is making reasonable progress toward its goals and can suggest ways in which the program can be improved to ensure that it ultimately meets its goals. However, it cannot adequately measure what matters most—the impact on the lives of the people the legislation seeks to serve. In recognition of this, in addition to providing the short-term evaluation that will be responsive to the legislative mandate, the IOM Committee is planning a long-term evaluation to determine whether PEPFAR has ultimately succeeded in improving the lives of the people in the focus countries by preventing infections, treating patients, and caring for people. We plan to publish the plan for a long-term study shortly after publication of the mandated report. This long-term evaluation plan will be informed by the Committee's fuller understanding of PEPFAR implementation and the challenging experience of evaluating it.

In the development of its plan, the Committee has consulted widely and remains open to receiving input from the broad range of parties interested in and affected by PEPFAR. To develop the plan, the Committee (and the additional subcommittee members) convened first in February 2005 and then again in April 2005 when the Committee was fully-formed to review documentation of and hear testimony about PEPFAR. The questions highlighted in the plan reflect the multiple data sources that the committee believes capture the primary components of PEPFAR implementation. The Committee has considered peer-reviewed literature on global efforts to combat HIV/AIDS in resource-limited settings, documentation provided by OGAC, and other program-related materials. The Committee has heard testimony from OGAC officials and PEPFAR Mission staff; global organizations such as the World Health Organization, UNAIDS, Global Fund, and World Bank; and numerous PEPFAR grantees and partners. In addition, one Committee member and one staff attended the PEPFAR Annual Meeting in Addis Ababa, Ethiopia in May 2005. Following these initial information–gathering activities and several phone conferences to further explore information specific to prevention, treatment, and care, the Committee met in July 2005 to outline the short-term evaluation plan (see Figure 1).

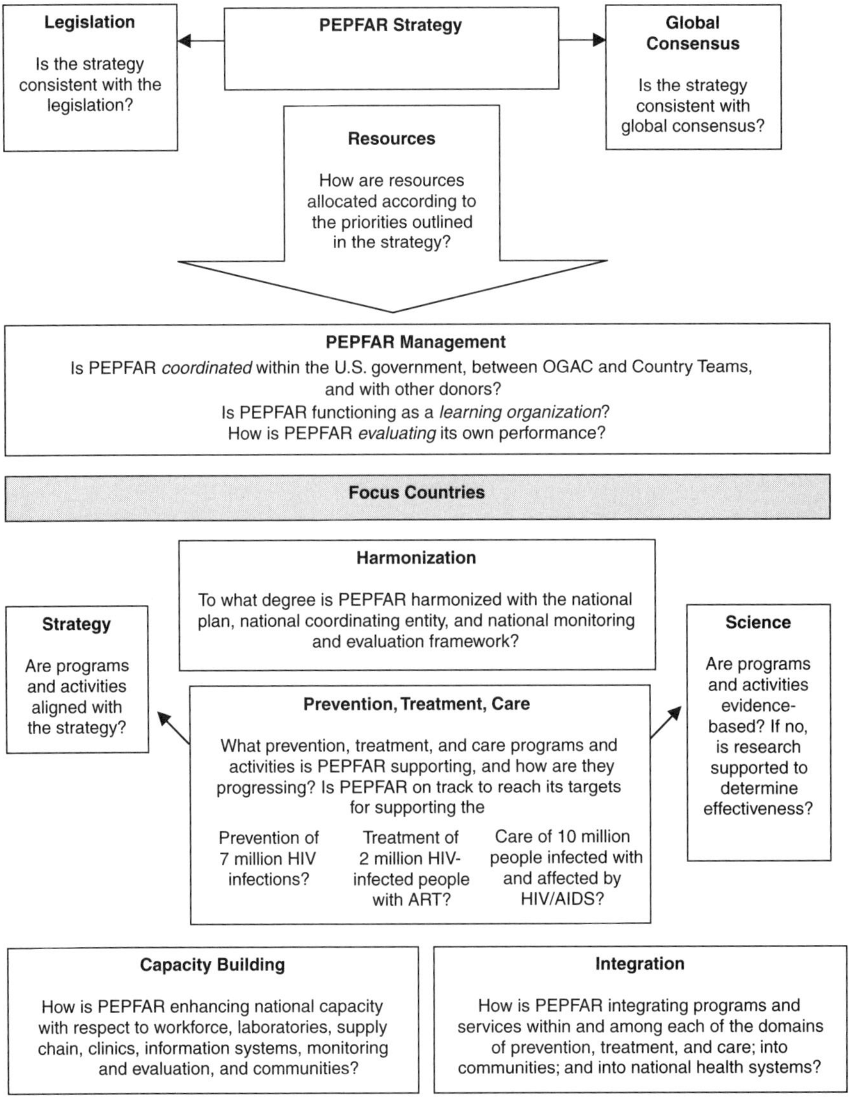

FIGURE 1-1 Short-term PEPFAR evaluation plan.

SHORT-TERM EVALUATION QUESTIONS

Strategy

Is the PEPFAR Strategy consistent with the Act and relevant global consensus?

The same section of the Act that mandates the IOM study also specifies the major elements that should be contained in the PEPFAR Strategy. In addition, the legislation calls for the U.S. to take a strong leadership position with respect to the global effort to combat HIV/AIDS and also to coordinate its efforts with the international donor community. The global HIV/AIDS community, led by organizations such as those of UNAIDS, has published guidelines outlining international consensus strategies for the development and implementation of prevention, treatment, and care programs.

- Does the PEPFAR strategy address the major elements of the Act such as:

—Developing specific objectives, approaches and strategies for activities related to HIV/AIDS prevention, treatment and care? (Sec. 101.a.1 & Sec.101.b.3.C)

—Focusing prevention funding, educational messages and activities on the reduction of HIV/AIDS behavioral risks? (Sec. 101.a.4 & Sec.101.b.3.C)

—Linking resources to program objectives and establishing of priorities for the distribution of resources based on factors such as population characteristics and needs as well as the existing infrastructure or funding levels? (Sec. 101.a.6 & 9 & Sec.101.b.3.M)

—Maximizing United States capabilities in the areas of technical assistance and training? (Sec. 101.a.8 & Sec.101.b.3.H)

—Improving coordination and reducing duplication among relevant executive branch agencies, foreign governments, and international organizations? (Sec. 101.a.3 & Sec.101.b.3.K & L)

—Focusing on strategies developed to meet the needs of women, orphans and families? (Sec. 101.b.3.E, G, R, & S)

—Promoting the development and implementation of strategies and programs designed to enhance the development of health care infrastructure, delivery systems and leadership capacity? (Sec.101.a.2 & Sec.101.b.3.C & D)

—Establishing monitoring and evaluating programs in order to measure success of the strategies, promoting successful models, and terminating unsuccessful programs? (Sec.101.b.3.B & N)

- Is the PEPFAR strategy consistent with best practices outlined in global consensus documents related to prevention, treatment and care of HIV/AIDS including:

—The Global Strategy Framework on HIV/AIDS (UNAIDS, 2001)

—Intensifying HIV Prevention (UNAIDS, 2005)

—A Public Health Approach for Scaling Up Antiretroviral (ARV) Treatment: A Toolkit for Programme Managers (WHO, 2003)

—The Framework for the Protection, Care and Support of Orphans and Vulnerable Children Living in a World with HIV and AIDS (UNAIDS and UNICEF, 2004)

—Joint ILO/WHO guidelines on health services and HIV/AIDS (ILO/WHO, 2005)

- Has OGAC modified the PEPFAR strategy to reflect insights gained and lessons learned during implementation?

Resources

How is PEPFAR allocating resources and what is the effect on implementation?

Both the Act and the PEPFAR strategy include guidance on the allocation of resources under the program. The legislation authorizes an annual appropriation for PEPFAR and outlines prioritization for resources in terms of program type (e.g., 20% for prevention, 55% for treatment, 15% for care, 10% for orphans and vulnerable children), and population and/or country characteristics (e.g., size and demographics of the HIV positive population, existing infrastructure). The PEPFAR strategy outlines allocation mechanisms including country allocations based on each country's five-year strategic plan and performance assessments related to reaching annual prevention, treatment, and care targets, as well as a central funding mechanism for regional activities. Although there are a number of constraints on resource allocation, OGAC leadership and country missions have discretion in the allocation of resources amongst agencies, countries, programs, and activities.

- How is PEPFAR allocating resources according to the priorities outlined in its strategy?
- How is PEPFAR managing congressional allocations in the context of harmonization?
- How do PEPFAR's funding mechanisms affect operations of programs?

- How is PEPFAR addressing the coordination of regulations for procurement among and within cooperating agencies?
- How is the Central Procurement Contract functioning?
- What kinds of technical assistance is PEPFAR providing and how is it distributed?

PEPFAR Management

How is PEPFAR coordinating its efforts, evaluating it progress, and improving its programs?

Coordination

Coordination is one of the key elements of PEPFAR implementation identified by the Act. More specifically, the stated objectives within the legislation include strengthening coordination among U.S. government agencies "to ensure effective and efficient use of financial and technical resources" and to foster greater dialogue and synchronization of efforts with foreign governments and international organizations. OGAC has emphasized its "new way of doing business" and has focused a great deal of effort on its role as "Coordinator" across U.S. government agencies and with other donors.

- How well are U.S. government agencies coordinating under the auspices of the Office of the Global AIDS Coordinator?
- How well coordinated are PEPFAR operations between headquarters and missions?
- How well coordinated is PEPFAR with other HIV/AIDS donors at all levels?

Monitoring and Evaluation

Measurement to assess progress, to improve programs, and for accountability is critical to the success of PEPFAR. With some unavoidable overlap, questions related to PEPFAR's support of the focus countries' monitoring and evaluation frameworks and capacity are emphasized in the harmonization and capacity building sections respectively. The questions emphasized in this section pertain primarily to PEPFAR's efforts to monitor and evaluate itself and demonstrate that it has achieved its goals.

- How is PEPFAR monitoring progress on the major components of its program?
    —Coordination

—Harmonization
—Intermediate Milestones for:
—Prevention of 7 million HIV infections
– Treatment of 2 million HIV-infected people with ART
– Care for 10 million people infected with and affected by HIV/AIDS
—Capacity Building
—Integration

- How is PEPFAR planning to evaluate its success in the long-term?
  —Prevention of 7 Million HIV Infections
  —Treatment of 2 Million HIV-infected People with ART
  —Care for 10 Million People Infected with and Affected by HIV/AIDS
  —Reduction of the HIV/AIDS Epidemic in the Focus Countries
  —Improved Survival and Quality of Life for People in the Focus Countries
  —Sustainable Programs and Systems
  —Enhanced Knowledge Base
- How does PEPFAR manage difficult monitoring and evaluation issues such as measurement of infections prevented and attribution of people treated or cared for?
- How does PEPFAR assure the quality of programs and services?
- What steps is PEPFAR taking to ensure that the necessary epidemiologic data and other information are available from the focus countries to assess the initiative's short-, as well as long-term impact?
- Is PEPFAR supporting programs to generate the information they need for on-going program improvement?

Learning Organization

PEPFAR is an acknowledged "emergency" response. By design, the initiative moved rapidly into implementation before all of the arguably necessary pieces were in place, and many foundational elements remain to be developed—for example, OGAC has yet to issue the majority of guidance documents that it has said are under development. In recognition of this, however, PEPFAR has committed to "learning-by-doing."

- Is PEPFAR functioning as a learning organization (Senge, 1990)?
- Does PEPFAR have an approach to *learning by doing* that allows them to generate and share evidence to improve programs?

Harmonization

How is PEPFAR harmonizing its efforts in the focus countries?

In April 2004, UNAIDS, the United Kingdom, and the United States co-hosted a high-level meeting at which donors reaffirmed their commitment to strengthening national AIDS responses to be led by the affected countries themselves. They endorsed the "Three Ones" as guiding principles to improve the country-level response (UNAIDS, 2004b):

- One agreed upon HIV/AIDS Action Framework that provides the basis for coordinating the work of all partners
- One National AIDS Coordinating Authority, with a broad-based multi-sectoral mandate
- One agreed upon country-level Monitoring and Evaluation System.

PEPFAR has expressed full commitment to the Three Ones, and although these principles were not formally in place at the time of the passage of the Act, the legislation calls for the U.S. to be coordinated with other donors, and thus PEPFAR's commitment to the Three Ones is consistent with the legislation. All of the PEPFAR focus countries have national AIDS authorities, and thus with this commitment, "Harmonization" with the Three Ones of each focus country became the centerpiece of the structure of PEPFAR. As such, it is central to the structure of the IOM evaluation.

- To what degree is PEPFAR harmonized with and what are the explanations for varying degrees of harmonization with the national plan, the national coordinating entity, and the national monitoring and evaluation framework?
- How do the goals that PEPFAR assigned to each country for number of infections prevented, number of people receiving treatment, and number of people cared for align with the country's goals?
- How does PEPFAR manage differences between its plan and the national plan?
- How has PEPFAR affected the development of national plans?
- How does PEPFAR manage varying degrees of participation in the national coordinating entity?
- How does PEPFAR manage differences between its data collection and reporting requirements and those of the national monitoring and evaluation framework?

Prevention, Treatment & Care

Are PEPFAR prevention, treatment and care activities aligned with its strategy and the best available science and how is implementation progressing?

Prevention, treatment and care activities are key components of an effective and comprehensive response to HIV/AIDS; helping to decrease risk, vulnerability, and impact of the epidemic (UNAIDS, 2001). The PEPFAR strategy identifies prevention, treatment and care programs as critical interventions, around which other PEPFAR strategies, such as strengthening health care systems, building capacity for long term sustainability of programs and the collection of strategic information, are structured (OGAC, 2004). The targets for PEPFAR-funded prevention, treatment and care programs—to support prevention of 7 million new HIV infections, treatment of 2 million HIV-infected people with ART, and care of 10 million people infected and affected by HIV/AIDS —were introduced in the State of the Union address given by President Bush in 2003, referenced in the Act, and later included in the PEPFAR strategy (OGAC, 2004).

- What programs and activities is PEPFAR supporting to address aspects of *Prevention* such as Behavioral Change, Blood Safety, Counseling and Testing, Post Exposure Prophylaxis, Prevention of Maternal to Child Transmission, and Safe Medical Practice?
- What programs and activities is PEPFAR supporting to address aspects of *Treatment* such as ARV Therapy, Clinical Laboratory Testing, and Prevention of Maternal to Child Transmission Plus?
- What programs and activities is PEPFAR supporting to address aspects of *Care*, particularly for Orphans and Vulnerable Children, such as Health Services and Social Support Services, Pain Management, and Prevention and Treatment of Opportunistic Infections?
- Are the programs and activities evidence-based?
- If evidence-base is incomplete or unclear, is PEPFAR supporting research to determine effectiveness?
- What programs and activities are focused on women and girls?
- How do programs and activities address stigmatization of and discrimination against people living with HIV/AIDS?
- How do programs and activities address issues of equity and human rights?
- How are prevention, treatment, and care programs and activities progressing?
- Has PEPFAR achieved the intermediate milestones established to measure progress in reaching its goals of supporting the prevention of 7

million HIV infections, treatment of 2 million HIV-infected people with ART, and care for 10 million people infected and affected by HIV/AIDS?

Integration

PEPFAR seeks to address prevention, treatment, and care in an integrated approach. The availability of these three interventions and effective linkages among them is expected to strengthen the effect of each intervention and have an impact that is greater than the sum of its parts. Integration of PEPFAR programs into the community and of HIV/AIDS programs into national health systems is intended to strengthen and enhance indigenous ownership and sustainability of these programs.

- How is PEPFAR integrating its programs and services and supporting integration with existing programs and services:
    —Within the domains of prevention, treatment, and care?
    —Among the domains of prevention, treatment, and care?
    —With communities?
    —With national health systems?

Capacity Building

In order to meet the goals of expanding and sustaining HIV/AIDS prevention, treatment, and care, PEPFAR must address the common barriers that affect progress in many countries: namely the scarcity of human resources and institutional capacity compounded by fragile health care systems (OGAC, 2005a). According to OGAC "supporting capacity development is the heart of the [PEPFAR] initiative" and more than $200 million of PEPFAR funding in 2005 is dedicated to capacity building efforts (Dybul, 2005). PEPFAR is committed to working predominantly with indigenous partners and believes that building capacity is necessary in order to enable national programs to achieve results, monitor and evaluate their activities, and sustain their programs over the long-term. (OGAC, 2004).

- How is PEPFAR enhancing the capacity necessary for the focus countries to have sustainable HIV/AIDS prevention, treatment, and care programs?
- Specifically, what is PEPFAR doing to support the building and strengthening of:
    —Human Resources?
    —Institutions?
    —Health Systems (including laboratories, clinics, supply chain)?
    —Communities?

—Information Systems?
—Monitoring and Evaluation?

- How does PEPFAR-funded technical assistance to national governments for activities such as policy development and dissemination of national strategies and guidelines contribute to the enhancement of national capacity?

APPROACH

In carrying out this evaluation plan, the Committee will use several approaches to examine PEPFAR's strategic development and programmatic implementation. In order to answer questions related to PEPFAR's strategy, the committee will compare the 5-year strategy with the authorizing legislation (P.L. 108-25) and relevant global consensus documents. To answer questions related to PEPFAR resource allocation, the committee will review and analyze budgetary and programmatic data provided by OGAC, PEPFAR Missions, and others. The Committee will examine the major aspects of program implementation including PEPFAR management; harmonization; prevention, treatment, and care programs and activities; capacity building; and integration through a wide variety of approaches including review of the scientific literature; analysis of PEPFAR guidance and other documents, national plans, and focus country reports; analysis of data from PEPFAR and other programs and donors; and discussions with OGAC staff, Mission staff, focus country officials, partners, program officials, community groups, and officials from other donor organizations.

Many of the aspects of program implementation that the Committee will be reviewing have a significant qualitative component, for example, Coordination. Thus, for example, in addition to examining whether there are structures and processes in place to facilitate coordination, the Committee will solicit the perspectives of all the major parties that are intended to be coordinated. We are attempting to create an environment in which individuals can speak frankly and toward that end have requested of OGAC that no OGAC staff be present when we hold discussions with Mission staff and that no PEPFAR staff be present when we visit sites that PEPFAR is supporting. The Committee will not attribute statements to individuals by name.

In order to facilitate consistency across discussions, the Committee is developing generic guides for each type of meeting or site visit to be conducted and plans to share them in advance with the parties involved so that they may be better prepared. These guides outline a standard set of issues to be addressed and also allow for additional issues to be explored, depending on the circumstance. These guides are intended to be tailored to the extent possible based on what the Committee is able to learn in advance about the particular people or program involved.

The Committee respects global efforts at harmonization of monitoring and evaluation—in which PEPFAR is a participant (Rugg et al. 2004)—and intends to rely on existing indicators and data sources to the greatest extent possible (OGAC 2005c, UNAIDS 2002, WHO et al. 2004). The Committee continues to review global monitoring and evaluation efforts already underway, systems/processes already in place, and existing data. The indicators developed by PEPFAR and others continue to evolve; the Committee plans to follow this evolution and also expects to contribute to it.

Focus Country Visits

As a result of PEPFAR's structure and commitment to harmonization, the majority of implementation activities are occurring in the focus countries. Thus, visits to the focus countries to directly observe implementation activities are a critical part of the Committee's evaluation plan. The Committee anticipates that these country visits will provide insight into the programmatic successes and challenges through concrete examples and first-hand accounts of how PEPFAR is working on the ground. In recognition of the unique nature of the HIV/AIDS epidemic and the country response to it in each of the 15 focus countries, PEPFAR has been designed to support national leadership and to adapt to the specific needs of each country. It is therefore important to observe how the conditions prevailing in each focus country affect the implementation of PEPFAR. The Committee—in small delegations—plans to visit all of the focus countries, although some visits may be precluded due to security concerns. The generic agenda that has been developed for the country visits will be tailored to the particular circumstances of each focus country in concert with PEPFAR staff, PEPFAR partners, national officials, other donors, community leaders, and others to provide as comprehensive on overview of PEPFAR implementation as possible in a short time. The Committee anticipates that follow-up by phone and email will be needed, not only because it will not be possible to accomplish everything in one visit, but also because it expects to learn from each visit and to discover themes emerging after several visits that will need to be explored further. The Committee is developing the country visits as a continuous learning process. Toward this end, it is creating flexible agendas to allow the visiting teams to adapt to what they learn as the visit progresses; a mechanism for the team that is currently on a country visit to provide feedback to the next team that is about to begin a country visit; and a cumulative, cross-visit analysis after each set of trips.

Limitations

A key and detailed source of information about PEPFAR programs and activities is the Country Operational Plan (COP) that each focus country Mission is required to develop each year. Because OGAC considers some of the information in the COPs to be sensitive and therefore not appropriate for the public domain, the Committee has been allowed access only to versions of the COPs that have been redacted. The Committee's work has been hampered by delays obtaining redacted versions of the fiscal year 2005 COPs, and we may encounter similar delays in obtaining the fiscal year 2006 COPs. Also, it may not be possible for the Committee to know the precise nature of the redacted information or its impact on our analysis. The Committee may encounter similar difficulties with respect to unpublished monitoring and evaluation data that PEPFAR has collected.

REFERENCES

Dybul M. 2005 (May 24). *Integrated Prevention, Treatment and Care: Network Systems.* Presentation at the PEPFAR Second Annual Field Meeting, Addis Ababa, Ethiopia.

ILO (International Labour Organization) and WHO (World Health Organization). 2005. *Joint ILO/WHO guidelines on health services and HIV/AIDS*: ILO.

Moloney-Kitts M. 2005 (April 19). *OGAC Presentation.* Presentation at the Second Meeting of the Institute of Medicine Committee for the Evaluation of PEPFAR Implementation, Washington, DC.

OGAC (Office of the Global AIDS Coordinator). 2004. *The President's Emergency Plan for AIDS Relief (PEPFAR): U.S. Five-Year Global HIV/AIDS Strategy.* Washington, DC: OGAC.

OGAC. 2005a. *PEPFAR First Annual Report.* Washington, DC: OGAC.

OGAC. 2005b. *Basic Requirements Under the President's Emergency Plan for AIDS Relief for All Bilateral Programs.* Washington, DC: OGAC.

OGAC. 2005c. *The President's Emergency Plan for AIDS Relief: Indicators, Reporting Requirements, and Guidelines for Focus Countries* (Revised for FY2006 Reporting) July 29, 2005

Rugg D, Peersman G, Carael M. 2004. *Global Advances in HIV/AIDS Monitoring and Evaluation.* Minneapolis, MN: Wiley Periodicals, Inc.

Senge P. 1990. The Fifth Discipline: The Art and Practice of The Learning Organization. [Online]. Available: http://www.infed.org/thinkers/senge.htm [accessed October 9, 2005].

UNAIDS (Joint United Nations Program on HIV/AIDS). 2001. *The Global Strategy Framework on HIV/AIDS.* Geneva, Switzerland: UNAIDS.

UNAIDS. 2002. *National AIDS Council's Monitoring and Evaluation Operations Manual*, Joint United Nations Programme on HIV/AIDS (UNAIDS) 2002.

UNAIDS. 2004a. *2004 Report on the Global AIDS Epidemic: 4th Global Report.* Geneva, Switzerland: UNAIDS.

UNAIDS. 2004b. "Three Ones" Key Principles. *Conference Paper 1, Washington Consultation of April 4, 2004.* Geneva, Switzerland: UNAIDS. [Online]. Available: http://www.unaids.org/NetTools/Misc/DocInfo.aspx?LANG=en&href=http://gva-doc-owl/WEBcontent/Documents/pub/UNA-docs/Three-Ones_KeyPrinciples_en.pdf [accessed August 25, 2005].

UNAIDS and UNICEF (United Nations Children's Fund). 2004. *The Framework for the Protection, Care and Support of Orphans and Vulnerable Children Living in a World with HIV and AIDS.* Geneva, Switzerland: UNAIDS.

WHO. 2003. *A Public Health Approach for Scaling Up Antiretroviral (ARV) Treatment: A Toolkit for Programme Managers.* [Online]. Available: http://www.who.int/hiv/toolkit/arv/en/index.jsp [accessed September 1, 2005].

WHO, UNAIDS, The Global Fund to Fight AIDS, Tuberculosis & Malaria, USAID, US Department of State, US Department of Health and Human Services, CDC, UNICEF and the World Bank. 2004. *Monitoring and Evaluation Toolkit HIV/AIDS, Tuberculosis and Malaria.*

APPENDIX 1

The Committee for the Evaluation of PEPFAR Implementation

The committee is composed of 13 members. Committee members were selected for their international experience in low- and middle-income countries, as well as their individual expertise in the following areas relevant to the committee's charge: behavioral science, bioethics, biostatistics, community nursing, community development, economics, epidemiology, infectious disease (adult), informatics, maternal and child health, modeling, monitoring and evaluation, operations research, professional training/education, public health program management, quality of care, and social services. Three advisory subcommittees comprised of 6-7 members each, are focused on prevention, treatment, and care. Additional members who serve only on the subcommittees provide expanded expertise in the following areas: child psychology/psychiatry, child welfare/services, demography, health communication, health education, infectious disease (pediatric), laboratory quality, logistics, palliative care, and pharmacology.

APPENDIX 2

PEPFAR Chronology

May 2003	PEPFAR authorizing legislation passed: "United States Leadership Against HIV/AIDS, Tuberculosis, and Malaria Act of 2003"
October 2003	Ambassador Tobias sworn in as first U.S. Global AIDS Coordinator
January 2004	First appropriation under the United States Leadership Against HIV/AIDS, Tuberculosis, and Malaria Act of 2003

February 2004	U.S. 5-year Global HIV/AIDS Strategy published: "The President's Emergency Plan for AIDS Relief (PEPFAR)"
March 2004	First year funds became available for obligation; grant and contract awards commenced; $350 million was provided to initial awardees
April 2004	The "Three Ones" endorsed as guiding principles to improve the global response to HIV/AIDS
June 2004	First PEPFAR Annual Meeting
September 2004	Majority of first year funding obligated
March 2005	First PEPFAR Annual Report published "ABC" Prevention Guidance published Palliative Care Guidance published
May 2005	Draft Guidance for Strategic Information published
May 2005	Second PEPFAR Annual Meeting
June 2005	Just over 50% of State Department authorized staff positions filled at OGAC. Additional staff on board included detailees from other US government agencies, contractors, fellows, and interns.
August 2005	Basic Requirements Under the President's Emergency Plan for AIDS Relief for all Bilateral Programs published
May 2008	United States Leadership Against HIV/AIDS, Tuberculosis, and Malaria Act of 2003 expires
2008	Goal of 2 million People with HIV/AIDS on Antiretroviral Therapy
2008	Goal of 10 million People Affected by HIV/AIDS Receiving Care
2010	Goal of Preventing 7 million HIV Infections

APPENDIX 3

Abbreviations

AIDS	Acquired Immunodeficiency Syndrome
ART	Antiretroviral Therapy
ARV	Antiretroviral Drug
CDC	Centers for Disease Control and Prevention
COP	Country Operational Plan
DoD	Department of Defense
DoL	Department of Labor

HHS	Health and Human Services
HIV	Human Immunodeficiency Virus
HRSA	Health Resources and Services Administration
ILO	International Labour Organization
NIH	National Institutes of Health
OGAC	Office of the Global AIDS Coordinator
PEPFAR	The President's Emergency Plan for AIDS Relief
UNAIDS	Joint United Nations Programme on HIV/AIDS
UNICEF	United Nations Children's Fund
USAID	U.S. Agency for International Development
WHO	World Health Organization

Note: *Individuals in italics serve only on the subcommittees.*

Committee for the Evaluation of PEPFAR Implementation

Chair—Jaime Sepulveda, M.D., Dr.Sc.
Vice Chair—Helen Smits, M.D., M.A.C.P.
Stefano Bertozzi, Ph.D., M.D.
James Curran, M.D., M.P.H.
William Holzemer, R.N., Ph.D., FAAN
Affette McCaw-Binns, Ph.D.
Charles Carpenter, M.D.
Geoff Garnett, Ph.D.
Ruth Macklin, Ph.D.
David Paltiel, Ph.D.
Priscilla Reddy, M.P.H., Ph.D.
David Ross, Sc.D.
Heather Weiss, Ed.D.
Mike Merson, M.D. (BGH Liaison)

Treatment Subcommittee

Chair—Charles Carpenter, M.D.
Hoosen Coovadia, M.B.B.S., M.D
Henry Fomundam Pharm.D.
David Paltiel, Ph.D.
Helen Smits, M.D., M.A.C.P.
Olaitan Soyannwo, M.Med., D.A., F.W.A.C.S., F.I.C.S.
Burton Wilcke, Ph.D.

Prevention Subcommittee

Chair—James Curran, M.D., M.P.H.
Stefano Bertozzi, Ph.D., M.D.
Geoff Garnett, Ph.D.
Paul Gertler, Ph.D.
Carl Latkin, M.S., Ph.D.
Priscilla Reddy, M.P.H., Ph.D.

Care Subcommittee

Chair—William Holzemer, R.N., Ph.D., FAAN
Maureen Black, Ph.D.
Affette McCaw-Binns, Ph.D.
James Ntozi, M.Sc., Ph.D.
James Sherry, M.D., Ph.D.
Heather Weiss, Ed.D.
Elena Nightingale, M.D., Ph.D. (BCYF Liaison)

APPENDIX D

Selected Bibliography for 25-Year Overview of Global HIV/AIDS

Cahn, P., and C. McClure. 2006. Beyond the first 25 years: The International AIDS Society and its role in the global response to AIDS. *Retrovirology* 3(85).

CDC (Centers for Disease Control and Prevention). 2006. Twenty-five years of HIV/AIDS, United States, 1981–2006. *Morbidity and Mortality Weekly Report* 55(21):585–589. http://www.cdc.gov/mmwr/preview/mmwrhtml/mm5521a1.htm (accessed January 30, 2007).

Cohen, J. 2006. HIV/AIDS: Latin America & Caribbean. *Science* 313(5786).

Cohen, P. 2006. 25 years with HIV. *The Scientist* 20(6). http://www.the-scientist.com/article/display/23586/ (accessed January 30, 2007).

Gallo, R. C. 2006. A reflection on HIV/AIDS research after 25 years. *Retrovirology* 3(72).

Gayle, H., R. Horton, M. Wainberg, A. Fauci, P. Piot, H. Broadbent, G. Gonsalves, and E. Madraa. 2006. *25 years of AIDS—Reflecting back and looking forward* (International AIDS Conference Session). http://www.aids2006.org/PAG/PSession.aspx?s=472 (accessed January 30, 2007).

Kaiser Family Foundation. 2006. *AIDS @ 25*. http://www.kff.org/hivaids/aidsat25.cfm (accessed January 30, 2007).

Poku, N. K., and A. Whiteside. 2006. 25 years of living with HIV/AIDS: Challenges and prospects. *International Affairs* 82(2):249–256.

Shao, Y. 2006. AIDS epidemic at age 25 and control efforts in China. *Retrovirology* 3(87).

The business of HIV/AIDS. 2006. *Lancet* 368(9534):423.

UNAIDS (The Joint United Nations Programme on HIV/AIDS). 2006. *25 years of AIDS.* http://data.unaids.org/pub/FactSheet/2006/20060428_FS_25YearsofAIDS_en.pdf (accessed January 30, 2007).

APPENDIX
E

Abbreviations and Acronyms

ABC	abstinence/be faithful/use condoms
AIDS	Acquired Immunodeficiency Syndrome
ART	antiretroviral therapy
ARV	antiretroviral medication
CD4	cluster of differentiation 4
CDC	Centers for Disease Control and Prevention
COPRS	Country Operational Plan and Reporting System
FDA	U.S. Food and Drug Administration
HIV	human immunodeficiency virus
IOM	Institute of Medicine
N/A	not available
NIH	National Institutes of Health
OGAC	Office of the U.S. Global AIDS Coordinator
OI	opportunistic infection
PEPFAR	President's Emergency Plan for AIDS Relief
TB	tuberculosis
UN	United Nations
UNAIDS	Joint United Nations Programme on HIV/AIDS
UNGASS	United Nations General Assembly Special Session
UNICEF	United Nations Children's Fund
USAID	U.S. Agency for International Development
WHO	World Health Organization

APPENDIX F

Committee and Staff Biographies

Jaime Sepúlveda, M.D., Dr.Sc. (*Chair*), is currently spending a sabbatical year as Visiting Professor at the University of California in San Francisco (UCSF), having received the 2007 Presidential Chair award at UCSF. Dr. Sepúlveda was appointed Director of the National Institutes of Health (NIH) of Mexico by President Vicente Fox in 2003. As Director, he was responsible for setting policy; planning and coordinating the programs and activities of the 12 NIH institutes as well as overseeing an intramural operational budget of close to $1 billion. Prior to this appointment, Dr. Sepúlveda was elected Director General of the National Institute of Public Health (INSP), 1 of the 12 NIH institutes in 1995, and reelected to a second term in 2000. He also served as the Dean of the National School of Public Health (NSPH), the first and most prestigious school in Latin America. As Director General of Epidemiology (1985–1991) and Vice-Minister of Health (1991–1994), he strengthened the country's Epidemiologic Surveillance System and founded the Universal Vaccination Program, which increased coverage for preschool vaccination from 45 to 94 percent in 2 years, and successfully eliminated poliomyelitis and diphtheria from Mexico. He was the founding chair of the National AIDS Committee (CONASIDA) and oversaw all AIDS prevention efforts in the country from 1986 to 1994. Among his many international responsibilities, he chaired the Advisory Committee to the Editors of the *Disease Control Priorities Project in Developing Countries* (2nd edition); a joint project between Fogarty International Center and the World Bank, the Bill & Melinda Gates Foundation, and the World Health Organization. He currently serves on the Harvard Board of Overseers (2002–2008). He was elected to the Institute of Medicine in 2004. Dr. Sepúlveda earned his M.D. at the National Autonomous University of Mexico (UNAM) in 1978, followed by an M.P.H. in 1980, an M.S. in Tropical Medicine in 1981, and a Ph.D. in Population Science in 1985, all from the Harvard School of Public Health.

Helen Smits, M.D., M.A.C.P. (*Vice Chair*), has just completed a Fulbright Lectureship in the new Masters in Public Health offered at the Faculty of Medicine of Eduardo Mondlane University in Mozambique. She also served as a Clinton Foundation volunteer working with the Mozambican Ministry of Health task force that developed a "business plan" to scale up AIDS treatment and prevention. During 2003 and the first half of 2004 she served on a volunteer basis as the Foundation's representative to the group of bilateral donors engaged in the Sector-Wide Approach with the Mozambican Ministry of Health. She is currently working with the Institute for Healthcare Improvement (Boston) and The Health Foundation (London) on quality improvement projects in Southern Africa. She has expertise in general health policy, with particular emphasis on quality monitoring. Dr. Smits served from 1993 to 1996 as the Deputy Administrator of the Health Care Financing Administration of the U.S. Department of Health and Human Services. She has served on several committees with the IOM, and was recently review coordinator for the IOM's publication *Scaling Up Treatment for the Global AIDS Pandemic*. She served from 1996 to 2000 as a member of the Board of Governors of the Clinical Center at the National Institutes of Health. She also served as co-chair of the Strategic Framework Board of the National Quality Forum, and is a former member and former Chair of the Board of Commissioners of the Joint Commission on the Accreditation of Health Care Organizations (JCAHO). Her most recent academic appointment was as Visiting Professor at the Robert F. Wagner Graduate School of Public Service at New York University. She has also been Professor of Community Medicine at the University of Connecticut and Associate Professor of Medicine and Public Health at Yale.

Charles Carpenter, M.D. (*Treatment Subcommittee Chair*), is Professor of Medicine and Director of the Brown University AIDS Center at Brown University. In 1962, Carpenter started the Johns Hopkins Cholera Research program in Calcutta, India, where he demonstrated the value of antibiotics and defined the fluid requirements essential for the treatment of cholera. At Johns Hopkins he built an infectious disease program focused on enteric pathogens; during his tenure as Chair of the Department of Medicine at Case Western Reserve Medical School he developed the first Division of Geographic Medicine within a Department of Medicine in the United States. Since moving to Brown University in 1986, he has focused on the global AIDS epidemic. He directed the Brown University International Health Institute from 1995 to 2001, and has worked with colleagues in the Philippines and India to prevent the spread of HIV in those nations. He is the director of The Lifespan/Tufts/Brown Center for AIDS Research (CFAR). He currently serves as a member of the Executive Committee of a Fogarty AIDS International Research and Training program that is based at Brown University. He has participated on numerous WHO Expert Advisory Committees on Infectious Diseases. He was a member of the founding Board of Directors of the International Center for Diarrheal Disease Research in Dacca, Bangladesh. He is a member of the Institute of Medicine and has served on seven National Academies committees.

James Curran, M.D., M.P.H. (*Prevention Subcommittee Chair*), Professor of Epidemiology and Dean of the Rollins School of Public Health at Emory University, has become Chair of the Board on Health Promotion and Disease Prevention of the IOM. Previously a Fellow at the Harvard Center for Community Health and Medical Care, Dr. Curran began his career with the Centers for Disease Control and Prevention and had a leadership position in HIV/AIDS from 1981 to 1995. He also is currently Director of the Emory Center for AIDS Research. He is a member of the IOM of the National Academy of Sciences. The Board on Health Promotion and Disease Prevention focuses on issues affecting the health of the public, including population-based public health measures and the public health infrastructure. In addition to his involvement with this Board, he has served on over 15 other National Academies committees.

William L. Holzemer, R.N., Ph.D., FAAN (*Care Subcommittee Chair*), is Professor and Associate Dean for International Programs, School of Nursing, University of California, San Francisco. His research focuses upon living well with HIV as a chronic illness, including dimensions of quality of life, adherence, stigma, and symptoms. One of his current projects is a study of the impact of stigma on quality of life for people living with HIV and on quality of worklife for nurses who care for people living with HIV in five African countries. Dr. Holzemer received a Ph.D. in Higher Education Administration from Syracuse University and a BSN from San Francisco State University. He has served on one previous National Academies committee.

Stefano M. Bertozzi, Ph.D., M.D., is the founding Director of the Division of Health Economics & Policy at Mexico's National Institute of Public Health (INSP). He directs its Masters Program in Health Economics, offered jointly with the Center for Economic Research and Teaching (CIDE) in Mexico City. He is a visiting faculty member at both CIDE and the

University of California, Berkeley. He is currently Chairman of the UNAIDS Reference Group on Economics, member of the Technical Evaluation Reference Group of the Global Fund to Fight AIDS, Tuberculosis and Malaria, member of the Editorial Boards of *AIDS* and *Cost Effectiveness and Resource Allocation*, former member of the Board of Trustees and of the Council on Scientific Affairs of the American Medical Association, and former member of advisory boards or steering committees of AIDSCAP, Synergy, ProCAARE, the International AIDS and Economics Network, and several international AIDS conferences and summits. Dr. Bertozzi's research focuses on a diverse range of projects in health economics and policy, the largest concentration of which is on the economic aspects of HIV/AIDS and on the health impact of large social programs. Before joining the INSP he worked with UNAIDS, the former WHO Global Programme on AIDS (GPA), the Government of Zaire, and the World Bank. He was responsible for overseeing the last year of GPA as its Acting Director and Director of Research and Intervention Development before moving to UNAIDS as Coordinator, Policy, Strategy, and Research. At the World Bank he worked with Mead Over on some of the first analyses of the impact of AIDS in developing countries. He has lived in and/or worked with developing countries in Africa, Asia, and Latin America since 1988 and speaks English, French, Spanish, and Italian. Dr. Bertozzi received his B.S. in Biology and Ph.D. in Health Policy and Management from MIT, his M.D. from UCSD, and residency training in internal medicine at UCSF.

Geoff Garnett, Ph.D., is Professor of Microparasite Epidemiology at Imperial College London. He has degrees in Zoology and Biological Computation from the University of Sheffield and University of York, studied the population biology of varicella-zoster virus for his Ph.D. at Sheffield University, and has held Wellcome Trust and Royal Society Fellowships at Oxford University and Imperial College London. He is currently Director of a Masters Programme in Epidemiology at Imperial College and is Leader of the Public and International Health Strategy in the Faculty of Medicine at Imperial College London. His major research goals are to integrate field and theoretical studies of the biological and behavioral patterns determining the incidence and prevalence of sexually transmitted infections (including HIV) and to understand the impact of interventions these infections. He is Chair of the UNAIDS Reference Group on Estimates, Models and Projections.

Ruth Macklin, Ph.D., is Professor of Bioethics in the Department of Epidemiology and Population Health at Albert Einstein College of Medicine. Her work focuses on ethics in research involving human subjects with a special interest in international collaborative research conducted in developing countries. Other areas of interest are HIV/AIDS and reproductive health, justice in global health, access to treatment, public health, assisted reproduction, and research involving embryos and stem cells. Dr. Macklin was elected to the Institute of Medicine in 1989. She serves on the Scientific and Ethical Review Group of the Human Reproduction Programme at the WHO and is a member of the Vaccine Advisory Group for HIV/AIDS vaccine research, also at WHO. She is a member of the Global Reference Group on Human Rights and HIV/AIDS at UNAIDS and chairs the external advisory committee of the Centers for Disease Control and Prevention (CDC). She is Co-director of a training program in research ethics in Latin America, sponsored by the Fogarty International Center of the NIH. Her latest book is *Double Standards in Medical Research in Developing Countries,* published by Cambridge University Press.

Affette McCaw-Binns, Ph.D., received her Ph.D. in Perinatal Epidemiology from the University of Bristol in England. She is a Professor in the Department of Community Health and Psychiatry at the University of the West Indies, Mona, in Kingston, Jamaica. Her research is concerned with the epidemiology of perinatal deaths and maternal mortality in the Caribbean, as well as antenatal and perinatal care in that region. She has recently published on "Strategies to prevent eclampsia in a developing country: I. Re-organisation of maternity services and II. Use of a maternal pictorial card" and "Skilled birth attendant competence: An initial assessment in four countries, and implications for the Safe Motherhood movement." Dr. McCaw-Binns has been a member of the Pan American Health Organization's Technical and Advisory Group of the Regional Plan for Action for the Reduction of Maternal Mortality in the Americas. She has served on one prior National Academies committee.

A. David Paltiel, Ph.D., is Professor of Public Health and Managerial Sciences at the Yale School of Medicine. He also holds a faculty appointment at the Yale School of Management. His research interests deal broadly with issues of resource allocation and decision making in health and medicine. An expert in the application of mathematical and economic simulation models to inform public choice and clinical practice, he has conducted numerous cost-effectiveness analyses of HIV/AIDS prevention, testing, and treatment interventions. He is a member of the Editorial Boards of both *Medical Decision Making* and *Value in Health*. He received his Ph.D. in Operations Research from Yale. He has served on one prior National Academies committee.

Priscilla Reddy, M.P.H., Ph.D., is Director of the Health Promotion Research and Development Unit at the Medical Research Council of South Africa. She has optained postgraduate qualifications from the United States and the Netherlands. She is one of the leading experts in South Africa on behavioral science of HIV, AIDS, and sexually transmitted diseases. She has been principal investigator on several NIH RO1 grants. She is also Visiting Associate Professor in the Department of Behavioral Science and Health Promotion at the Rollins School of Public Health at Emory and Georgetown University. She is a member of the South African Academy of Science and serves on the council. Dr. Reddy has served on one prior National Academies committee.

David Ross, Sc.D., is Director of the Public Health Informatics Institute. He became the Director of All Kids Count in 2000, a program of the Institute supported by the Robert Wood Johnson Foundation (RWJF), and subsequently began the Institute in 2002, also with funding from RWJF. His experience spans the private health care and public health sectors. Before joining the Task Force, Dr. Ross was an executive with a private health information systems firm, a Public Health Service officer with CDC, and an executive in a private health system. Dr. Ross holds a doctoral degree in operations research from Johns Hopkins University (1980) where he was involved in health services research. After serving as Director of the Health Service Research Center, Baltimore USPHS Hospital, he became Vice President for Administration with the Wyman Park Health System. In 1983, he joined the CDC's National Center for Environmental Health. During his career at CDC, he worked in environmental health, CDC's executive administration, and public health practice. Dr. Ross was founding director of the Information Network for Public Health Officials (INPHO), CDC's national initiative to improve the information infrastructure of public health. His research and programmatic interests reflect those of the Institute: the strategic application of information technologies to improve public health practice.

Heather Weiss, Ed.D., is the Founder and Director of Harvard Family Research Project (HFRP) and is a Senior Research Associate and Lecturer at the Harvard Graduate School of Education. From its beginning in 1983, the HFRP's mission has been to help create more effective practices, interventions, and policies to support children's successful development from birth to adulthood. Dr. Weiss writes, speaks, and advises on programs and polices for children and families and serves on the advisory boards of many public and private organizations. She is a consultant and advisor to numerous foundations on strategic grant making and evaluation. Her latest publications include several articles reporting on her longitudinal study of ways family involvement in children's learning promotes development and school success, a book about how to involve families and communities in children's learning and development, papers on how to measure and to encourage youth participation in after school and youth programs, and a paper on the use of data and evaluation in democracies. Dr. Weiss received her doctorate in Education and Social Policy from the Harvard Graduate School of Education and she was a postdoctoral research fellow at the Yale Bush Center in Child Development and Social Policy.

Subcommittee Members, Liaisons, and Study Consultants

Maureen Black, Ph.D., is the John A. Scholl Professor of Pediatrics at the University of Maryland School of Medicine. She also holds an appointment in the Division of Endocrinology, Diabetes, and Nutrition in the Department of Medicine and is an adjunct professor in the Center for Human Nutrition, Johns Hopkins Bloomberg School of Public Health and the Department of Psychology, University of Maryland Baltimore County. Dr. Black is the director of the Growth and Nutrition Clinic and chief of the Consortium on Child Development and Neurosciences. Dr. Black is a pediatric psychologist and completed her training at Emory University and the Neuropsychiatric Institute of UCLA. She has been the President of the Society of Pediatric Psychology and the Division of Children, Youth, and Family Services of the American Psychological Association. She is a member of the Psychosocial Risk and Disease Prevention Study Section of NICHD and has served on several committees for UNICEF and WHO. Dr. Black specializes in intervention research related to children's nutrition, health, and development. She has worked on projects in Bangladesh, India, Peru, and Ethiopia. She is an Associate Editor of the *Journal of Pediatric Psychology,* on the Editorial Board of four other journals, and has published over 150 articles and chapters.

Hoosen Coovadia, M.B.B.S., M.D., is a pediatrician and expert in perinatal transmission. Dr. Coovadia was the Head of the Department of Pediatrics at the University of Natal until 2000, and is now the Victor Daitz Professor for HIV/AIDS research at the University of Natal. He has made a substantial contribution in pediatric diseases, including the definitive work on nephrosis in South African black children, malnutrition and immunity, and measles, particularly the effect of vitamin A supplementation on children with measles and other infections. He is internationally recognized for his groundbreaking research in HIV/AIDS transmission from mother to child, especially through breastfeeding and is the Protocol Chair for HIVNET 023 and HPTN 046. He is particularly committed to developing research capacity, having supervised over 40 postgraduate students and taught in the medical, nursing, and allied health professions for more than 20 years. He is also a Fellow of the University of Natal and was awarded the Star of South Africa by President Nelson Mandela for his contribution to democracy in

South Africa. In 1999, he was awarded the Silver Medal by the Medical Research Council for his achievements in medical research. Dr. Coovadia is a member of the Institute of Medicine in the National Academies.

Henry Fomundam, Pharm.D., is a Public Health/Pharmaceutical Care Consultant with several years of international experience. Dr. Fomundam graduated from Howard University, Washington, DC, with a doctorate in Pharmaceutical Care and did a postdoctoral fellowship at the National School of Public Health (HIV/AIDS management) in South Africa and subsequently worked in the Southern, Eastern, and Central African region for the last 6 years. He is currently a Regional Director at Howard University/PACE Centre for the ROADS, HIV/AIDS Pharmaceutical Care Project in Eastern and Central Africa. Prior to working in Africa, he worked in several facilities in Washington, DC, as a pharmaceutical care clinician for Clinical Pharmacy Associate and a faculty member at Howard University international programs.

In Africa he served as the Director of Pharmacovigilance, National HIV/AIDS Program in South Africa and as Coordinator of an HIV/AIDS public health training program at the National School of Public Health in South Africa. He supervised HIV/AIDS community-based research projects in South Africa, Botswana, Namibia, Swaziland, and Lesotho. In South Africa he also worked as a research consultant on three major HIV/AIDS research projects at the HSRC; HIV/AIDS clinical trial project (Project Phidisa in the SA military in collaboration with NIH, SA and U.S. Departments of Defense); Medicines Control Council of South Africa to review Nevirapine use in the first 18 pilot sites. At the National HIV/AIDS Directorate he served as one of the consultants to oversee the implementation of the HIV comprehensive plan countrywide, Pharmaceutical Care Consultant for UNDP Regional Service Centre in South Africa, and a consultant for the HIV/AIDS Treatment Program for the Family Planning Association of Kenya.

He has served on several national and international committees including the National Clinical Trials Committee in South Africa, Pharmacovigilance Committee, Nelson Mandela Foundation HIV/AIDS Committee, CIOMS/WHO Clinical Trials Committee, WHO/TDR Product Research Evaluation Committee and Federal Employee Program, BCBS National P and T in the United States. He is the author of an HIV/AIDS pharmacovigilance handbook in South Africa and also published research/commissioned work.

Paul Gertler, Ph.D., is Professor of Economics, Haas School of Business; Professor of Health Services Finance, School of Public Health; and Faculty Director, Graduate Program in Health Services Management at the University of California, Berkeley. Historically, his research has focused on the link between health, education, and poverty. He has spent recent years studying the Mexican anti-poverty program PROGRESA, a conditional cash transfer anti-poverty program that significantly reduced childhood illness, increased the health of babies and pregnant mothers among the Mexican participants, and indicated that proper health care can help end the poverty cycle among the poor. He previously served for the RAND Corporation as senior economist, and as an assistant professor at Harvard University and State University of New York at Stony Brook. He has experience in consulting and policy making with international agencies such as the World Bank, United Nations, and WHO, as well as governments in Latin America and Asia and private corporations.

Carl A. Latkin, M.S., Ph.D., is a Professor in the Department of Health Policy and Management, Division of Social and Behavioral Sciences, at the Johns Hopkins School of Public Health with a joint appointment in the Department of Epidemiology. He has published over 100 peer review papers. Dr. Latkin has served as consultant on expert panels at CDC and NIH in developing and evaluating community-based HIV prevention interventions. He is currently serving as the Chair of the NIH and National Institute of Allergies and Infectious Diseases first international behavioral intervention. Currently Dr. Latkin is the principal investigator of HIV prevention projects in Baltimore, India, and Russia, and is co-investigator or consultant on projects in South Africa, India, Thailand, Congo, and China.

James Ntozi, M.Sc., Ph.D., is a medical demographer and statistician who has extensive experience in conducting and coordinating qualitative and quantitative monitoring and evaluation studies. Dr. Ntozi holds a bachelor's degree in Statistics and Economics, a master's in Statistics and Demography, and a doctorate in Medical Demography. For 18 years he held top managerial and administrative positions in Uganda and Africa, including being a Census Commissioner (1979–1984), Head of Department of Population Studies (1984–1989), and Director of the Regional Institute of Statistics & Applied Economics, Makerere University (1989–1997). He was a team leader of international and national study teams in Rwanda (HIV/AIDS Prevalence Survey in 1997/1998 funded by the World Bank), Tanzania (Evaluation of Reproductive Health Training Project in 1999 by USAID and INTRA), and Uganda (adolescent baseline study for PEARL/UNFPA in 1999/2000, evaluation for UNFPA in 2000, situation analysis in 2001 for AYA/Consult (U), baseline study in 2001 for UNICEF, and preparation of Uganda Human Development report in 2002 (for Uganda Government and UNDP). Dr. Ntozi has researched in the area of HIV/AIDS in Uganda for over a decade and published and presented over 100 scientific papers including over 30 on HIV/AIDS, written 6 books, and co-edited 4 books on HIV/AIDS in Africa. He has also helped develop indicators for UNFPA, UNDP, UNECA, and UNICEF.

James Sherry, M.D., Ph.D., is currently Professor of Global Health, School of Public Health and Health Services at The George Washington University, Washington, D.C. Prior to this appointment, he was Vice President of Policy, Research and Advocacy for the Global Health Council. Before joining the Global Health Council, Dr. Sherry was based in Geneva, Switzerland, serving as UNAIDS Director of Programme Development and Senior Advisor to its Executive Director, Dr. Peter Piot. There he played a crucial role in the global strategy, organizational development, and UN system reform. Earlier assignments with UNICEF headquarters included Senior Advisor to Programme Strategy, Chief of Health, and Senior Fellow at the Harvard Institute for Population and Development Studies. As a U.S. Foreign Service Officer in India, Dr. Sherry served as Director of Biomedical Research and Technology Development with USAID. He also worked as Chief of Staff for U.S. Rep. Sander M. Levin of Michigan. A graduate of Oakland University, Sherry earned a doctorate in biochemistry from Carnegie Mellon University and received his M.D. from the University of Michigan School of Medicine.

Olaitan Soyannwo, M.Med., D.A., F.W.A.C.S., F.I.C.S., is a Professor of Anesthesia and a Consultant Anesthetist at the College of Medicine at the University of Ibadan in Nigeria. Her principal fields of interest are pain education, manpower development, and public information. She is also active in advocating pain management and treatment in developing countries. She has served as a consultant to the National Health Development Project in Gambia, a council member of the West African College of Surgeons, President of the Society of Anesthetists of West Africa, and Dean of Clinical Sciences, College of Medicine, University of Ibadan. At the national level, she served as a member of the HIV/AIDS Palliative Care Guidelines Working Group and Consultative Committee on Cancer Control. She is the immediate past President, Society for the Study of Pain, Nigeria, a council member of the International Association for the Study of Pain, and a member of the Board of Trustees for the African Palliative Care Association. She is a Fellow of the Nigerian Academy of Science.

Burton Wilcke, Jr., Ph.D., is currently the Chair of the Department of Medical Laboratory and Radiation Sciences at the University of Vermont College of Nursing and Health Sciences. Previously Dr. Wilcke had been Director of the Divison of Health Surveillance at the Vermont Department of Health (1995–2002), where he was also Laboratory Director from 1998 to 1995.

As past President of the Association of Public Health Laboratories and immediate past Chair of its Leadership Development Task Force, Dr. Wilcke regularly presents to national audiences on public health issues. He was senior author for APHL on the Centers for Disease Control Mortality and Morbidity Report on Core Functions of Public Health Laboratories, and also lead the laboratory infrastructure development team in Zimbabwe as part of the CDC/APHL initiative to fight AIDS in South Africa. He received his Ph.D. in Microbiology and Immunology at the Temple University School of Medicine in Philadelphia, and completed a postdoctoral fellowship in medical and public health microbiology at the California Department of Health. He has no prior experience with the National Academies.

Michael Merson, M.D. (*Board on Global Health Liaison*), is the founding Director of the Global Health Institute at Duke University. Prior to this appointment he was the Dean of Public Health and Chairman of the Department of Epidemiology and Public Health Director of the Center for Interdisciplinary Research on AIDS at Yale University. Dr. Merson graduated from Amherst College (B.A.) and the State University of New York Downstate Medical Center. After serving as a medical intern and resident at Johns Hopkins Hospital, he spent 3 years in the Enteric Diseases Branch at the Centers for Disease Control and Prevention in Atlanta, GA, and then served as the Chief Epidemiologist at the Cholera Research Laboratory in Dhaka, Bangladesh. In 1978, he joined the World Health Organization's Diarrheal Disease Control Programme in Geneva, Switzerland, and served as Director of the Programme from 1980 until 1990. In 1987, he was also appointed Director of the WHO Acute Respiratory Infections Control Programme. He was appointed as Director in 1990 and later as Executive Director in 1993 of the WHO Global Programme on AIDS, which was the agency initially responsible for mobilizing and coordinating the global response to the AIDS pandemic. Dr. Merson received two Commendation Medals from the U.S. Public Health Service, the Arthur S. Flemming Award, the Surgeon General's Exemplary Service Medal, and two honorary degrees. He has served on various NIH review panels, advisory committees, and institutional boards, and has been elected to the Connecticut Academy of Science and Engineering and the American Epidemiological Society.

Elena Nightingale, M.D., Ph.D. (*Board on Children, Youth, and Families Liaison*), is a Scholar-in-Residence at the IOM, and Adjunct Professor of Pediatrics at both Georgetown University Medical Center and George Washington University Medical Center. For more than 11 years she was Special Advisor to the President and Senior Program Officer at Carnegie Corporation of New York, and Lecturer in Social Medicine at Harvard University. She retired from both positions at the end of 1994. Dr. Nightingale earned an A.B. in Zoology, summa cum laude, from Barnard College of Columbia University, a Ph.D. in Microbial Genetics from the Rockefeller University, and an M.D. from New York University School of Medicine.

Dr. Nightingale is a member of the IOM and the Academies' Report Review Committee. She is a Fellow of the American Association for the Advancement of Sciences, the New York Academy of Sciences. In her role as Scholar-in-Residence, Dr. Nightingale serves as advisor to the President and Executive Officer of the IOM. In that role she coordinated the IOM Board self-assessment process. She is also a member of the Board on Children, Youth, and Families. Her interests are in genetics and child and adolescent health, and currently she is working on strategies for increasing participation of under-represented minorities in the work of the IOM. In 2006 Dr. Nightingale was awarded the IOM's McDermott Medal for Distinguished Service.

Julia Coffman (*Consultant*), is a Washington D.C.-based consultant specializing in evaluation, strategy, and communications. Since 1996 she has worked with the Harvard Family Research Project (HFRP), a research and evaluation organization at the Harvard Graduate School of Education that for over 20 years has helped develop and evaluate strategies to promote the well being of children, youth, families, and their communities. Ms. Coffman leads HFRP's evaluation work, which includes helping organizations use evaluations to learn about and improve their strategies. HFRP conducts evaluations in areas of particular interest (typically large-scale complex initiatives), and publishes *The Evaluation Exchange*, a quarterly periodical on emerging evaluation theory, methods, and resources.

Thomas N. Denny, M.Sc. (*Consultant*), is Research Associate Professor and Chief Operating Officer at the Duke Human Vaccine Institute and Center for HIV/AIDS Vaccine Immunology, Duke University Medical Center, Durham, North Carolina, and has 25 years of immunology experience studying host defense mechanisms. As part of the HIV clinical trials program, he has served on numerous committees for NIH over the last two decades. Previously, he served on an expert panel for CDC helping to establish clinical laboratory guidelines for using T-cell immunophenotyping in patients with HIV disease. In 1997, he received an NIH HIV Innovative Vaccine Grant award to study a new method of vaccine delivery. He is the principal investigator of the NIH-NIAID Division of AIDS Immunology Quality Assurance Program. Mr. Denny was a 2002–2003 Robert Wood Johnson Foundation Health Policy Fellow at the IOM. As a Fellow, he served on the U.S. Senate Health, Education, Labor and Pensions Committee with legislation/policy responsibilities in global AIDS, bioterrorism, clinical trials/human subject protection and vaccine-related issues. He has extensive international experience and is a consultant to the U.S. CDC for the PEPFAR project to oversee development of an HIV laboratory network in Guyana. In early 2004, he was awarded a Fogarty International HIV Grant for a project in Burkina Faso. In September 2004, IOM appointed him as a consultant to its Board on Global Health Committees studying the options for overseas placement of U.S. health professionals. Previously, Mr. Denny helped establish a small laboratory in the Republic of Kalmykia (former Soviet Union) to improve the care of children with HIV/AIDS. As a Board Member of the Children of Chernobyl Relief Fund Foundation, Mr. Denny focused on donor recruitment, program planning and assessment, and medical mission/training for Ukrainian physician scientists. Mr. Denny has authored or co-authored more than 75 peer-reviewed papers and serves on the Editorial Boards of *Clinical and Diagnostic Laboratory Immunology, Communications in Cytometry,* and *Clinical and Applied Immunology Reviews.* He holds an M.Sc. in Molecular and Biomedical Immunology from the University of East London. In 1991 he completed a course of study in Strategic Management at The Wharton School, University of Pennsylvania. In 1993, he completed the Program for Advanced Training in Biomedical Research Management at the Harvard School of Public Health.

Mr. Denny is active in his community gaining additional experience from two publicly elected positions. In 1994, he was elected to the Cranford Board of Education, a K–12 district of more than 3,000 students and a budget exceeding $30 million. He served in various capacities before being elected Vice-president of the Board in 1995. In 1996, Mr. Denny was elected to his first term on the Cranford Township Committee (municipal governing body) and re-elected to a second term in 1999 followed by a term as Mayor of Cranford. In 2000, Mr. Denny was selected by the New Jersey League of Municipalities to serve on the New Jersey Community Mental Health Citizens' Advisory Board and Mental Health Planning Council.

Florencia Zulberti, M.P.H. (*Consultant*), is Assistant Director for Global Health at the National Institutes of Health (NIH) of Mexico. Prior to joining the Mexican government in 2004, she was an HIV/AIDS Consultant to the World Food Programme based in Rome, Italy, and the Major Gifts Officer for the New York office of Médecins Sans Frontières. In 2000, she managed the financial, administrative, and human resource operations of a local technology access center located in East Palo Alto, California, called Plugged In and served as a human resource consultant for Impact Networks, an Internet provider in the Philippines. From 1997 to 2000 Ms. Zulberti worked for the Boston-based public health consultancy firm, John Snow Inc., where she backstopped several USAID/World Bank-funded projects, mainly in Morocco and Venezuela, before heading to Zambia to support the JSI Family Planning and HIV/AIDS project. Ms. Zulberti began her professional career as a Camp Sadako Volunteer for the United Nations Commissioner for Refugees in Chiapas, Mexico, where she worked on a human rights and reproductive health project with Guatemalan refugees. Ms. Zulberti received her MPH in International Health with an emphasis on reproductive health, family planning, and HIV/AIDS prevention programs from Boston University in 1997. In 1996 she received her B.A. in Psychology and Health from Queens University in Canada.

IOM Staff

Patrick W. Kelley, M.D., Dr.P.H., joined the Institute of Medicine in July 2003, serving as the Director of the Board on Global Health and the Board on African Academy Science Development. Previously he served in the U.S. Army for more than 23 years as a physician, residency director, epidemiologist, and program manager. In his last Department of Defense (DoD) position, Dr. Kelley founded and directed the presidentially-mandated DoD Global Emerging Infections Surveillance and Response System (DoD-GEIS). This responsibility entailed managing approximately $42 million of emerging infections surveillance, response, training, and capacity-building activities undertaken in partnership with numerous elements of the federal government and with health ministries in over 45 developing countries. He also designed and established the DoD Accessions Medical Standards Analysis and Research Activity, the first systematic DoD effort to apply epidemiology to the evidence-based development and evaluation of physical and psychological accession standards. Dr. Kelley is an experienced communicator having lectured in over 20 countries and authored over 50 scholarly papers and book chapters. He also designed and served as the specialty editor for the two volume textbook entitled *Military Preventive Medicine: Mobilization and Deployment*. Dr. Kelley obtained his M.D. from the University of Virginia and his Dr.P.H. from the Johns Hopkins School of Hygiene and Public Health.

Rosemary Chalk is the Director of the Board on Children, Youth, and Families and the Committee on Adolescent Health and Development, both of which are joint efforts of the National Research Council and the Institute of Medicine. Ms. Chalk is a policy analyst who has been a study director for the National Academies since 1987. She has directed or served as a senior staff member for over a dozen studies within the Institute of Medicine and the National Research Council, including studies on vaccine finance, the public health infrastructure for immunization, family violence, child abuse and neglect, research ethics and misconduct in science, and education finance. From 2000 to 2003, Ms. Chalk also directed a research project on the development of child well-being indicators for the child welfare system at Child Trends in Washington, D.C. She has previously served as a consultant for science and society research projects at the Harvard School of Public Health and was an Exxon Research Fellow in the Program on Science, Technology, and Society at the Massachusetts Institute of Technology. She was the program head of the Committee on Scientific Freedom and Responsibility of the American Association for the Advancement of Science from 1976 to 1986. Ms. Chalk has a B.A. in foreign affairs from the University of Cincinnati.

Michele Orza, Sc.D., is a scholar with the IOM's Board on Global Health where she is Study Director for the President's Emergency Plan for AIDS Relief (PEPFAR) Evaluation. Currently, she is also serving as Acting Director of IOM's Board on Health Care Services. Previously, she has served as Assistant Director of the Health Care Team at the Government Accountability Office where she was responsible for managing study teams evaluating a wide range of federal programs. For several years she also served as Director of Science and Research at the American College of Cardiology (ACC) where her department was responsible for supporting the college's evidence-based medicine activities including clinical guidelines, performance measures, data standards, and quality improvement projects. Prior to coming to Washington, D.C., she worked as a research assistant in the Technology Assessment Group at the Harvard School of Public Health. While there she worked on a wide variety of methods for and applications of systematic reviews and meta-analysis and other tools to promote and support evidence-based public health. Dr. Orza received both her M.S. in Health Policy and Management and her Sc.D. in Program Evaluation from the Harvard School of Public Health and received the first B.A. in Women's Studies from Harvard/Radcliffe University.

Kimberly A. Scott, M.S.P.H., joined the IOM's Board on Global Health in September 2005 as the Senior Program Officer for the PEPFAR evaluation. She has worked in public health for nearly 20 years with an emphasis on service planning, delivery, and evaluation related to community mental health and to HIV/AIDS care, prevention, and treatment. She has also been a national trainer and consultant for many topical issues in public health, including HIV/AIDS, diabetes management, and cultural competence in the provision of clinical and social services in public health settings. Prior to IOM, she was an analyst on the health care team at the U.S. Government Accountability Office focusing on public health programs and policies including childhood obesity in the United States and evaluation of the PEPFAR program. Prior to returning to graduate school, she worked at Duke University's Center for Health Policy, Law, and Management as an agency coordinator to integrate mental health services into the continuum of care for people living with and affected by HIV/AIDS in 54 counties in North Carolina. She has also served as Executive Director of a Ryan White-funded HIV/AIDS consortium that developed a comprehensive ambulatory care system for 21 mostly rural counties in North Carolina. She has also served on a number of advisory committees to the Governor of North Carolina as well as the Secretary of NC DHHS for programmatic and policy issues related to HIV care, prevention, and treatment in North Carolina. She received her undergraduate degree in Psychology from the University of Virginia as well as an M.S. in Public Health with a concentration in health policy analysis from the University of North Carolina at Chapel Hill.

Lucía Fort, M.P.H., M.P.A., joined the IOM's Board on Global Health in November 2005 as a program officer for the PEPFAR evaluation. Before coming to IOM, she was a health care analyst with the U.S. Government Accountability Office (GAO), where she planned and conducted reviews of the internal operations of individual government agencies and multi-agency programs. Her work at GAO included a review of per capita medical care spending and coverage policies provided for populations served by the Indian Health Service and an assessment of the expenditure and obligation of funds awarded by CDC for bioterrorism preparedness. She was a consultant with the Dominican Network of People Living with HIV in Santo Domingo and with Family Care International's Latin America and Caribbean Division. She also coordinated community outreach programs for young adults and Latina women at Whitman-Walker Clinic, a large AIDS service organization in Washington, D.C. She received her M.P.A. from the School of International and Public Affairs and her M.P.H. from the Mailman School of Public Health, both at Columbia University.

J. Alice Nixon, M.A., recently joined the IOM's Board on Global Health in July 2005 as a program officer for the Committee for the Evaluation of PEPFAR Implementation. Prior to coming to the Board, Alice focused on health care utilization and international health program evaluation. She worked as a project manager at the Agency for Healthcare Research and Quality (AHRQ) examining urban/rural differences in health care expenditures and access to care using AHRQ's Medical Expenditure Panel Study (MEPS). Most recently, she was a health care analyst at the GAO conducting research related to U.S.-funded international public health programs and initiatives, including evaluations of U.S. global malaria control initiatives and PEPFAR. Ms. Nixon has a degree in Sociology with a minor in Fine Arts from Goucher College as well as a master's in Medical Sociology from the University of Maryland.

Angela Mensah joined the IOM's Board on Global Health in June 2005 as Senior Program Assistant and is currently providing support to the PEPFAR evaluation. Over the past 13 years, Angela has been involved primarily in business and project management serving as a small business advisor with Empretec Ghana Foundation (a United Nations Project), Administrative Assistant at the American College of Cardiology, Project Manager with a Private Events and Project Management Firm implementing national projects and private initiatives in Ghana, and Office Manager at a private medical practice at the Washington Hospital Center in Washington, D.C. She also served as a member of Ghana's delegation to South Africa to understudy the National Job Summit held in South Africa in October 1998, Lead Coordinator and Organizer of the first Business Support Services Expo in Ghana, and President of the Soroptimist International, Kumasi Club (Ghana), an international charity organization for women in the various professions that championed amongst other projects an Aids Orphans Project. Ms. Mensah graduated from the University of Science and Technology in Ghana with an associate degree in Data Processing and Office Management and Secretarial Duties from East London Polytechnic, respectively. She is currently pursuing a Certificate Program in Project Management at Kaplan University.

Kimberly Weingarten was Senior Program Assistant for the study evaluating PEPFAR in the Board on Global Health until September 2006. In May of 2004 she returned from Zambia where she served for over 2 years with the Peace Corps. As a Community Action for Health Volunteer, Kimberly focused primarily on HIV/AIDS sensitization, education, and outreach. Prior to her Peace Corps service, she volunteered with various organizations such as the American Red Cross and NOVAM (Northern Virginia AIDS Ministry). She graduated from San Francisco State University in 2000 with a B.A. in Psychology and a minor in Human Sexuality Studies.

APPENDIX G

Information-Gathering Meeting Agendas

COMMITTEE FOR THE EVALUATION OF PEPFAR IMPLEMENTATION

February 23–25, 2005
Baltimore, Maryland

Wednesday, February 23, 2005

10:30 a.m.– 12:30 p.m. **PEPFAR Program Description**

Joseph F. O'Neill, M.D., M.S., M.P.H.
Deputy Coordinator
Office of the U.S. Global AIDS Coordinator

Question and Answer Session

Kathy Marconi, Ph.D., M.S.
Director of Monitoring, Evaluation, and Strategic Information,
Office of the U.S. Global AIDS Coordinator

Question and Answer Session

12:30–1:30 p.m. **Lunch Break**

1:30–3:30 p.m. **PEPFAR Agencies and Participants Panel**

Ms. Nobayeni Dladla
Health Attaché, Embassy of South Africa

Richard A. Shaffer, Ph.D., M.P.H.
Director, HIV/AIDS Prevention Program
U.S. Department of Defense

Carl C. Stecker, Ed.D., M.P.H.
Senior Program Director and Chief of Party
AIDSRelief ART Project
Catholic Relief Services

Constance Carrino, Ph.D.
Director, Office of HIV/AIDS, Global Health Bureau
U.S. Agency for International Development

Question and Answer Session

3:30–3:45 p.m. **Afternoon Break**

3:45–4:45 p.m. **Public Comment**

Thursday, February 24, 2005

8:30–11:45 a.m. **Global Monitoring and Evaluation Programs Panel**

Daniel Low-Beer, Ph.D. (by phone)
Deputy Director, Strategic Information & Evaluation
The Global Fund

Ties Boerma, M.D., Ph.D. (by phone)
Director, Department of Measurement and Health Information Systems
Evidence and Information for Policy Cluster
World Health Organization

Joseph Valadez, Ph.D., M.P.H., Sc.D.
Senior M&E Specialist, Global HIV/AIDS Program
World Bank

Paul R. DeLay, M.D. (by phone)
Director, Monitoring & Evaluation
Joint United Nations Programme on HIV/AIDS

11:45 a.m.–12:30 p.m. **U.S. Department of Health and Human Services**

Bill Steiger, Ph.D.
Director, Office of Global Health Affairs
U.S. Department of Health and Human Services

12:30–1:30 p.m. **Lunch**

1:30–3:30 p.m. **U.S. Department of Health and Human Services (continued)**

Deborah Rugg, Ph.D.
Associate Director for Monitoring and Evaluation
U.S. Department of Health and Human Services/ Centers for Disease Control and Prevention
Global AIDS Program

Q & A with
Kathy Marconi, Ph.D., M.S.
Director of Monitoring, Evaluation, and Strategic Information
Office of the U.S. Global AIDS Coordinator

COMMITTEE FOR THE EVALUATION OF PEPFAR IMPLEMENTATION

Tuesday, April 19–21, 2005
Washington, DC

Tuesday, April 19, 2005

10:15–10:30 a.m. **Chair's Introduction**

Jaime Sepúlveda, M.D., Dr.Sc.
Director, National Institutes of Health, Mexico

10:30 a.m.– 1:00 p.m	**Office of the U.S. Global AIDS Coordinator Update**
	Ambassador Randall L. Tobias *Office of the U.S. Global AIDS Coordinator*
	Michele Moloney-Kitts *Director, Program Services* *Office of the U.S. Global AIDS Coordinator*
1:00–2:00 p.m.	**Lunch Break**
2:00–3:30 p.m.	**PEPFAR Partners Panel Presentations**
	Phyllis J. Kanki, D.V.M., S.D. *Principal Investigator* *AIDS Treatment Care and Prevention Initiative* *Harvard PEPFAR*
	Peter Lamptey, M.D., Dr.P.H. *President, Institute for HIV/AIDS* *Family Health International*
	Jean W. Pape, M.D. *Director, GHESKIO* *(Haitian Group for the Study of Kaposi's Sarcoma and Opportunistic Infections)*
	Stacy Rhodes, J.D., M.A. *Director, HIV/AIDS Unit* *Save the Children*
	Jeffrey Stringer, M.D. *Associate Professor and Director* *University of Alabama, Birmingham* *Centre for Infectious Disease Research in Zambia (CIDRZ)*
	Cathy Wilfert, M.D. *Scientific Director, PMTCT* *Elizabeth Glaser Pediatric AIDS Foundation*
3:30–3:45 p.m.	**Afternoon Break**

3:45–5:15 p.m. **PEPFAR Partners Panel Q&A**

5:15–6:00 p.m. **Public Comment**

Wednesday, April 20, 2005

Closed Committee Meeting

Thursday, April 21, 2005

8:00–9:00 a.m. **Conference Call with CDC-GAP Field Staff**

Chiefs of Party

Tim Mastro, M.D., Acting Director
Division of HIV/AIDS Prevention, National Center for HIV, STD and TB Prevention, CDC, Atlanta, GA

Peter Kilmarx (Botswana)
Okey Nwanyanwu (South Africa)
Jono Mermin (Uganda)
Mitch Wolfe (Vietnam)
Shannon Hader (Zimbabwe)
Karen Hawkins-Reed (Democratic Republic of Congo)

9:00–10:00 a.m. **Office of the U.S. Global AIDS Coordinator Update**

Kathy Marconi, Ph.D., M.S.
Director, Strategic Information
Office of the U.S. Global AIDS Coordinator

10:00–10:15 a.m. **Morning Break**

10:15 a.m.–12:30 p.m. **Office of the Global AIDS Coordinator Update (continued)**

Kathy Marconi, Ph.D., M.S.
Director, Strategic Information
Office of the U.S. Global AIDS Coordinator

Michele Moloney-Kitts
Director, Program Services
Office of the U.S. Global AIDS Coordinator

12:30 p.m. Adjourn

COMMITTEE FOR THE EVALUATION OF PEPFAR IMPLEMENTATION

Thursday, September 15, 2005
Washington, DC

9:30–10:30 a.m. Legislative History and Context

Allen Moore, M.B.A.
Senior Fellow, Global Health Council
Senior Associate, Center for Strategic and International Studies
Former Deputy Chief of Staff and Policy Director for Senator Bill Frist

Nancy Stetson, Ph.D.
Senior Professional Staff Member, Senate Foreign Relations Committee
Senior Foreign Policy Advisor to Senator John Kerry

10:30 a.m.– 12:30 p.m. Perspectives on the PEPFAR Focus Countries

Ambassador Johnnie Carson
Senior Vice President
National Defense University
Former Ambassador to Kenya and Uganda

Ambassador Cameron Hume
Deputy Inspector General
U.S. Department of State
Former U.S. Ambassador to Algeria and South Africa

Ambassador Princeton Lyman, Ph.D.
Ralph Bunche Senior Fellow and Director of Africa Policy Studies
Council on Foreign Relations
Former U.S. Ambassador to South Africa and Nigeria

	J. Stephen Morrison, Ph.D. *Executive Director, Task Force on HIV/AIDS* *Director, Africa Program* *Center for Strategic and International Studies*
12:30–1:30 p.m.	**Lunch Break**
1:30–3:30 p.m.	**Office of the U.S. Global AIDS Coordinator Update**
	Mark Dybul, M.D. *Deputy U.S. Global AIDS Coordinator*
	Carolyn Ryan, M.D., M.P.H. *Senior Technical Advisor, Prevention*
	Kenneth Schofield *Budgetary Planning and Reporting Officer*
	Kathy Marconi, Ph.D., M.S. *Director, Strategic Information*
3:30–3:45 p.m.	**Break**
3:45–5:15 p.m.	**PEPFAR Implementing Partners**
	Helen Cornman, M.S.W. *HIV/AIDS Technical Advisor, Community REACH Program Pact*
	Madhuvanti Deshmukh, M.A. *Director, HIV/AIDS Unit* *CARE International*
	Susan Purdin, R.N., M.P.H. *Senior Technical Advisor, Reproductive Health* *International Rescue Committee*
5:15–5:45 p.m.	**Public Comment**

Index

A

D

G

H

I

Q

R

S

U

V

W